This book is to be returned on or before
the last date stamped below.

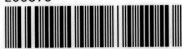

Psychological disorders in obstetrics and gynaecology

To Mary and Ursula

Psychological disorders in obstetrics and gynaecology

Edited by

R. G. Priest, MD, FRCP(Edin), FRCPsych
Professor of Psychiatry, Academic Department of Psychiatry, St. Mary's Hospital Medical School,
London, UK

Butterworths
London Boston Durban Singapore Sydney Toronto Wellington

First published 1985

© **Butterworth & Co. (Publishers) Ltd 1985**

British Library Cataloguing in Publication Data

Psychological disorders in obstetrics and gynaecology.
    1. Gynecology—Psychosomatic aspects
    2. Obstetrics—Psychosomatic aspects
    I. Priest, R.G.
    618   RG103.5

    ISBN 0-407-00373-8

Library of Congress Cataloging in Publication Data

Main entry under title:

Psychological disorders in obstetrics and gynaecology.
    Includes bibliographies and index.
    1. Gynecology--Psychological aspects. 2. Obstetrics
    --Psychological aspects. 3. Women--Mental health.
    I. Priest, Robert G. [DNLM; 1. Genital Diseases,
    Female--psychology. 2. Psychophysiologic Disorders--
    in pregnancy. WP 140 P9735]
    RG103.5.P773   1985   618'.01'9   85-7887

    ISBN 0-407-00373-8

Photoset by Butterworths Litho Preparation Department
Printed in England by Garden City Press Ltd, Letchworth, Herts.

Foreword

Every obstetrician and gynaecologist knows that the proper practice of this specialty demands consideration not only of the physical disorders with which the patient presents, but her emotional reaction to them. Most obstetrical and gynaecological patients are fortunately so well adjusted that the psychological aspects of their cases play merely a minor part, and although this always requires the sympathetic attention of the doctor, little more is called for. But the emotional reaction of some women to reproduction and its disorders is profound and may be much more of a problem in management than the physical state which it accompanies. All experienced obstetricians and gynaecologists have encountered such patients and have attempted, to the best of their ability, to deal successfully with them, but most have wished to have a deeper insight into serious psychological reactions of this kind and better guidelines for management.

Such are what this book provides. It deals with psychiatric disease associated with menstruation including the vexed question of the premenstrual syndrome, childbirth and its difficulties, abortion, sterilization, abnormalities of sexual function, surgery, and disorders of the menopause and climacteric. These aspects of human reproduction require emotional adjustment by all women, although authoritative accounts of these problems are few. This text, compiled by authors experienced in the field, is therefore most welcome especially since the approach is essentially a practical one which aims to give guidance to the busy obstetrician and gynaecologist on recognition and management of the many important conditions which may be encountered. The international team of contributors has been admirably chosen and the approach of each to the task in hand is to be highly commended. I wish this valuable text every success.

Sir John Dewhurst
Queen Charlotte's Hospital for Women,
Goldhawk Road,
London W6 0XG, UK

v

Preface

It is a paradox that some psychological problems in women are more likely to take them to the gynaecologist than to the psychiatrist. For example, pelvic pain of psychological origin is a common symptom seen in gynaecological patients, and a very difficult one for the gynaecologist to treat, but patients rarely go with such a complaint to the psychiatrist's consulting room. The same is true of some sexual disorders. Medical practitioners, nurses and other members of the helping professions are faced with the challenge of trying to aid such patients and sometimes do not know what way to turn. Patients whose symptoms take an apparently physical or bodily form are often reluctant to accept psychiatric help. This may be because they fear that an organic disease is being overlooked, or because they resent the implication of some mental weakness. If they accept referral to a psychiatrist, the answers may still not be found. The education and training of psychiatrists traditionally pays little attention to this area and the psychiatrist may be as baffled as the gynaecologist. This book is designed to be of value to all those who are concerned with helping these distressed women.

I would not have been happy in editing such a book if we had been short of facts. I have a horror of vast tomes full of verbiage, of pontification, of vain theorizing or speculation that has no empirical basis. I have some sympathy with those who suspect psychiatric and related books of being high on words and low on data. I know that psychosomatic medicine in particular is commonly viewed as being a soft subject, with little of the hard science about it. However, factual knowledge has been growing and consolidating, and as far as possible that is what this volume is filled with. The authors give as little space as possible to classifying and theorizing, and as much space as possible to stating what is known about the subject, quoting their sources as they do so.

That is not to say they have all the answers. Some of you will find, as readers, that your favourite theory is demolished and that nothing is put in its place. That is how it has to be if we are to reflect, as faithfully as possible, the present stage of knowledge. For the most part, however, there are practical treatments that are available for the maladies of our patients, and not necessarily treatments that take years on the analyst's couch. Our hope is that after reading this book you will have a clear idea of what is known and what is not known.

As an editor I have been fortunate in that the authors who have agreed to contribute are not only experts in their own particular fields, but are also clear and articulate writers. I hope that you will find that the style is a pleasure to read and that the text is high in information. Above all, I shall be gratified if the contents attract and keep your interest. The aim of the book is to inform and teach, and the reader will learn better if he finds what he is reading to be intriguing and absorbing.

I would like to acknowledge with gratitude the help of Dr Joe Herzberg in the preparation of the Index.

ROBERT G. PRIEST

Contributors

Barbara L. Andersen, PhD
Associate Professor of Psychology, The University of Iowa, Iowa City, Iowa 52242, USA.

C. Barbara Ballinger, BSc MB ChB MRCP FRCPsych
Consultant Psychiatrist, Dundee Psychiatric Services, Royal Dundee Liff Hospital, Dundee DD2 5NF, Scotland, UK.

A. J. Cooper, MD FRCPsych DPM DipPharmMed
Director of Research, St. Thomas Psychiatric Hospital, St. Thomas, Ontario, Canada; Associate Professor, University of Western Ontario, Canada

Sir John Dewhurst, FRCS FRCOG
Professor of Obstetrics and Gynaecology, Queen Charlotte's Hospital for Women, Goldhawk Road, London W6 0XG, UK.

Lynne M. Drummond, MB ChB MRCP MRCPsych
Senior Registrar in Psychiatry, St. Mary's Hospital, Praed Street, London W2 1NY, UK.

D. Gath, DM FRCP FRCPsych
Clinical Reader in Psychiatry, University Department of Psychiatry, Warneford Hospital, Oxford OX3 7JX, UK.

P. C. Olley, MB ChB BSc MRCPsych DIP(Psych)
Consultant Psychiatrist, Grampian Health Board Psychiatric Services, The Ross Clinic, Cornhill Road, Aberdeen AB9 2ZF, Scotland, UK; Clinical Senior Lecturer in Mental Health, University of Aberdeen, Aberdeen AB9 1FX, Scotland, UK.

Gisela B. Oppenheim, MB ChB FRCPsych DPM
Consultant Psychiatrist, Charing Cross Hospital (Fulham), Fulham Palace Road, London W6 8RF, and Queen Charlotte's Hospital for Women, Goldhawk Road, London W6 0XG, UK.

R. O. Pasnau, MD
Professor of Psychiatry and Director of Adult Psychiatry Clinical Services, UCLA Neuropsychiatric Institute, Center for the Health Sciences, 760 Westwood Plaza, Los Angeles, California 90024, USA.

B. M. N. Pitt, MD BS FRCPsych DPM
Consultant Psychiatrist, Department of Psychological Medicine, St. Bartholomew's Hospital, West Smithfield, London EC1A 7BE, UK.

R. G. Priest, MD FRCP(Edin) FRCPsych
Professor of Psychiatry, Academic Department of Psychiatry, St. Mary's Hospital Medical School (University of London), Norfolk Place, London W2 1PG, UK

N. D. B. Rose, MB ChB DObs RCOG MRCPsych
Clinical Lecturer in Psychiatry, University Department of Psychiatry, Warneford Hospital, Oxford OX3 7JX, UK.

S. Soldinger, MD
Assistant Clinical Professor, UCLA Neuropsychiatric Institute, Center for the Health Sciences, 760 Westwood Plaza, Los Angeles, California 90024, USA.

C. M. Tonks, MB, ChB FRCP FRCPsych DPM
Consultant Psychiatrist, St. Mary's Hospital, Praed Street, London W2 1NY, UK.

Contents

Chapter 1

Sexual dysfunction and infertility

Alan J. Cooper

The first part of this chapter deals with sexual disorders; the second with infertility.

Sexual disorders

Types of sexual disorder

Sexual disorders, which have been estimated to have a prevalence approximating 25% (Masters and Johnson, 1970; Crown and D'Ardenne, 1982), may be broadly divided into the following three types: general unresponsiveness; orgasmic dysfunction; vaginismus.

GENERAL UNRESPONSIVENESS

General unresponsiveness manifests with low, or absent, libido and arousal even when stimulation from a partner is technically adequate. Such women usually lack sexual curiosity and tend to be relatively indifferent to erotic films, conversations, literature, or other commonly exciting stimuli. They rarely have intense sexual fantasies, or masturbate, and are often astonished to hear that other women do, and more so, that they enjoy it.

ORGASMIC DYSFUNCTION

Orgasmic dysfunction exists when, despite the presence of libido and arousal, orgasm is absent or infrequent to the point where a complaint of sexual inadequacy is voiced. High levels of sexual tension not culminating in orgasm, especially when stimulation is prolonged, may result in pelvic congestion, frustration, irritability or depression.

VAGINISMUS

These disorders, which are best conceptualized along a continuum of severity, are not mutually exclusive. For instance, women with vaginismus may also suffer from low libido and be generally unresponsive. Therefore, it is essential to take a comprehensive history to define precisely the extent of the problem.

Causes of a sexual disorder

It is useful to further categorize sexual disorders as primary or secondary. Primary refers to a condition present from the first experience; secondary indicates previous competence. The latter have generally been seen to have better prognoses (Masters and Johnson, 1970), but this is not invariable. In the individual case, the specific psychodynamics and, particularly, the quality of the relationship or the extent of any inhibitory emotions, such as anxiety or disgust, may be more important than the type of disorder *per se*. The development and manifestations of sexual dysfunction in homosexuals takes the same form as in heterosexuals; the treatment is also essentially similar (Masters and Johnson, 1979). However, only the latter will be considered here.

A meaningful evaluation of a sexual disorder demands a great deal of patience and skill. It requires a flexible, non-judgmental approach, with an awareness that aetiology may be protean, encompassing organic, psychosocial, constitutional and biological elements which might overlap to a greater or lesser degree. The physician must assess the many possible factors in perspective, make a valid diagnostic formulation, and then tailor treatment to the individual. *Tables 1.1* and *1.2* summarize the main causes of female sexual dysfunction. These may be conveniently considered in four arbitrary groups: (1) organic, (2) psychosocial and (3) constitutional (probably mainly genetic) and (4) biological.

TABLE 1.1. Classification of main causes of female sexual disorders

Organic	Psychological	Constitutional (mainly genetic)	Biological

Debilitating physical illness (such as diabetes) and side effects of drugs, e.g.
    antidepressants
    sedatives
    hypotensives
    tranquillizers
    anticholinergics
    alcohol
	Anxiety
	Personality and relationship problems
	Hostility
	Anger
	Disgust
	Inhibition
	Sexual inversion
	Sexual ignorance
	Faulty stimulative techniques
	Male sexual disorders, e.g.:
	    prematurity;
	    impotence
	Depression
	Dyspareunia
	Pelvic pain
		Probably determines the strength of sex-drive and the upper limits of arousability
		
		Low sex-drive may minimize sexual learning during adolescence and early adulthood and thus compromise adult proficiency
		
		Weak or absent glandipudendal reflex
			Pregnancy and post-partum
			Aging
			Menopause
			Menstrual cycle

The ubiquity of sexual dysfunction and the need to approach the subject holistically is now well established; thus an exhaustive review of the many aetiological possibilities will not be undertaken. However, in the light of some recent research findings with therapeutic implications, the following possibilities are worthy of special note.

TABLE 1.2. Organic disorders and physical causes associated with female sexual dysfunction*

Organic disorders	Other physical causes

Genito-urinary:
  Cystitis
  Endometriosis
  Fibroids
  Laceration of broad ligament
  Urethritis
	Side effects of the following drugs:
	  Alcohol
	  Amitriptyline (and other tricyclics)
	  Amphetamines
	  Atropine
	  Benperidol
	  Bethanidine
	  Chlordiazepoxide
	  Chlorpromazine (and other major tranquillizers)
	  Guanethidine
	  Methantheline bromide
	  Pesticides
	  Reserpine

Infections:
  Candida albicans
  Endometritis
  Genital tuberculosis
  Gonorrhoea
  Syphilis
  Trichomonas	

Neurological:
  Amyotrophic lateral sclerosis
  Multiple sclerosis
  Parkinsonism
  Peripheral neuritis
  Tabes dorsalis
  Temporal lobe lesions
  Transection of the cord
	Anatomical:
	  Congenital deformities
	  Episiotomy scar
	  Hydrocoele
	  Hysterectomy
	  Intact hymen
	  Sympathectomy

Vascular:
  Haemorrhoids
  Pelvic irradiation
  Thrombosis of aortic bifurcation
	Interference with sensitivity reactions:
	  Condoms
	  Douches
	  Pessaries

Cardiorespiratory:
  Angina
  Emphysema
  Myocardial infarction	

Endocrine:
  Acromegaly
  Addison's disease
  Adrenal neoplasms
  Chromophobe adenoma
  Diabetes
  Infantilism
  Myxoedema
  Obesity
  Thyrotoxicosis	

* With the exception of diabetes and the side effects of certain drugs, all are rare or in many cases debatable.

ORGANIC FACTORS

It is probable that organic factors make a greater contribution than was hitherto believed. Although most of the work to date has been on impotent men, in whom up to 20% have been found to have significant organic pathology, and since in almost every respect the factors mediating arousal and response are similar for both sexes, it is likely that organic disorders will turn out to be equally important in the female.

The most common physical disorders likely to be associated with a female sexual dysfunction are set out in *Table 1.2*. Diabetes, other endocrinopathies, and side effects of prescription drugs are the most important but, as can be seen, there are many other possibilities.

TABLE 1.3. Some clinical features distinguishing a secondary organic from a secondary psychogenic dysfunction*

Psychogenic dysfunction	*Organic dysfunction*
Acute onset	More likely insidious onset
More likely to be a time relationship to a specific stress, e.g. bereavement, marital problem, depression, fatigue, anxiety; sexual trauma, and a history of previous emotional problems	Develops in association with previously diagnosed organic condition, without significant antecedent stress; or follows use of certain medications
More likely to be selective intermittent and transient, the disorder being present on some occasions and situations but not others, and with some sexual partners but not others	More likely to be persistent and progressively worsening, although some degree of fluctuation, especially in the early stages, is common
Evidence of potential to respond erotically, e.g. the active pursuit of alternative sexual outlets to orgasm, such as masturbation, and other sexual partners, and the retention of erotic desire, e.g. libido, in sexual situations. Unless alternative sexual activities continue to be regularly indulged, libido generally declines	Glandipudendal reflex most likely to be absent or weak
	Evidence of progressive generalized waning of sexual interest and activities, e.g. the absence of, or only rarely practised, alternative sexual outlets, and diminished fantasies and erotic desire in sexual situations

* Primary anorgasmia and general unresponsiveness are more likely to have a significant constitutional (mainly hereditary) element, but both psychological and organic factors may be important.

Table 1.3 summarizes some clinical and developmental features which may be relatively helpful in distinguishing organic dysfunctions from those primarily of psychosocial origin. It should be stressed, however, that the former are seen only rarely in pure culture. Secondary anxiety, inhibition and feelings of inadequacy are common, and may exacerbate or variably complicate the clinical picture. However, generalized waning of libido and arousability, developing in close temporal proximity to an organic disorder, should suggest the possibility of an aetiological relationship and prompt appropriate investigations.

Unwanted drugs effects
Many drugs are stated to have adverse effects on sexual response. In a few instances, these are well documented and might have been predicted from pharmacological knowledge. In others, the evidence is vague and inconclusive. This is especially so for contraceptive hormones. In some women, after starting on the 'pill' there may be an increase of libido and enjoyment during coitus, possibly because they might feel secure against an unwanted pregnancy. In others, apprehension about reported side effects, especially depression, anorgasmia and thrombosis, result in negative consequences. In fact there are no real data for an effect on sexual responsiveness either way, but individuals may experience enhanced or dimished libido, coincidently. The subject has been well surveyed by Weissman and Slaby (1973).

All hypnotics, narcotics and tranquillizers may impair libido and sexual response, if large enough doses are taken. However, paradoxical effects are sometimes observed depending on the emotional state of the user and the social milieu at the time. Adrenergic-blocking agents, such as the older hypotensives guanethidine and bethanidine, may diminish or inhibit orgasm, as might some major tranquillizers (including thioridizine and chlorpromazine) and the tricyclic antidepressants. The pharmacological bases for these effects, which may be extremely variable, remain largely unclarified.

Clinically, the important point is to be aware of the possibility that drugs prescribed for other purposes (e.g. hypertension) may inhibit, or limit, sexual response, and to make pertinent enquiries to allow an assessment of any aetiological significance. Thereafter, if feasible, and if the patient is motivated for improved sexual functioning, it may be possible to reduce the dose of a particular drug without incurring unacceptable medical risks, or to recommend an alternative without the sexual side effects. However, each case must be judged on its merits. Unfortunately, at present, it is not possible to predict either a drug's likely causal contribution to sexual dysfunction or the effects of discontinuing it. This can be determined only by cautious trial and error.

PSYCHOSOCIAL FACTORS

The importance of psychological influences on sexual functioning is now well recognized. However, it is possible that in the past these influences have been over-emphasized. It should be stressed again that they are just some of numerous possibilities, which should be adduced positively and in perspective. If operating, they should be elicitable in all cases during a searching examination, even if subtle and disguised. The main causes which may need to be explored are indicated in *Table 1.1.*

Personality and relationships
Since the early days of Masters and Johnson, as the limitations of predominantly physiological treatment became more apparent, there has been an increasing tendency for personality and relationship factors to be given greater weight in diagnoses and management. This is nothing more than redressing the psychodynamic–behavioural balance resulting from the positions taken by iconoclasts of the psychoanalytical and behaviourist schools. A return to perspective was long overdue and most thoughtful practitioners, untrammelled by dogma, have come to realize the pivotal importance of the relationship. Generally, if this is seriously flawed, then no amount of 'practical' treatment is likely to be of much help. In such cases, a great deal of exploration and remedial counselling may be necessary before the sexual problem, *per se,* can be tackled. Therefore, these couples may require marriage guidance or more sophisticated psychotherapy.

Disgust
This is a common cause of sexual malfunctioning and may be extremely intractable to treatment. For this reason, it is important to distinguish it from other inhibitory emotions such as anxiety, anger or depression. For many individuals, this is a particularly sensitive subject, and the presence of disgust may be denied or disguised. Therefore, the physician will need to be subtle in his examination, which should include a sympathetic exploration of the woman's attitudes and perceived

emotional response to menstruation, childbirth, sex-play, especially self- and partner-masturbation and her own and partner's genitalia.

High levels of disgust about sexual matters may be associated with obsessional traits and over-concern with orderliness, cleanliness and self-restraint, and a dislike of or even phobias about dirt, contamination and loss of control. Careful observation will usually allow the physician to assess the causal significance of disgust. This seems to be more common in cases of vaginismus.

Problems in the male partner

Faulty or inadequate stimulation, based on ignorance, misinformation or simply thoughtlessness, may play an important role in all types of female sexual dysfunction. Detailed questioning about preparatory love-play and coital techniques is mandatory.

Frank dysfunction in the male, especially premature ejaculation or impotence, or a marked disparity between the sex-drives of the partners, obviously may be expected to contribute to an inadequate response or dissatisfaction in the female and, if present, will need to be treated concurrently (Masters and Johnson, 1970).

Attention should also be directed to the environment in which sexual behaviour takes place (e.g. the time, place and circumstances), to ensure that this is as propitious as possible. Some couples, out of ignorance or lacking initiative, may have been operating suboptimally for years, and simple rectifying advice may improve things dramatically.

Promiscuity

This is more likely to be encountered in teenagers, especially those away from home such as university students. Promiscuity can result in psychological and physical disasters; more so, in those who are relatively unstable and immature. The commonest sexual manifestation is probably orgasmic inadequacy, but emotional difficulties, including loss of self-esteem and depression, are not unusual. Often these girls trade sexual favours for status and popularity or because they believe it is 'adult'. They are likely to be sexually exploited by predatory males, and to suffer multiple rejections and humiliations which further compromise an already fragile personality and tend to exacerbate the sexual problem.

Promiscuous adolescents also run high risks of contracting venereal disease, notably gonorrhoea. Except in extreme cases, this is generally less deleterious than the effects on personality, especially the capacity to form stable, mutually rewarding and respecting relationships with the opposite sex, which may be irreparably damaged. Typically, these unfortunate girls need long-term support and psychotherapy. Sexual maturity, when it occurs, tends to do so *pari passu* with personality growth. However, this is a time-consuming and daunting therapeutic undertaking which is best left to a suitable psychotherapist. If depression is severe, appropriate medication may be indicated.

Psychogenic sexual pain: dyspareunia and pelvic pain

Non-organic dyspareunia may be found in both sexes, but is commoner in the female. It may be caused by poor lubrication, as a consequence of clumsy, or inadequate, stimulation. However, anger, anxiety or disgust may inhibit full arousal and cause intercourse to be painful or impossible. Careful questioning usually indicates the essential psychodynamics.

Pelvic, as opposed to genital, pain is a ubiquitous gynaecological symptom. In a sizable minority of women, in whom it is judged to be psychosomatic, it may mask an underlying sexual problem. It should be diagnosed on positive psychological grounds and not by the absence of an organic lesion, although, of course, this may settle the question.

In order to get an accurate assessment of family interactions, which are usually important in the genesis of the condition, a home visit by a social worker may be useful. Alternatively, the physician may choose to undertake the task himself in the outpatients clinic.

Typically, the complainant projects herself as bravely putting up with her pain, but it is frequently obvious that she feels 'sorry for herself', and expects sympathy and concessions from others. She may express guilt about being unable to fulfil her sexual obligations to her spouse. He is often described as sympathetic and understanding; never making demands if these occasion discomfort – but his attitude may harden later. Although the pain may be almost constant, it fluctuates in severity, tending to be worse during sexual activity. Initially, it might have functioned as a 'protection' against coitus, but with time it may become incorporated into a life-style and acquire diverse secondary gain characteristics.

In some cases, it is clear that the symptom is being used to manipulate aspects of a relationship – especially to satisfy a variety of dependency needs. The essential psychogenesis may be revealed when, despite her complaints, the woman is able to continue to do something personally important such as keeping a job or socializing. A sizable proportion of complainants manifest other neurotic symptoms, especially anxiety and emotional instability (Beard *et al.*, 1977).

Longstanding psychological pelvic pain is a daunting problem. Many of these women patients have undergone numerous prior laboratory investigations, and even laparotomy, at the hands of many different clinicians. They remain convinced that their pain is organic and express a willingness to go to any (physical) lengths to seek a remedy. Repeated laboratory investigations may serve to reinforce their conviction. They rationalize: 'If there is nothing organically wrong with me, why am I having so many tests?' Unwittingly, or even collusively, surgeons may perpetuate the symptom. Indeed, the bulky gynaecological notes on many patients, full of essentially normal laboratory tests, may have labelled the pain as psychological; yet, more investigations have been ordered. It is probable that many gynaecologists are quite aware of the nature of their patient's pain, but do not know how to deal with it. The patients may be described as manipulative, aggressive or hysterical. For some, the barely disguised threat of 'trouble' (e.g. litigation), should something physical be missed, provides sufficient reason to order yet another test.

Unless the physician is knowledgeable about psychodynamics and personality structure, pelvic pain is best handled by a suitable psychiatrist. Pain of short duration, especially in a setting of somatic tension, may respond to relaxation training, superficial psychotherapy and, later, a more direct behavioural approach to the sexual dysfunction (Weissman and Slaby, 1973). In chronic cases, in which the original cause may long since have been denied or repressed and the symptom integrated into the personality, significant change may not be possible.

Depending upon the circumstances and chronicity, interpretative psychotherapy may be directed primarily at the woman with the hope of giving her insight as to the nature of her pain and a desire to 'relinquish' it. In longstanding and recalcitrant cases, the aim may be simply to allow the patient an opportunity of abreacting and also to provide reassurance and support. This may suffice to ease the lot of a spouse or other dependant. Again, when indicated, interpreting the patient's symptoms to family members may be justified and even desirable. Each case must be judged on merit. A cure, with complete freedom from pain, is relatively unusual, but is more likely in acute onset cases of short duration.

CONSTITUTIONAL AND BIOLOGICAL FACTORS

An unusually low sex-drive, determined constitutionally, may significantly contribute to a sexual dysfunction as well as limit a therapeutic response. Although 'constitutional' usually implies an important hereditary component, inhibitory psychological influences during development might also be involved. The importance of a low sex-drive is frequently overlooked, as it is often assumed that all women are endowed with an equal capacity to become aroused to sexual stimulation. This is not so, and a woman with an excessively low sex-drive may simply not have sufficient need (motivation) to seek out, or engage in, sexual experiences during the critical stages of growth during adolescence and early childhood, in comparison with her more active peers. Accordingly, the requirements of optimal learning cannot be satisfied and sexual stimulus–responses patterns are not laid down, or are inadequate. It is conceivable that the importance of learning in the acquisition of sexual arousal and response has been understated (Mead, 1949; Marshall, 1971; Eysenck and Wilson, 1979).

Clinically, it is important to distinguish the inhibited woman who is unable to let herself go because of constraining attitudes from the woman who is 'just not interested'. Generally, the former are better treatment prospects.

Recent research has delineated a specific spinal reflex (glandipudendal), which appears to be an essential component of both male and female orgasm. In the woman, the normal receptor field is the glans clitoris and the responding muscles, which are supplied by the pudendal nerve, lie in the perineum. The reflex can be demonstrated electromyographically, and it may be elicited in its phasic form by pinching the glans and scrutinizing and palpating the perivaginal musculature and the anal sphincter.

Brindley and Gillan (1982), who described this reflex, found it to be absent in a substantial proportion of patients with primary anorgasmia. They speculated that this was based on a structural defect in the spinal cord present from puberty or before. They further conjectured that the defect may be no more than the extreme of a continuous range of efficiency in a group of spinal reflexes that are rather variable. However, they acknowledge that psychological factors can also make a contribution to a weak or absent glandipudendal reflex, since a few of their patients became orgasmic after mainly behavioural treatment resolved the issues in question. These issues were usually simple and obvious, especially ignorance, with the patient not knowing what stimulus was necessary to induce an orgasm, and lack of confidence arising from unsuccessful attempts. Brindley and Gillan were unable to demonstrate any of the often imputed 'deeply seated fears and complex psychopathology' so dear to many sex therapists.

Their work has important practical implications. Examination of the reflex is a simple, easily learned technique suitable for an outpatients clinic and which is capable of yielding important prognostic information. Women who lack it very rarely respond to currently available treatment methods.

DIAGNOSTIC FORMULATION

After a measured assessment of all relevant aetiological considerations, the next step is to make a diagnostic formulation. This is a prerequisite of optimal treatment. The majority of therapists usually combine a number of principles in varying permutations according to the features in the individual case (*Table 1.4*).

TABLE 1.4. Common treatment ingredients

Male and female co-therapists
Partners treated together
Contract and compromise
Ban on coitus and sensate focus
Provision of optimal sexual stimulation
Homework assignments
Relaxation training
Progressive self- and partner-exploration and dilatation of vagina
Desensitization and imagination *in vivo*
Self- and partner-masturbation including use of vibrator
Kegal's muscle-shaping exercises
Drugs including anxiolytics and androgens
Teaching interpersonal sexual skills
Enhancing client motivation
Conditioning techniques
Disinhibition of sexuality including therapist disclosure
Sexual education including use of books and films
Psychotherapy appropriate to circumstances

Treatment concepts

GENERAL MEASURES

The maintenance of a good overall standard of health, hygiene and sensible habits, and an attractive appearance, are commonsense measures for patients with sexual problems. If appropriate, a weight-reducing programme under the auspices of a dietitian should be arranged and modest exercise prescribed.

Masters and Johnson's original format called for different sex co-therapists. However, current research does not support their notion that two are better than one. A single therapist, of either sex, is generally adequate (Mathews *et al.*, 1976; Crowe, Gillan and Golombok, 1981). However, in women who previously might have been abused, raped or the victim of male incest, a female therapist is sometimes to be preferred, and patients should be given this option. A woman is also generally better in cases of severe vaginismus, especially when this is associated with immaturity and emotional fragility – a fairly common eventuality.

The partners should be encouraged to attend together from the outset. Not only does this allow for an accurate assessment of the relationship, which is essential, but it also avoids unnecessary repetition and misunderstandings. Furthermore, the axiom 'there is no such thing as an uninvolved partner in a sexual problem' (Masters and Johnson, 1970) is invariably true.

Sensate focus
Prohibiting intercourse tends to reduce performance anxiety and facilitate the implementation of sensate focus exercises and optimal sexual stimulation. The

essential details of these exercises, which were developed by Master and Johnson (1970), are as follows.

The couple are instructed to engage in mutual bodily pleasuring initially in non-erogenous zones, and later to explore and test out each other's erotic potential using more specific stimulations. There is nothing to prove; they should just let themselves go without there being any predetermined goal (e.g. coitus or orgasm). No attempt should be made to force arousal since this is a physiological impossibility; it is most likely to occur when an individual is warm, relaxed and comfortable, and receiving appropriate stimulation in a smooth continuous manner from an involved, caring partner.

In the majority of cases, a measure of sexual arousal often develops from non-genital caresses, whether intended or not, which may lead naturally to more overtly sexual stroking, which may become imperative. The watchword, however, is gradualness; coitus is deferred by mutual consent until arousal is maximum and confidence has been boosted to the point where the couple feel success is likely. During this mutual pleasuring, the partners are instructed to communicate their precise needs and, if conducive, to guide each other's hands to sensitive areas. Mutual expressions of emotion and endearments further heighten arousal and are strongly encouraged.

Specific sensate focus tasks and progressively more intense sexual exchanges, short of coitus, worked out between the physician and the couple are scheduled as 'homework' and are an important aspect of the treatment contract. Essentially, the couple agree to complete the behavioural assignments on time, while the therapist promises to arrange a set number of sessions to achieve the stated goals.

Sensate focus and optimal stimulation is an integral part of therapy in *all* types of sexual dysfunction.

Enhancing subject motivation
Positive and sustained motivation is crucial for success, and some practitioners require a written daily record from the couple, which details every aspect of their sexual behaviour and thus provides continuous feedback. If necessary, this enables immediate treatment adjustments to be made. Although preparation of the record is time consuming, many couples welcome the procedure which is frequently perceived as a measure of the physician's commitment. This may sharpen their own sense of responsibility to the programme, which increases the likelihood of a favourable outcome.

Enhancing subject's arousal
When the female fails to become sexually aroused by her partner, conditioning techniques focusing either on masturbation, other sex-play or intercourse with him, may be useful. For example, during masturbation, the woman is instructed to focus her imagination on any erotic stimuli that she finds arousing. Just prior to climax, she switches to fantasies of sexual activity (masturbation or coitus) with her partner. The unconditioned stimulus of a previously exciting fantasy and the unconditioned response of sexual arousal and orgasm are thus paired with the presently neutral stimulus of sexual activity with the partner. If successful on subsequent occasions, the woman is told to turn to partner fantasies earlier until these become a conditioned stimulus for sexual arousal, and the artificial stimuli previously required become redundant.

Teaching interpersonal skills
Many couples with sexual problems have difficulty expressing their emotions, in initiating and refusing sexual advances and assertively communicating their likes and dislikes to the other in a frank but empathic manner. These deficits may be addressed through therapist modelling and patient role-playing. This procedure, practised and learned first in the clinic, can then be incorporated into the 'homework' tasks. For instance, a woman might complain to her husband that he initiates sexual activity in a crude, alienating non-arousing manner. In this case, the failure is twofold because she has not told him *what* she desires. The therapist models verbal initiation of sexual activity and expressions of tender emotions, which the couple copy and later extend during the sessions at home. Being able to voice sexual likes and dislikes without being perceived as being condescending or critical may foster understanding and increase self-esteem, and also improve sexual activities (Kaplan, 1974).

Disinhibiting sexual response
A non-orgasmic woman may be instructed to role-play an orgasm (Lobitz and LoPiccolo, 1972). This is not to deceive her partner, but to disinhibit herself about losing control and displaying intense excitement. Orgasmic role-playing may be especially useful with intellectual, rigid and inhibited women, who are ashamed and embarrassed about the muscular contractions, involuntary sounds and the various physical contortions which may accompany (and probably augment) high levels of sexual tension and climax. Mackay (1977), who refers to such individuals as 'emotionally constipated', has also used disinhibitory training to advantage.

Therapist self-disclosure
This somewhat controversial procedure may be used in an attempt to disinhibit an overly controlled individual. For example, admissions about masturbation, oral sex and 'failure', have all proved useful. However, such revelations should be withheld until the couple have got to know, and feel comfortable with, the therapist. Possibly because of cultural differences, the technique has attracted more attention in the USA (Lobitz and LoPiccolo, 1972), but has some advocates in the UK (Hawton, 1982).

PRACTICAL MEASURES

Relaxation training
Training in progressive muscular and concomitant mental relaxation is a non-specific measure which may benefit a patient manifesting high levels of anxiety, regardless of the type of disorder. Its use is based on the assumption that anxiety (or other distressing emotion) can cause, perpetuate or exacerbate a sexual dysfunction, and that relaxation, by inhibiting these states reciprocally, may facilitate the optimal implementation of more specific treatment ingredients (Wolpe, 1958).

Current methods include simple antenatal-type relaxation training, as well as more psychologically sophisticated procedures like progressive visual desensitization (while being fully relaxed), to imagined sexual activity, provided the individual is capable of such fantasy – starting with less threatening situations (e.g. non-genital caressing) and proceeding in a stepwise manner to more intimidating ones, culminating in coitus (Wolpe, 1958; Lazarus, 1963). Actually, sensate focus is desensitization *in vivo*.

Physiological desensitization
Following a vaginal examination to exclude a physical cause and demonstrate patency to the woman, digital self-exploration and progressive dilatation while being fully relaxed, using erotic fantasy (if this helps), is an essential early step in the treatment of vaginismus. Women who are unwilling (or unable) to perform these simple manoeuvres, whatever the stated reason, often harbour deeply seated feelings of digust which complicates therapy. As desensitization proceeds and tolerance increases, the procedure should be repeated by the sexual partner until the woman can accommodate 2 or 3 fingers without undue distress. The male partners of women with vaginismus are frequently timid and passive. They may have to be instructed specifically by direct example or anatomical charts. Successful resolution of vaginismus, which is relatively easy, does not necessarily result in a concomitant improvement in libido, responsiveness or orgasmic capacity (Malleson, 1942; Friedman, 1962).

Masturbation
Self- and partner-masturbation has proved especially effective in orgasmic dysfunction, for which it is the core practical intervention. It is also of prime importance in vaginismus. Failure to respond to manual stimulation calls for the use of a battery vibrator which, in some instances, will be successful. Unfortunately, some couples consider this aid unnatural and are loath to use it. If there is serious resistance, the issue should not be forced. The following sequence, described by Riley and Riley (1978), is recommended:

Step 1. The patient is encouraged to explore her vulva and vagina in private (husband not present).
Step 2. She continues to explore her external genitalia, increasing the duration of manual contact. She is asked to find, by trial and error, specific areas (e.g. the clitoris) that give pleasure when touched. Simultaneously, the obligatory use of fantasies or anything else (e.g. pictures, literature, voluntary muscle contractions, rapid breathing) which might increase arousal is advocated. If she remains dry, or experiences discomfort, lubricant jelly is prescribed.
Step 3. Manipulation of the genitalia is continued for up to 30 min, while peak sexual tension is maintained.
Step 4. If orgasm has not been reached, the patient is provided with a battery vibrator and encouraged to experiment with it privately, until orgasm occurs.
Step 5. After a few successes, and provided both partners agree, she uses the vibrator with her husband in the room.
Step 6. The husband is encouraged to stimulate his wife with the vibrator. It is recommended that at first they should both hold the instrument so that it can be guided to the position of maximum feeling.
Step 7. The couple are advised to engage in intercourse in the female superior sitting position, while the wife continues to stimulate herself with the vibrator.
Step 8. The couple engage in coitus in any position they wish. Stimulation with the vibrator is stopped prior to orgasm and the husband manually stimulates her during intercourse.

Step 9. The use of the vibrator is stopped progressively earlier in the sexual act. Later, if mutually desired, vibrator stimulation can be incorporated into the couple's permanent sexual repertoire.

Muscle control

Some women discover that, by 'will-power', they can induce and control contractions of the perivaginal musculature (Kegal, 1952). This capacity, which may be augmented by regular practice, can enhance sensory appreciation, with overall beneficial effects on arousal. 'Bearing-down' exercises may have a similar effect.

Sexual education

Relevant sexual information should be given, as required, to rectify beliefs or fill any gaps in knowledge. This is particularly important in the previously sexually inexperienced. A common stumbling-block is the notion that certain sexual practices are innately abnormal and, therefore, taboo (e.g. oral sex). It should be stressed to both partners that any variety of stimulation which is mutually pleasurable and emotionally acceptable should be valued and can be indulged without fear or guilt. It is equally important to make clear the corollary: that being unable to perform certain activities does not make the patient abnormal or prudish. Although partners should be encouraged to experiment and gradually to be more adventurous in their lovemaking, they should not be pushed into stimulative techniques beyond their emotional resources. If they find any activity too stressful, they should revert to a familiar, less demanding one, until they feel confident enough to proceed further.

Many sexually ignorant individuals can benefit from sensible advice found in volumes like *The Book of Love* (Delvin, 1974) or *The Joy of Sex* (Comfort, 1975). Drawings, photographs, slides and films may also be a boon to selected couples. However, the optimal use of such aids in sexual therapy, especially those which are mildly pornographic, remains to be determined (Gillan and Gillan, 1976).

Drugs

Unless the sexual dysfunction is clearly secondary to a treatable medical illness (e.g. diabetes, endogenous depression) medication should never be the main ingredient. Rarely, it has an adjunctive role with sensate focus or other physiological measures in certain cases. For example, in a women with high levels of anxiety it may be helpful to prescribe a small dose of a benzodiazepine such as diazepam 5–10 mg to be taken orally 30 min, or lorazepam 1–2 mg sublingually 5 min, before a coital attempt. Intravenous barbiturates have also been used with fantasy desensitization for the same type of patient (Cooper, 1964; Friedman, 1968).

There is some evidence that small doses of androgens (e.g. methyl testosterone 5 mg b.i.d.) may be beneficial in some patients with general unresponsiveness and low libido (Carney, Bancroft and Mathews, 1978), but the results are not very convincing at present (Mathews, 1981). However, it would seem reasonable to give it on a trial basis for up to 12 weeks, carefully assessing the outcome and any unwanted effects (e.g. hirsutism).

Psychotherapy

Psychotherapy is the essential catalyst of treatment and practitioners who believe that sex therapy consists only of a series of behavioural tasks will in most cases be disappointed. However, the key is perspective. For instance, in the case of a young, sexually inexperienced woman, with an adequate sex-drive, presenting with anxiety and anorgasmia, recently married to a similarly naive male, psychotherapy should mainly be concerned with providing factual information relating to the anatomy, physiology and psychology of sexual arousal and sensate focus, relaxation training and stimulative techniques. To boost confidence, successes are praised, failures analysed and appropriate counter-measures prescribed. Such counselling requires no great sophistication, but rather common sense and empathy.

On the other hand, if the problem is symptomatic of grave personality and relationship difficulties, then *a priori* these will need to be resolved sufficiently before a substantial practical component can be introduced. These problems generally require a greater awareness of psychodynamics, especially the nuances and ambiguities of communication (both verbal and behavioural), as well as the significance of various mental defence mechanisms including projection, denial and rationalization. These cases, which are difficult, are best handled by an experienced psychotherapist.

Treatment is a dynamic process and, as it evolves in the light of new information derived from increasing knowledge of the couple or of amelioration or exacerbation of symptoms, it should be constantly reappraised and, if indicated, changes in emphasis made. Inertia or reluctance in one or both partners, which may suggest reduced motivation or a deteriorating relationship, may be countered by clarification, confrontation or interpretation, which may help to crystallize important matters after which momentum may pick up (Sandler, Holder and Dare, 1970; Dare and Holder, 1970). Sometimes it may become clear that fundamental incompatibilities and conflicts are irreconcilable and separation or divorce may become a legitimate subject for discussion. Surprisingly, this may be welcomed by both partners.

Generally, most sex therapists recommend 10–15 sessions as the initial commitment. These may be spread weekly or monthly; the results appear equivalent in each case (Carney, Bancroft and Mathews, 1978; LoPiccolo, 1979; Mathews, 1981). If, at the end of this time, the sexual dysfunction remains essentially unchanged, the situation should be carefully reviewed and the next course of action decided. This may be termination by mutual agreement, or continuing short-term or longer term psychotherapy to improve non-sexual facets of the relationship. Again, specific goals and a timetable should be carefully worked out and followed.

SUMMARY OF TREATMENT CONCEPTS

1. In the first session each partner is seen separately (for history taking), then jointly for about 30 min. Both should receive a thorough physical examination augmented by appropriate laboratory tests, if indicated. Once a diagnosis has been formulated, intercourse is generally prohibited and detailed instructions are given on sensate focus and more specific techniques, e.g. masturbation for anorgasmia and vaginismus, vaginal self- and partner-exploration for vaginismus, etc. Home assignments are set, and the importance of strict adherence is stressed. These should be carried out at least 3 times a week for 30–60 min, or more frequently if the partners wish, provided on each occasion *all* the stipulations are satisfied. Any factual gaps in sexual knowledge are filled. If there are reasons to believe the couple might 'forget or misunderstand' what is required of them, especially regarding specific stimulations, the information should be provided in writing.

2. At subsequent meetings, the couple are always seen together. The sessions are devoted to discussing the extent to which previously agreed behavioural goals have been attained. Relevant sexual attitudes are explored and attempts made to modify them, if appropriate. For instance, one or other of the partners might be inflexible about the time of day and location of intercourse, or be dogmatic about who should initiate it. It may be possible to negotiate a change in such attitudes with a resultant increase in the novelty of sexual exchanges, which might increase arousal and overall enjoyment.

3. Channels of communication are promoted between the couple, who are encouraged to express themselves both verbally and emotionally.

4. New behavioural goals are set in hierarchical fashion until, by mutual agreement, coitus is attempted, on average after 4–6 sessions.

5. Once successful, variations in technique are introduced to enhance enjoyment and consolidate the sexual gains.

6. If, after the agreed number of sessions, there is no improvement in the sexual problem the situation is reviewed and treatment is either terminated by mutual agreement or different goals set.

Prognostic factors in sexual dysfunction

Approximately 60% of women with a sexual dysfunction will derive significant benefit from the therapeutic methods described. Provided the partners are honouring their side of the treatment contract, some measure of improvement should be apparent after 4–6 sessions, which augurs well for the final outcome. Failure to respond by this time should prompt a searching review. Lack of progress may indicate persisting low sexual drive of mainly constitutional (e.g. hereditary) origin, or complex subconscious or disguised motives and diverse interpersonal difficulties which thwart the optimal implementation of the practical regimens. Indeed, the treatment process itself may bring the hindrances into sharp focus; they may turn out to be irreconcilable and separation may follow.

There is very little objective data on prognostic factors in female sexual dysfunction, but *Table 1.5*, derived from the literature (Cooper, 1970; Marks, 1981; Hawton, 1982), offers some guidance. However, in a subject of such complexity, these relationships may not hold in all instances and cases should be considered individually. Vaginismus (and non-consummation) has generally been seen to have the best outcome, cures in excess of 75% being claimed (Friedman, 1962; Ellison, 1968), with the 100% claim of Masters and Johnson (1970) standing out. This disorder is usually considered to be 'superficial' often with a 'transparent' causation (Malleson, 1942; Friedman, 1962; Ellison, 1968). On the other hand, orgasmic dysfunction and general unresponsiveness are represented as being more pervasive and deeply seated and require correspondingly more complicated and time-consuming management (Friedman, 1962). There is probably some truth in this assertion, since the successful resolution of vaginismus may reveal a relatively intractable, orgasmic dysfunction, or generalized unresponsiveness (Malleson, 1942; Friedman, 1962).

The longer a disorder has persisted, the worse is the outcome. This probably relates to motivation for therapy which, typically, is inversely related to the duration of the problem. In women with longstanding disorders, libido declines progressively and, as apathy replaces anxiety, sex may become no longer important. These patients are often strongly motivated to retain the status quo (usually abstinence, or a much reduced coital frequency) rather than to embark on a treatment course perhaps involving a level of sexual communication and experimentation which may be distressing or irrelevant. Comfort's aphorism 'if you don't use it, you *will* lose it' is apt (Comfort, 1975). On the other hand, in disorders of recent onset, libido remains undiminished and the woman is more likely to seek a remedy to restore an experience she both misses and values, and which at this time is probably equally important to her spouse.

TABLE 1.5. Relationship of some variables to treatment response

Variable	Significantly related to a better treatment outcome
Type of disorder	Vaginismus has best outcome
Time of onset	Secondary disorders have better outcome
Duration of disorder	Recent onset disorder has better outcome
Strength of sex-drive	Strong libido has better outcome
Direction of sex-drive	Preferentially heterosexual has better outcome
Premarital coitus	Experience of physically and emotionally fulfilling premarital coitus has better outcome
Premarital orgasm (from any source)	Experience of premarital orgasm has better outcome, especially in cases of anorgasmia
Sexual attitudes	Positive attitude about own and partner's genitalia and sexual experimentation has better outcome
Feelings towards male partner	Positive feeling towards partner has better outcome
Personality	Stable personality has better outcome; extreme immaturity, oversensitivity and other features of the hysterical personality are bad pointers
Marital happiness	Good relationship has better outcome
Sexual arousal	Positive arousal to coital and other sexual activities has better outcome
Sexual fantasies	Capacity to experience exciting and pleasurable sexual fantasies has better outcome
Sudden stress	Presence of specific stress, such as marriage, bereavement, pregnancy, etc., has better outcome
Reason for seeking treatment	Self-referral for a personally important 'sexual reason' has better outcome
Attendance at therapy and adherence to programme details, e.g. homework	Regular attendances and conscientious application to programme has better outcome

Secondary disorders have generally proved to be better treatment prospects, especially if the woman had derived satisfaction from sexual experiences during adolescence and early adulthood, when heterosexuality normally crystallizes and consolidates. Habitual behaviours, especially longstanding ones, are apparently more resistant to change or eradication.

A woman's attitudes and feelings about sex may have an important bearing on the outcome of therapy. Generally, the more positive these are, the better (*Table 1.5*).

Sex-drive (libido), which has two dimensions (strength and direction), influences outcome; heterosexually oriented females having high drives do better. This appears to be mainly due to a significantly higher level of motivation for seeking therapy. These women are likely to have referred themselves and have a primary sexual reason for seeking advice. On the other hand, those whose attendance is instigated by a spouse, mother or girlfriend, or who are primarily concerned with non-sexual matters such as appeasement, do less well.

Personality and relationship issues are probably the single most important factor in therapy. Unless there is genuine commitment, based on mutual affection, and willingness to compromise, then optimal therapy cannot be provided. Longstanding rancour and conscious or unconscious deployment of the dysfunction punitively against the partner is particularly unfortunate (Gutheil, 1959).

The question of male potency *per se*, which is often stated to be crucial in therapy, needs to be viewed in perspective. It would seem that, provided he is able to accomplish full penetration and delay ejaculation for approximately 2–3 min, the emotional status of the female, the extent and quality of the preparatory sex-play and the smooth and uninterrupted nature of the coitus are more significant in influencing female responsiveness. The practice of intermittent thrusting, with the aim of delaying his orgasm so that both partners may climax simultaneously, is more likely to inhibit the female and cause frustration and irritability. This is based on the fallacy that females are innately slower in their sexual responses; actually, the sexes are equally quick provided that stimulation is uniform and optimum for each (Kinsey, Pomeroy and Martin, 1948, 1953; Masters and Johnson, 1970).

Conclusions

A treatment package for sexual dysfunction may consist of a number of variably weighted ingredients (*Table 1.4*), depending on the key features in the individual case. Currently, all assume the presence of various anxieties and inhibitions, which are believed to have adverse effects on arousal and responsiveness, it being further held that the latter will improve if the former can be remedied. Generally, in a case in which it is judged that anxiety, ignorance and inexperience are dominant, there is a tendency for the treatment to have a straightforward, largely educational and behavioural content. On the other hand, a disorder considered to be secondary to relationship and personality issues – and which may be more complicated, not always being what it seems – probably requires a greater analytical, psychotherapeutic content. Moreover, without wishing to detract from the importance of psychopathology, biological influences must also be acknowledged. These may be crucial in determining the strength of libido and ultimately may limit the response to a treatment modality, which assumes a dominant psychogenesis.

Kinsey's statistical data indicate that sexual drive is normally distributed across populations, some individuals being innately more interested and active than others (Kinsey, Pomeroy and Martin, 1948, 1953). Malleson, a clinician, believed that there was a sizable minority of women (up to 25%) who are simply physiologically incapable of responding to the point of orgasm, despite being psychologically normal and involved in a mutually rewarding love relationship with their partner. Malleson points out that to imply the presence of inhibitions or some other emotional aberration is to misunderstand the nature of the dysfunction and also to do a grave disservice to the women concerned (Malleson, 1942).

Clearly, not everyone benefits from therapy. Non-responders appear more often to have either low sex-drives and limited potential for arousal or personality disorders and serious relationship problems. The most important matter confronting the subject in its present state is to learn how to use the various components more efficiently.

Infertility

The relevance of psychosocial factors in infertility is less well established and more conjectural than in sexual dysfunction. However, there is a strong clinical impression that these may be important in the individual case. Therefore, a middle-of-the-road analysis of some of the more creditable work on the subject will be attempted here, and some practical suggestions on assessment and treatment will be offered.

Much of the earlier, somewhat fanciful, literature written by psychiatrists will not be reviewed here. Instead, the opinions of practising obstetricians and gynaecologists, experienced in infertility, are drawn together and an essentially psychosomatic argument is presented. This does not imply of course that all, or even the majority, of cases are necessarily psychogenic, or that psychological therapy is always necessary. It should be recalled that psychogenic and organic factors are not mutually exclusive. Both may, and frequently do, overlap and complicate each other to varying degrees, and optimal management requires recognition of this fact.

TABLE 1.6. **Clinical syndromes which may be associated with infertility**

Male	Female
Impotence	Non-consummation (vaginismus, more rarely pelvic pain)
Ejaculative incompetence	Tubal spasm and 'hypogonadism'
Premature ejaculation	Spontaneous abortion
Retrograde ejaculation	Hyperemesis and physiological vomiting
	Pre-eclamptic toxaemia
	Amenorrhoea and anovulation
	Anorexia nervosa

Infertility, although best considered as a problem which involves husband and wife inextricably, may be due to clinical disorders affecting one or other, or both. *Table 1.6* lists the main syndromes which may lead to infertility and which, to some extent, are believed to be caused by psychosocial factors. For completeness, male dysfunctions are listed, but are not considered further.

Non-consummation

The commonest psychosomatic disorder resulting in non-consummation is severe vaginismus. However, in a small number of women with personality disorders, non-consummation may result from wilful refusal without pain or cramps, and this should be excluded. A good description of vaginismus may be found in Friedman's book *Virgin Wives* (Friedman, 1962): 'When these patients are examined the mere attempt or actual touch of the labia may produce spasm and pain. The introitus may become so constricted that it entirely prohibits the entrance of the tip of the finger (or during coitus the penis). The spasm may involve the perineal muscle alone or may constrict the levator ani right up to the vaginal fornices. Accompanying the spasm, there is a marked adduction of the thighs, even a cramplike spasm of the adductor muscles.' These muscles have been called the 'pillars of virginity': 'Invariably the lumbar spine is extended in the position of lordosis; frequently, the posture is one of opisthotonus with the head bent backward. These symptoms are not only present during coitus, but can be witnessed during the attempted examination.'

Vaginismus 'protects' the patient from penetration and its consequences (i.e. coitus and pregnancy), and is usually caused by various permutations of fear or guilt or revulsion. Thus, in two series of 100 cases each (Friedman, 1962; Ellison, 1968), ignorance and misinformation acquired during adolescence, or before, were seen in over 90%. The following were particularly common: (a) feelings that menstruation was unhygienic or disgusting; (b) the assumption that sex was for men only; (c) the belief that rupture of the hymen must inevitably be accompanied by pain and bleeding; (d) a conviction that they were 'too small'; (e) a conviction that sex was dirty or messy.

In many cases, an examination of the fantasies or dreams of such women reveal that coitus is viewed as exploitation and degrading. The penis is often symbolized as a knife, or a large snake, and intercourse is visualized fearfully as 'painful'. Some describe the act, with obvious distaste, as 'animal'.

Commonly, such attitudes can sometimes be traced to a hostile mother who, hating sex herself, paints a frightening picture to her young and impressionable daughter. An attitude of sexual negativism acquired by contagion may persist and consolidate into the latter's adult life, and history repeats itself. The family constellation most frequently found in non-consummation is the 'S.D.S. complex', consisting of a submissive father, dominant mother and submissive husband (Ellison, 1968). Possibly, timid husbands are chosen assortively because these women think that a gentle person would hurt them less. Friedman (1962), reiterating this view, also points out the subconscious collusion between a husband and wife, who both fear the aggressiveness of sexuality. However, the woman may also use her symptom manipulatively to get her own way. It is equally true, however, that it suits some men psychologically to be the 'underdog'.

It is interesting that almost without exception patients with severe vaginismus believe it to be due to physical abnormality. They may see themselves as too small, although some think the problem is hormonal or infective – vaginal discharge being common. The husbands may present with potency problems including premature ejaculation and pain in the penis and testes. Psychodynamically, both have a strong need to maintain the sexual status quo (i.e. non-consummation). Depending on the extent and nature of the psychopathology, treatment may be directed initially at the female alone or, preferably, at both marital partners.

First, a search for the origins of the emotional tension underlying the 'self-protective' perineal and vaginal spasm must be made. During this early exchange, great efforts should be taken to win the patient's confidence; this is a vital prerequisite for optimum therapy. She is encouraged to express her attitudes about menstruation, her sex organs, lovemaking and childbearing; also her feelings about her husband's genitalia, as well as any memories of early psychosexual trauma.

At an early stage, a vaginal examination is essential, which can be used to demonstrate to the patient the psychosomatic nature of her complaint. Even with a careful single-finger penetration, muscular cramps may be induced; however, by retaining the finger *in situ* it is possible to talk most into relative relaxation, when the contractions and pain wane and finally disappear. Following this examination, the patient is encouraged to explore her own genitalia with one or more fingers while being fully relaxed; additionally, self-dilatation may be taught using graduated dilators. Using this sort of approach, up to 80% of patients consummate within 10 hours' treatment.

Treatment is more likely to succeed in women showing only mild degrees of immaturity of personality or neurosis. Patients with more severe personality abnormalities are probably better dealt with by a psychiatrist, as are those in which the psychodynamics are complex or obscure. If the husband has a disorder of potency, treatment of this will need to be integrated into an overall programme (Masters and Johnson, 1970). Sometimes, a more directive approach may be necessary to overcome a therapeutic impasse.

The following illustrative case, in which the husband was actively incorporated in therapy, shows how failure was transformed into success. The case also demonstrates the 'subconscious collusion' which may exist between such couples, and which tends to perpetuate the sexual dysfunction (Cooper, 1969).

CASE REPORT

The patient, an attractive 21-year-old, presented with non-consummation since her marriage 1½ years previously. Her reason for seeking advice was a desire to be pregnant. She had come on her own initiative, her husband apparently being unconcerned with her problem (incidentally, a bad prognostic sign!).

Prior to marriage, she had engaged in and enjoyed petting with her fiancé, but had been unable to tolerate penetration of her vagina because of severe pain. Following marriage, despite numerous attempts, coitus had not been possible; mutual masturbation (clitoral stimulation in her case) to orgasm usually followed these abortive attempts. The patient always apologized tearfully to her husband, expressing distress at her inability to allow penetration. He had been tolerant and sympathetic, and reassured her that he would never purposefully do anything to hurt her.

Clinically, the patient appeared to be a pleasant, co-operative woman, who had a well-developed phobia of penetration based on the belief that her husband's penis was too big. She described her husband as sympathetic and gentle.

The diagnosis was non-consummation, due to severe vaginismus, which had probably been maintained and consolidated by the submissive and sexually compliant attitudes of the patient's spouse. The symptom (vaginismus), present prior to marriage, seemed to be due to a marked fear of, and a desire to avoid, the pain she associated with coitus. Thus, the mechanism was solely self-protective in nature; there was no evidence that it was symptomatic of marital conflict or was part of a personality disorder or was otherwise subserving unconscious motives. Because of this fact, and despite the husband's apparent apathy, the prognosis was considered favourable.

Treatment consisted of initial vaginal examination, followed by gradual dilatation using plastic dilators of progressively increasing size while the patient was fully relaxed (and well lubricated). Simultaneously, she was encouraged to express her fantasies and these were interpreted as being related to her overriding fear of pain. At the end of each session, the patient was invited to examine and then to pass the dilators herself; thereby, to gain confidence about the obvious adequacy (for coitus) of her vagina. She was also shown that with mental and concomitant muscular relaxation the spasms could be controlled. She was advised to practise masturbation at home.

After six sessions, she was able to tolerate the largest dilator in comparative comfort, and said she felt sufficiently confident to attempt coitus. She was advised to tell her husband that, following sensate focus exchanges, he should be prepared to rouse her fully, with prolonged foreplay; also that he was to ignore any protests from her, since any pain would diminish as sexual tension increased and coitus became imperative.

After 4 weeks, she reported that despite great efforts and co-operation from her husband, penetration had not been achieved. On each occasion they had tried, muscular spasm had developed and her husband had found it impossible to proceed further, since he could not bring himself to hurt her.

The couple were invited to attend the clinic together. Her husband was told that he was oversensitive to his wife's discomfiture, and by 'colluding' with her not to go beyond minimal penetration was jointly responsible for the failure of therapy. It was asserted that full sexual arousal was incompatible with pain, which would diminish reciprocally as his wife became excited. The importance of ignoring his wife's reservations were re-emphasized as was the necessity for persistent and skilful aggressive techniques to overcome her resistance to full penetration. Furthermore, he was warned that the customary clitoral stimulation to the exclusion of coitus, with the obvious reinforcement for its repetition which orgasm must bring, was likely to diminish in her any desire for change. He was told that his wife's vagina was more than able to accommodate his penis, and that it was not possible to cause any physical damage through (normal) coitus. The essentially 'protective' nature of the spasms were pointed out. The husband was then shown the dilators which had been previously used, and was persuaded to pass them into his (relaxed) wife's vagina. He was surprised to find that she was able to accommodate the largest (considerably bigger than an erect penis) without pain. Finally, he was advised that if a contraction developed during penile penetration he was not to withdraw, but should remain *in situ* until the spasm and pain waned, whereupon he was to continue penetration in a leisurely, but determined, manner.

Shortly following this joint interview the marriage was consummated, although the patient failed to reach orgasm. After 10 months, despite fairly frequent and sustained coitus (up to 7 min) from which she derived pleasure, the patient had still not climaxed. She was pleased with her new-found ability to allow full penetration but felt disappointed about not reaching orgasm. However, she felt that with continuing experience, this would become possible. After 1 year, she had her greatest wish fulfilled, when she became pregnant.

The case exemplifies the submissive personality of the male partner and the collusive psychopathology that may exist between such couples, which tends to retain the status quo.

In a minority of cases arising out of persisting severe spasms, impotence or ejaculative failure (Brindley, 1981), artificial insemination–husband (AIH) may be the only feasible and acceptable means of achieving pregnancy. If possible, this is best performed at home, using a small plastic syringe. However, if the wife is unable to tolerate this, appropriate hospital intervention may be the only recourse. In the event of recalcitrant vaginismus, AIH should be considered sooner ιather than later in those seeking pregnancy, especially older women. It should be cautioned, however, that with grossly neurotic, or otherwise psychologically disturbed, marital partners who insist on pregnancy, some thought should be given to the possible consequences. Sandler (1968) reminds us that some such couples are psychologically ill-equipped to deal with the associated responsibility and stresses. Fortunately, this question of great moment confronts the gynaecologist only rarely. When it does, he may choose to look at it collaboratively with a psychiatrist.

Tubal spasm and hypogonadism

An association between stress, tubal spasm and hypogonadism has been imputed by several investigators, but notably by Sandler (1968). He examined 268 consecutive patients in a subfertility clinic and was convinced that stress was causally important in approximately 25%. Two main categories were recognized – abnormal attitudes to parenthood, and tubal spasm.

ABNORMAL ATTITUDES TO PARENTHOOD

In many instances, Sandler believed he was able to bring into consciousness the underlying psychopathology which, although diverse, had the common theme of 'wishing to avoid conception'. Points from two of his cases tend to bear this out:

Case 1. A woman, aged 34, had been sterile for 10 years. She had undergone numerous curettages and other investigations without benefit. She was referred by an orthopaedic surgeon who could find no physical explanation for her severe hip pain and suspected some kind of sexual maladjustment. She owned a dancing-school and was ambivalent about becoming pregnant, because having a child would mean giving up her career and having to adjust to a lower standard of living. Following appropriate counselling the patient gained sufficient insight into her unconscious rejection of pregnancy to face her conflict, which centred on whether or not to close the school. She decided to do so and conceived the next month without any other treatment.

Case 2. A 26-year-old woman, with a rather immature personality, derived little pleasure from sexual intercourse. She was introspective, suffered from colitis, and was unable to stand up for herself against a dominant and argumentative mother-in-law who always sided with her son. Each serious altercation was followed by an attack of diarrhoea. Psychotherapy in this case aimed to help the woman gain insight into the interpersonal nature of her problems, and to learn assertiveness. Gradually, she became more self-assured and happier, and shortly after she conceived.

The question confronting the physician in such cases is: does the patient really wish to be pregnant, and is she mature enough for motherhood? There is no doubt that in some emotionally disturbed women sterility can be a defence.

Often the relationship between stress and a failure to conceive may be obvious, as might be the role of psychological therapy. For instance, if it is established that there is serious marital conflict, referral to an appropriate counsellor may be extremely helpful and is always worthy of trial.

TUBAL SPASM

According to Sandler, the 'hypgonadal' uterus is frequently associated with tubal spasm, and suitable cases may respond to psychological intervention with increased fertility. He describes the tubal insufflation of a young woman referred for the investigation of infertility. Emotionally labile and over-reactive, she was extremely tense and nervous during the examination, and showed apparent occlusion with a pressure of 200 mmHg. Sandler concluded anxiety to be causally implicated in this case and, following training in relaxation techniques, conception occurred some months later. He sums up the situation as follows: 'To look at the cervix and forget the patient is to be in the same position as the man who looks at the mouth of a terrified woman, notes that it is excessively dry, and then proceeds to prescribe a mouth wash. The irrationality of such treatment is self-evident, when the sign is a dry mouth; it is not perhaps so obvious when a douche is prescribed for the dry cervix of a tense patient.'

A sizable proportion of tense and anxiety-prone women may be sexually unsatisfied. They may receive continuous sexual stimulation without orgasmic release. This can lead to chronic pelvic congestion – one of the commonest causes of the non-receptivity of cervical mucus (Sandler, 1968; Masters and Johnson, 1970).

Sandler's opinions are based on uncontrolled clinical observations; therefore, they do not carry the weight of scientific pronouncements. However, his holistic approach to infertility is laudable. He looks in depth for both psychological and organic causes, which are assessed in perspective. Accordingly, his treatment programmes often consist of various permutations of physical and psychological procedures.

Sandler also examined the effects of emotion on infertility by studying conception rates in 3 groups of sterile patients. The first group consisted of those who had reached a decision to adopt, the second was suffering from a variety of organic diseases and the third from 'stress'. Treatment considered appropriate to the presumed aetiology was prescribed and the conception rate plotted as a function of time for each group. The curves were remarkably similar in the adoption and 'stress' groups, which was in contrast to the organic group (in which conception rates were slower to peak). Sandler argues that the close accord in the outcome of the 'stress' and adoption series suggested a common factor, which he postulated as being 'relief of emotional tension'.

These findings are impressive, but other workers have found no relationship between 'a decision to adopt' and an increase in infertility (Fisher, 1973). In general, it would seem reasonable to conclude that, for some women, deciding to adopt does represent a fundamental resolution of psychological conflicts about motherhood, which may possibly have a beneficial effect upon fertility. Unfortunately, the subject is of such complexity that generalizations cannot be made.

One of the most searching questions a sterile woman can be asked is: why does she want a child? If she answers: to be like other women, to spite her mother, or in some such manner, then further enquiries will usually reveal her as immature and beset with neurotic conflicts. Both of these factors may be contributing to her infertility. Psychotherapy may be worthy of trial in these cases.

Repeated abortion

There are few references in the literature on this subject, but the investigations of Michel-Wolfromm (1968) are noteworthy. She studied 60 (20%) out of 300 cases of repeated aborters in which she felt psychogenic factors might be operating. However, organic disease was also present in 50%. She divided her cases into the following.

ACUTE EMOTIONAL TRAUMA

Acute situation stress was believed to be important in 30% (e.g. sudden severe anxiety).

NEUROTIC DISORDER

Forty-three women were judged as 'markedly neurotic', having been prone to suffer from a number of hysterical symptoms throughout their adult lives. Pregnancy phobia was extremely common. This phobia reflects both fear and desire. The woman both desires to be pregnant, to become a mature woman, while at the same time (being immature) she fears it.

UNSTABLE MARITAL RELATIONSHIP

Thirty-three women did not get on well with their husbands. Three main psychopathological themes were found. First was the woman who controls and dominates her husband, while at the same time being servile. For example, she will not take a pill unless he brings her a glass of water, or eat a meal unless he cooks it.

Second was the woman whose main defence is denial. Smiling bravely throughout, she insists that 'everything is fine', but nevertheless demands that her husband identify with her and share all of her anxieties and miseries. Third was the woman who, openly hostile to her spouse, blames him for making her pregnant. The reason for her having the child may be to avoid separation or divorce.

CONFLICTING ATTITUDES TOWARDS MOTHERHOOD

Forty-four of Michel-Wolfromm's cases were ambivalent towards motherhood. Although overlap was common she identified four clinical profiles:

1. The cowardly woman who passionately protests a desire for pregnancy, yet refuses all procedures that might assist in achieving this aim.
2. The unhappily married woman who thinks that the birth of a child will stabilize a precarious relationship, which she needs to maintain for prestige or security reasons.
3. The 'posterity' woman who consents to have a child purely to satisfy her spouse's need for an heir. For her, having it represents a great personal sacrifice.
4. The narcissistic woman whose rationale for having a baby is to boost her own ego and to flaunt it as a 'possession'.

Michel-Wolfromm is unduly sceptical about her therapeutic usefulness in the cases described which, despite evidence to the contrary, she tends to demean. However, it is not too difficult to understand her frustration. Psychological causes are rarely as obvious as organic ones; neither can they be confirmed by laboratory tests.

Nevertheless, with experience and an increasing realization of the psychodynamics of stress and the importance of this in individual cases, it becomes possible to improve one's diagnostic acumen. Practically, the most rewarding corroboration of a correct formulation is in the response to treatment (psychotherapy). In all but the most psychiatrically disturbed patients, this is best performed by the gynaecologist, together with any medical measures that might be necessary. Thus, a detailed exploration of the patient's attitudes towards pregnancy, sexual behaviour, her husband and the unborn child should be undertaken in an empathic but searching manner. Initially, the emphasis should be on listening rather than talking, since once confidence and trust has been gained, this becomes a great source of relief to the patient. Strenuous efforts should be made to convert pessimism into optimism. This can best be achieved by providing factual information, support and reassurance. It should be remembered that these patients are often acutely perceptive and over-responsive; therefore, scepticism or hostility in the physician might be noticed, with the risk of adverse sequelae.

Psychotherapy, which should be tailored to the individual's needs, is based mainly on common sense. Michel-Wolfromm's words are illustrative: 'The doctor has much greater influence if he is a good listener and has an acute sense of responsibility towards his patient. One should listen patiently to all complaints and fears. This way it is possible to help her solve any problem that may occur. It would be silly to try to trace its origin. The most effective means of a psychotherapy of total involvement is identification with the patient, taking on with her almost in her stead responsibility for the birth.'

Using this approach, Michel-Wolfromm claims 45% success (i.e. reaching full term). Other workers are apparently more successful, with success rates of up to 100% (Mann, 1957; Tupper and Well, 1962; Sandler, 1968).

Once a psychotherapeutic commitment has been made by the physician, it must be honoured throughout the pregnancy, or until the baby is lost. The frequency of meetings is usually a compromise between the patient's needs and the doctor's availability. However, as a rough guide, about 20 min every 2–3 weeks may be adequate. Attention to the home environment may also be required, and a social work visit should be arranged.

The use of psychoactive drugs during pregnancy is contentious. In general, for a number of reasons avoidance is the best course; however, acute overwhelming stress may call for the short-term administration of a benzodiazepine or other anxiolytic agent. Clearly, each case should be judged carefully on its merits.

Hyperemesis and physiological vomiting in pregnancy

The incidence of vomiting in pregnancy, severe enough to warrant hospitalization, is extremely low (Tylden, 1968). It is not known whether the condition differs in some fundamental way from physiological vomiting, or is merely a more severe form of it. Both are probably multifactorial, involving hormonal, physiological and psychological factors.

Fairweather (1958) studied hyperemesis nationally, and found a greatly increased prevalence of previous pregnancy wastage (31–40% by miscarriage and neonatal death). Tylden (1968), who was mainly interested in examining current methods of treatment, examined 3 groups of patients. Forty-seven were hyperemetics, 40 presented with anxiety and physiological vomiting, and 44 had anxiety without vomiting. The incidence of previous pregnancy loss was approximately the same for each group, up to 40%. The hyperemetics differed significantly from the other groups in the number of previous 'operations, major illnesses, and major emotional stresses' such as loss of a parent, homelessness, imprisonment, desertion, divorce, etc.

Rejection seems very common in these women; there may be a history of disturbed upbringing, especially chronic exposure to familial hostility. Typically, they lack self-confidence and, being constantly reminded of their shortcomings, they tend to develop into extremely vulnerable personalities. Generally, they are over-responsive, even to the mildest criticism. They often have unstable and turbulent marriages; being immature, they frequently crave a level of support that the spouse may be unable, or unwilling, to provide.

Vomiting and hyperemesis are probably not disease entities *per se*, but are symptomatic of more pervasive physical or psychological disorders in a susceptible group of pregnant women. These have a high incidence of abnormal pregnancy and labour, and have suffered more miscarriages than the general population. As in many psychosomatic conditions, the symptom of vomiting may represent a 'cry for help', which should be sympathetically and comprehensively explored.

The old psychoanalytic belief that vomiting symbolizes (oral) rejection of the unborn child, which is followed by actual fetal expulsion, is no longer tenable. On the contrary, there is some evidence that vomiting in this group of women actually reduces the neonatal and perinatal death rate.

Tylden (1968) points out how the attitude of some nursing and medical attendants, far from helping hyperemetics, can actually worsen them. Characteristically, the patient is seen as being attention-seeking, 'bloody-minded' or merely a nuisance, and is brusquely told to 'pull herself together'. The doctor may be unable, or unwilling, to provide the sympathetic understanding and support that these vulnerable women need. In these circumstances, whatever the original cause, vomiting may become conditioned as a hostile counter-response to authority. Thus, whenever she is criticized, she vomits, inviting more abuse which provokes further vomiting. So, the vicious circle is completed, and the symptom perpetuated.

In the treatment of these personality-disordered hyperemetics, it is crucial to avoid confrontation, even if this seems what the patient wants. It may well be that she is testing the relationship (e.g. inviting rejection by the doctor!), thereby confirming her view that nobody understands her. Many of these women are grossly immature, suspicious and neurotic, and require a great deal of tact and reassurance. It is essential to be accepted by the patient and not, as is so often the case, be seen as a punitive or authoritarian figure.

Using supportive psychotherapy, it may be possible to suppress, or at least reduce, the frequency of the vomiting and carry the woman to term. Clearly, however, this is palliation and will do little to change the underlying personality abnormality or neurotic diathesis. These problems may need to be addressed long term by a psychiatrist.

Pre-eclamptic toxaemia

Although the literature on the subject is sparse, several authorities consider pre-eclamptic toxaemia (PET) to be a psychosomatic condition (Garret, 1950; Dieckmann, 1952; Coppen, 1958). Coppen's work is especially noteworthy. He hypothesized there would be 'bodily and psychological differences' between a group of pre-eclamptic and a control group of women attending the same antenatal clinic. In summary, he found the following significant differences (Coppen, 1958).

PERSONALITY FACTORS

The PET group showed high rates of (a) emotionally disturbed menarche, (b) premenstrual tension, (c) poor sexual adjustment, (d) disturbed attitudes towards pregnancy, (e) psychiatric symptoms and (f) anxiety proneness.

Coppen concluded that women who develop toxaemia are likely to have difficulties in adjusting psychologically to the 'feminine role'. He advised considering abortion or adoption in especially disturbed patients.

PHYSIQUE

Coppen found an abnormal discriminate androgyny score in the PET group (3 × bi-acromial–1 × bi-iliac diameter), with a tendency towards androgyny (i.e. maleness – as evidenced by broader shoulders and narrow hips).

His research, which surprisingly does not appear to have been repeated, is important. It has prognostic and therapeutic implications. Thus, it may prove possible by studying the psychological and physical characteristics of pregnant women to predict those at risk for developing PET. It would also be of great interest to examine the contribution of psychotherapy in treatment.

Amenorrhoea

Secondary amenorrhoea can be precipitated by acute stress, or be symptomatic of various psychiatric illnesses (e.g. marital problems, change of environment or occupation, anxiety, depression, schizophrenia).

At present, it is not clear why some women, under stress, become amenorrhoeic, and others do not. It is probable that this might be determined mainly by genetic factors which render some but not other organ systems vulnerable.

The sudden onset of amenorrhoea following an emotional shock suggests an aetiological relationship, and the patient often shows other signs of being anxiety prone. However, thorough physical and endocrine examinations are essential to establish an accurate formulation; management is that of the underlying conditions. Amenorrhoea due to acute stress is usually self-limiting, but supportive treatment consisting of psychotherapy, with or without minor tranquillizers, may facilitate resolution. Reassurance is doubly important since some of these women are convinced that they are suffering from 'serious organic disease'. In a number of secondary amenorrhoeics, causation may never be established.

Anorexia nervosa

It is rare for a patient with anorexia nervosa to be referred initially to a gynaecologist. Generally, the emaciation or bulimia will have suggested the nature of the illness to the family physician, who will have instigated a psychiatric evaluation. Sometimes, however, amenorrhoea presents before weight loss becomes too noticeable and may obfuscate the condition. However, at a time when anorexia nervosa is becoming more prevalent, even minimal weight loss in a young female should alert the physician to its possibility. The diagnosis can be made with confidence only following lengthy discussions, both with the patient and appropriate family members. The latter are especially important since anorexics, who are often vivacious and active, typically deny any illness. Apart from the almost invariable dread of becoming fat and ugly (Crisp, 1970), the psychopathology may be diverse. For example, some patients, terrified of physical maturity, try to suppress the development of secondary sexual characteristics by stringent dieting; their desperate need is to remain 'a little girl'. Fear of losing control is a recurring theme, and anorexics may show other manifestations of compulsive behaviour.

In summary, the anorexic is generally unable to face the responsibilities of being adult. The physical manifestations of her psychopathology, such as extreme emaciation and physical immaturity, are pathognomic. The cessation of the menses in anorexia nervosa is probably due to extreme weight loss and, in particular, carbohydrate starvation; however, in some cases, it may possibly be caused by psychological factors. Treatment, especially if food restriction has been great, is best begun in hospital. Initially, it consists in restoring the weight to around average for the patient's age and height, together with appropriate psychotherapy. Sometimes, depression will coexist and be severe enough to warrant specific drug treatment.

Following early weight gain, sufferers may enter a 'convalescent phase' of intermittent overeating and obesity before stabilizing. Ovulation and regular menstrual bleeding are likely to be re-established within 1 year following the restoration of a stable weight and more normal feeding habits. Persuading the patient to eat is relatively easy and is the least of her problems. Whether or not she can become a mature, childbearing women is another matter. Crisp (1970), who treated and followed up 21 anorectics for up to 42 months, reported pregnancy in 1 case. The overall prognosis in anorectics is guarded. Unequivocal anorexia nervosa, which occurs in approximately 1–2% of adolescent girls (but certain groups run special risks, up to 10%), will rarely be seen in an infertility clinic. A gynaecologist is probably more likely to encounter patients with secondary anorexia, amenorrhoea and sterility.

Psychopathologically, these women should be investigated in a broadly similar manner as repeated aborters. Treatment will be on psychosomatic lines, recognizing that both physical and psychological anomalies may coexist.

Conclusions

Although at present the precise relevance of psychosocial factors in contributing to infertility is arguable, nevertheless there is a wealth of clinical observation worthy of consideration. It is restressed that organic and psychological aetiologies (and treatment) are not mutually exclusive. Each may overlap and complicate the other to varying degrees. The difficulty of perspective is well illustrated by Michel-Wolfromm (1968), a psychodynamically oriented gynaecologist who, if she finds psychological and physical factors in a patient, tends to ignore the former. Her position is both arbitrary and contradictory, since she uses psychotherapy in her treatment programmes and claims a success rate in 'emotionally determined cases' of up to 45%.

The main reasons why many physicians have difficulty in accepting psychogenic factors are as follows. First, unlike organic lesions, the diagnosis cannot be confirmed by curettage or laparotomy (i.e. scientifically). However, provided a full history is obtained, the relevance of such elements can be adduced positively and not by default (e.g. the absence of organic causes), which so often is the approach. The second problem relates to treatment. It is far easier to perform surgery, or administer a drug, than give psychotherapy. Not only is it usually less demanding on the physician, but it is generally more acceptable to the patient and the results are easier to assess. On the other hand, psychotherapy is fraught with difficulties. At best, it is an uneasy marriage between art and science; at worst, an intervention which, far from helping, can actually worsen the patient's condition.

From the gynaecologist's point of view, perhaps the most difficult thing of all is the acceptance of a role which is in sharp contrast with that of a traditional mechanistic surgical approach. Psychotherapy demands an empathic and sensitive physician, who is a skilful prober, good listener and an accomplished educator. Above all, he must be able to separate psychological relevance from irrelevance, and to advise accordingly. This is not as daunting as it might sound. There is no need for an in-depth knowledge of psychopathology or the more subtle aspects of personality and interpersonal interactions; rather, a basic appreciation of the psychosomatic significance of stress and the fundamental tenets of simple supportive counselling is necessary. If more is required, collaboration with a psychiatrist experienced in the field may be worth while.

References

BEARD, R. W., BELSEY, E. M., LIEBERMAN, B. A. and WILKINSON, J. C. M. (1977) Pelvic pain in women. *American Journal of Obstetrics and Gynecology*, **128**, 566–570

BRINDLEY, G. S. (1981) Electroejaculation: its technique, neurological implications and uses. *Journal of Neurology, Neurosurgery and Psychiatry*, **44**, 9–18

BRINDLEY, G. S. and GILLAN, P. (1982) Men and women who do not have orgasms. *British Journal of Psychiatry*, **140**, 351–356

CARNEY, A., BANCROFT, J. and MATHEWS, A. (1978) Combination of hormonal and psychological treatment for female sexual unresponsiveness. *British Journal of Psychiatry*, **132**, 339–346

COMFORT, A. (1975) *The Joy of Sex*. London; Quartet

COOPER, A. J. (1964) Behaviour therapy in the treatment of bronchial asthma. *Journal of Behaviour Research and Therapy*, **1**, 351–356

COOPER, A. J. (1969) An innovation in the behavioural treatment of a case of nonconsummation due to vaginismus. *British Journal of Psychiatry*, **115**, 721–722

COOPER, A. J. (1970) Frigidity: a clinical and statistical study of some factors which influence the short-term prognosis. *Journal of Psychosomatic Research*, **14**, 133–147

COPPEN, A. J. (1958) Psychosomatic aspects of pre-eclamptic toxaemia. *Journal of Psychosomatic Research*, **2**, 241–265

CRISP, A. H. (1970) Anorexia nervosa 'feeding disorder', 'nervous malnutrition' or 'weight phobia'. *World Review of Nutrition and Dietetics*, **12**, 452–504

CROWE, M. J., GILLAN, P. and GOLOMBOK, S. (1981) Form and content in the conjoint treatment of sexual dysfunction: a controlled study. *Behaviour Research and Therapy*, **19**, 47–54

CROWN, S. and D'ARDENNE, P. (1982) Controversies, methods, results: symposium on sexual dysfunction. *British Journal of Psychiatry*, **140**, 70–77

DARE, C. and HOLDER, A. (1970) Basic psychoanalytic concepts: III Transference. *British Journal of Psychiatry*, **116**, 667–672

DELVIN, D. (1974) *The Book of Love*. London; New English Library

DIECKMANN, W. J. (1952) *The Toxaemias of Pregnancy*. London; Henry Kimpton

ELLISON, C. (1968) Psychosomatic factors in unconsummated marriage. *Journal of Psychosomatic Research*, **12**, 61–65

EYSENCK, H. J. and WILSON, G. (1979) *The Psychology of Sex*. London; Dent

FAIRWEATHER, D. V. I. (1966) Hyperemesis gravidarum. *M.D. thesis*, Univ. of St. Andrews, Scotland

FISHER, S. (1973) *The Female Orgasm*. London; Allen Lane

FRIEDMAN, D. (1968) The treatment of impotence by Brietal relaxation therapy. *Behaviour Research and Therapy*, **6**, 256–261

FRIEDMAN, L. J. (1962) *Virgin Wives*. London; Tavistock Publications

GARRET, S. S. (1950) Etiology of eclampsia. *Western Journal of Surgery, Obstetrics and Gynecology*, **58**, 229–235

GILLAN, T. and GILLAN, P. (1976) *Sex Therapy Today*. London; Open Books

GUTHEIL, E. H. (1959) Sexual dysfunctions in men. In *American Handbook of Psychiatry*, Vol. 1 (Arieti, S., Ed.). New York; Basic Books

HAWTON, K. (1982) The behavioural treatment of sexual dysfunction. *British Journal of Psychiatry*, **140**, 94–101

KAPLAN, H. S. (1974) *The New Sex Therapy*. London; Baillière, Tindall

KEGAL, A. H. (1952) Sexual functions of the pubococcygeus muscle. *Western Journal of Surgery, Obstetrics and Gynecology*, **60**, 521

KINSEY, A. C., POMEROY, W. B. and MARTIN, C. E. (1948) *Sexual Behaviour in the Human Male*. Philadelphia; Saunders

KINSEY, A. C., POMEROY, W. B. and MARTIN, C. E. (1953) *Sexual Behaviour in the Human Female*. Philadelphia; Saunders

LAZARUS, A. A. (1963) The treatment of chronic frigidity by systemic desensitization. *Journal of Nervous and Mental Disorders*, **136**, 272–278

LOBITZ, W. C. and LOPICCOLO, J. (1972) New methods in the behavioural treatment of sexual dysfunction. *Journal of Behaviour Therapy and Experimental Psychiatry*, **3**, 265–271

LOPICCOLO, J. (1979) *Sexual Dysfunction in Behavioural Medicine: Theory and Practice* (Pomerleau, O. F. and Brady, J. P., Eds). Baltimore; Williams & Wilkins

MACKAY, D. (1977) Emotional constipation. *British Journal of Sexual Medicine*, **4**, 14–17

MALLESON, J. (1942) Vaginismus: its management and psychogenesis. *British Medical Journal*, **2**, 213–218

MANN, E. C. (1957) The role of emotional determinants in habitual abortion. *Surgical Clinics of North America*, **37**, 447–458

MARKS, I. M. (1981) Review of behavioural psychotherapy, II: sexual disorders. *American Journal of Psychiatry*, **138** (6), 750–763

MARSHALL, D. S. (1971) Sexual behaviour on Mangaia. In *Human Sexual Behaviour – Variations in the Ethnographic Spectrum* (Marshall, D. S. and Suggs, R. C., Eds.). Basic Books; New York

MASTERS, W. H. and JOHNSON, V. E. (1970) *Human Sexual Inadequacy*. London; Churchill

MASTERS, W. H. and JOHNSON, V. E. (1979) *Homosexuality in Perspective*. Boston; Little Brown and Company

MATHEWS, A. M. (1981) Treatment of sex dysfunction: psychological and hormone factors. In *Learning Theory Applications in Psychiatry* (Boulougouris, J. C., Ed.). New York; Wiley

MATHEWS, A., BANCROFT, J., WHITEHEAD, A., HACKMAN, A., JULIER, D., BANCROFT, J., GATH, C. and SHAW, P. (1976) The behavioural treatment of sexual inadequacy: a comparative study. *Behaviour Research Therapy*, **14**, 427–436

MEAD, M. (1949) *Male and Female*. New York; William Morrow

MICHEL-WOLFROMM, H. (1968). The psychological factor in spontaneous abortion. *Journal of Psychosomatic Research*, **12**, 67–71

RILEY, A. J. and RILEY, E. J. (1978) A controlled study to evaluate directed masturbation in the management of primary orgasmic failure in women. *British Journal of Psychiatry*, **133**, 404–409

SANDLER, B. (1968) Emotional stress and infertility. *Journal of Psychosomatic Research*, **12**, 51–59

SANDLER, J., HOLDER, A. and DARE, C. (1970) Basic psychoanalytic concepts: II The treatment alliance. *British Journal of Psychiatry*, **116**, 555–558

TUPPER, C. and WELL, R. J. (1962) The problem of spontaneous abortion. The treatment of habitual aborters by psychotherapy. *American Journal of Obstetrics and Gynecology*, **83**, 421–424

TYLDEN, E. (1968) Hyperemesis and physiological vomiting. *Journal of Psychosomatic Research*, **12**, 85–93

WEISSMAN, M. M. and SLABY, A. E. (1973) Oral contraceptives in psychiatric disturbance. *British Journal of Psychiatry*, **123**, 513–518

WOLPE, J. (1958) *Psychotherapy by Reciprocal Inhibition*. Stanford, USA; Stanford University Press

Chapter 2

Psychological problems and gynaecological surgery

Dennis Gath and Nicholas Rose

This chapter deals with psychiatric problems occurring in relation to gynaecological surgery. The chapter is in two main parts. The first is concerned with psychiatric problems specific to gynaecology; the second with psychiatric problems associated with surgery in general. An example of a specifically gynaecological problem is the extent to which psychiatric factors should influence selection for hysterectomy or sterilization. An example of a general problem in surgery is how to assess and manage a patient who becomes muddled and disorientated a few days after an operation.

Psychiatric problems specific to gynaecological surgery

There are three gynaecological operations with which psychiatric problems are commonly said to occur – hysterectomy, sterilization and oophorectomy. They are also the operations that have been most studied by psychiatrists. For both reasons this part of the chapter focuses on these three procedures, but similar principles apply to them and to other gynaecological surgery.

Psychiatric aspects of hysterectomy

Until a few years ago, hysterectomy was often said to be a common cause of psychiatric disorder, particularly depression. As evidence for this belief, numerous studies were quoted in which high levels of psychiatric morbidity had been found among women at varying intervals after hysterectomy. Unfortunately, these early studies did not justify any conclusions about the possible role of hysterectomy as a cause of subsequent psychiatric disorder. Such conclusions were not warranted because of serious limitations of research method, which can be illustrated by three examples.

First, the early psychiatric studies examined women at some time after hysterectomy, but not before the operation. Such an approach can tell us nothing about the effects of hysterectomy, because there is no way of knowing whether any psychiatric morbidity detected after the operation was already present before the operation or whether it started after the operation. In short, the *post hoc* approach does not justify a *propter hoc* conclusion.

Secondly, the early studies used unsatisfactory methods for defining and identifying psychiatric disorders. For example, psychiatric disorders were sometimes defined in terms of referral to a psychiatrist, or the prescribing of anti-depressant medication by the general practitioner. Such indirect criteria cannot give accurate estimates of levels of psychiatric morbidity.

Thirdly, the selection of hysterectomy patients for research purposes was often unsatisfactory. For example, a common mistake was to study heterogeneous samples, such as patients undergoing hysterectomy for mixed gynaecological indications, including dysfunctional uterine bleeding, prolapse and cancer. If the aim is to study the psychiatric effects of removal of the uterus uncontaminated by other factors, there is no point in studying such mixed samples. Thus, little can be learned about hysterectomy from studying patients with malignant disease, because greater psychiatric problems may be caused by cancer than by the operation.

These earlier studies will not be reviewed further here, but a detailed account of them can be found in a recent review (Gath and Cooper, 1982). Instead this chapter will focus on two recent studies which aimed to avoid the above limitations of method in three ways: by assessing patients before hysterectomy as well as after it; by using standardized psychiatric measures of known reliability and validity; and by selecting patients undergoing straightforward hysterectomy for menorrhagia of benign origin.

The first study was carried out in Oxford (Gath, Cooper and Day, 1981; Gath et al., 1981). The research sample consisted of 156 women undergoing hysterectomy for menorrhagia of benign origin (fibroids; endometriosis; dysfunctional uterine bleeding). These patients were assessed psychiatrically 4 weeks before hysterectomy, and 6 months and 18 months after the operation. Several standardized psychiatric measures of known reliability were used. Among these, the main measure was the Present State Examination (PSE) (Wing, Cooper and Sartorius, 1974; Wing, 1976), a standardized psychiatric interview which makes it possible to classify patients into psychiatric 'cases' and 'non-cases' for research purposes, using clearly specified criteria. Using the PSE, the Oxford group found that 90 patients (58%) were psychiatric cases before hysterectomy, while postoperatively the numbers fell significantly to 38 (26%) at 6-month follow-up, and 43 (29%) at 18 months.

By using the PSE, it is possible to chart the distribution of severity of psychiatric morbidity in groups of patients. As shown in *Figure 2.1,* preoperatively the distribution of severity of psychiatric morbidity in the hysterectomy group was half-way between that of women in the general population and that of psychiatric patients (the differences from both being significant). After the operation, the hysterectomy group was much closer to the general population, but still differed from it significantly.

Since patients were assessed psychiatrically before hysterectomy, it was possible to tell how many new psychiatric cases emerged after the operation. Of the 66 patients who were psychiatrically well before surgery (PSE non-cases), only 9 were PSE cases at the 18-months follow-up – less than one-quarter of all the PSE cases (i.e. 43) detected at that follow-up. This finding pointed strongly to the conclusion that hysterectomy seldom leads to psychiatric disorder. Furthermore, there was some evidence that the operation may have alleviated pre-existing psychiatric disorder – of 90 women who were PSE cases preoperatively, as many as 51 (57%) were non-cases at follow-up.

Numerous other psychiatric and social measures pointed to a generally good outcome after hysterectomy. An example is provided by measures of psychosexual functioning. At the 6-month follow-up, the reported frequency of sexual

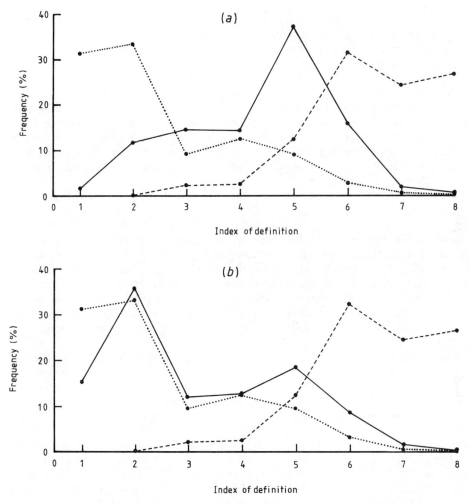

Figure 2.1. (a) PSE index of definition, preoperative (●———●, preoperative hysterectomy sample, n = 156; ●----●, psychiatric inpatients and outpatients, n = 148; ●····●, general population sample, n = 237); (b) PSE index of definition, postoperative (●———●, 18 months postoperative hysterectomy sample, n = 148; ●----●, psychiatric inpatients and outpatients, n = 148; ●····●, general population sample, n = 237)

intercourse was increased in 56% of patients, unchanged in 27% and decreased in 17%. In the sample as a whole, the frequency of sexual intercourse was very significantly increased. Reported enjoyment of sexual intercourse showed equally satisfactory improvements. At the 18-month follow-up the findings were much the same. Such findings are sharply at odds with the reports of earlier research.

The second recent study was carried out in St Louis, USA (Martin *et al.*, 1977; Martin, Roberts and Clayton, 1980). A standardized psychiatric interview was used to assess 49 women admitted to hospital for non-malignant conditions. The investigators used different diagnostic categories from those usually employed in the UK. Nevertheless, the proportion of patients given a psychiatric diagnosis preoperatively (57%) was virtually the same as the proportion of psychiatric cases (58%) in the Oxford sample preoperatively. The 44 patients examined at 1-year follow-up were found to have fewer psychiatric symptoms than preoperatively. The investigators concluded that their findings did not support the hypothesis that hysterectomy is followed by an excess of psychiatric symptoms.

The findings of the Oxford and St Louis studies were encouraging, since they indicated that hysterectomy seldom leads to psychiatric disorder. Nevertheless, sizable proportions of patients were psychiatrically unwell at postoperative follow-up. In the Oxford study, for example, over one-quarter of the patients were psychiatric cases at the 6-month and 18-month follow-ups. For this reason, it is important to look for gynaecological, psychiatric and other factors that might be associated with a poor psychiatric outcome.

In the previous literature, it was reported that psychiatric outcome was worse in patients with no demonstrable pathology in the uterus (dysfunctional uterine bleeding) than in patients with organic pathology such as fibroids and endometriosis (Barker, 1968; Richards, 1973). However, in the Oxford study no significant differences between dysfunctionals and organics were found in psychiatric status before or after hysterectomy (and no differences in previous psychiatric history, or in the personality dimension of neuroticism).

No association was found between psychiatric outcome and any other gynaecological variable, including the patients' self-reports of the severity of their menstrual problem, the use of abdominal or vaginal surgery, or any postoperative complications.

It is sometimes stated that a poor psychiatric outcome is commoner in women aged under 35, those with no or few children, and those who are unmarried, divorced or widowed. There is no convincing evidence for any of these reported associations. Nor is there any evidence that social class is relevant.

By far the most consistent finding is that psychiatric disorder *after* hysterectomy is much more frequent in women who have had psychiatric disorder at any time *before* the operation. This association was found in retrospective studies by Lindemann (1941), Melody (1962), Patterson and Craig (1963), Barker (1968) and Richards (1973). The finding was strongly confirmed in the two prospective studies described above. In the USA, Martin *et al.* (1977) and Martin, Roberts and Clayton (1980) found that virtually all patients receiving psychiatric treatment after hysterectomy had received similar treatment before the operation. In the Oxford study, psychiatric outcome after hysterectomy was significantly positively associated with preoperative mental state, a history of psychiatric referral at any time in the patient's life, and the personality dimension of neuroticism.

We have seen that, in the two studies in which patients were examined before hysterectomy, levels of psychiatric morbidity were remarkably high preoperatively (57% in St Louis, 58% in Oxford). These findings are consistent with those of a survey by Ballinger (1977) in Dundee. In this survey, levels of psychiatric morbidity in gynaecological patients aged 40–55 were found to be much higher than in the general population, or in patients consulting their GP, or in patients admitted to a medical ward. Furthermore, among the gynaecological patients, psychiatric morbidity was particularly high in those complaining of excessive menstruation; within the latter group, morbidity was even higher among those subsequently selected for hysterectomy.

These findings suggest a possible explanation for the excess of psychiatric morbidity detectable preoperatively among patients selected for hysterectomy. It may be that the combination of psychiatric disorder and complaints of excessive menstruation plays a part in the processes whereby the patient decides to consult the GP, the GP decides to refer the patient to the gynaecologist, and the gynaecologist decides to recommend hysterectomy. This is, of course, only speculation, since we do not know the distribution of psychiatric disorder among patients with similar menstrual complaints who do not pass through this chain of decision-making.

If it is true that psychiatric disorder is sometimes a determinant of selection for hysterectomy, it may be possible to explain why half the patients with pre-hysterectomy psychiatric disorder remain psychiatrically unwell after the operation. For this purpose we need to turn to research on the relationship between menstrual blood loss as objectively measured and the patient's own estimate of menstrual loss. In a study of 92 women with complaints of heavy but regular periods for which no cause could be found, Chimbira, Anderson and Turnbull (1980) measured menstrual blood loss objectively during two consecutive menstrual periods, using the method first described by Hallberg and Nilsson (1964). No significant correlation was found between measured menstrual loss and the patients' judgements of their menstrual loss. Particularly important was the finding that, among menstrual periods rated by the women as heavy, as many as 47% were below 80 ml, the level generally regarded as defining menorrhagia (Nilsson and Rybo, 1971; Haynes, Anderson and Turnbull, 1979). Moreover, no significant relationship was found between measured menstrual loss and the number of days of menstrual bleeding, or the number of sanitary towels and pads used. The authors concluded that the methods used to assess menstrual loss are unsatisfactory in many women.

The evidence suggests that women with psychiatric disorder before hysterectomy may fall into two groups:

1. Women who would be found to have 'true' menorrhagia on objective measurement. In this group, it is likely that psychiatric disorder is secondary to menorrhagia. Heavy periods may be distressing and handicapping, and it is psychologically understandable that they may lead to psychiatric disorder. It is equally understandable that psychiatric disorder may be alleviated by surgical relief of heavy periods.
2. Women who would be found to have normal or light periods on objective measurement. In this group, it seems likely that preoperative psychiatric disorder is primary; that is, not induced by menstrual symptoms. Complaints of excessive menstruation may be secondary to psychiatric disorder, which could, for example, reduce the patient's tolerance to a previously well-tolerated level of menstruation. It is therefore understandable that hysterectomy makes no difference to mental state. It is possible that patients in this group would benefit more from psychiatric treatment than from hysterectomy.

All this is speculative, and at present it is not known whether such groups can be identified, and how large they are likely to be. Further research is needed to answer these questions. In the meantime, the following suggestions can be made about the relevance of psychiatric factors to the selection of patients for hysterectomy for complaints of excessive periods.

If the patient is free from psychiatric disorder before hysterectomy, then the postoperative psychiatric outcome is likely to be good, and there are no implications for selection.

If the patient has a psychiatric disorder before the operation, the chances of a good psychiatric outcome are about 50%. In the present state of knowledge it cannot be firmly said that psychiatric factors should play a part in deciding for or against hysterectomy. However, it may be useful to bear the following points in mind. Clinical evaluation of the patient's menstrual complaints should be as thorough as possible; if available, objective measurement of menstrual loss might be helpful. An attempt should be made to determine how far the psychiatric disorder is primary; that is, induced by factors other than menstrual symptoms. For this evaluation, an assessment should be made of any current problems in the patient's life (in marriage, family, work, housing and so forth), and of the previous psychiatric history. If it seems that the patient may not have 'true' menorrhagia, and may have a primary psychiatric disorder, then the possibility of psychiatric referral is worth considering as a first alternative to hysterectomy.

Psychiatric aspects of sterilization

In the past 10–20 years, the practice of sterilization has changed substantially in the UK. It has become much more frequent – in some centres the frequency increased tenfold in a decade (Bledin, Beral and Ashley, 1978). In addition, sterilization has become increasingly an elective interval procedure and has been performed more on younger women and on those with fewer children.

For these reasons, there is no point in reviewing the pre-1970 literature, although it is worth noting that several early studies reported high rates of psychiatric morbidity after sterilization. These studies have been reviewed by Schwyhart and Kutner (1973) and by Gath and Cooper (1982).

Among the more recent studies, several had the same limitations of method as the hysterectomy studies reviewed above; that is, patients were not assessed before the operation, methods of assessment were not clearly defined or standardized, and samples were mixed. Two recent studies have avoided these methodological problems, and both found no evidence that sterilization led to adverse psychological sequelae in the samples studied.

The first of these two studies was carried out by Cooper et al. (1981, 1982) in Oxford. Nearly 100 women undergoing elective interval sterilization were interviewed on three occasions. A few months before sterilization the proportion of PSE cases was just over 10%, which is no greater than the proportion to be expected among women in the general population. Six months after sterilization the proportion fell significantly to under 5%, and 18 months after the operation it had risen to just under 10%.

Among the 180 patients who had been psychiatrically well (PSE non-cases) before the operation, only 12 (6.7%) became PSE cases after the operation. This strongly suggested that sterilization did not lead to psychiatric disorder in this sample.

In contrast to many earlier studies (all retrospective) the Oxford study found that both frequency and enjoyment of sexual intercourse were increased after sterilization, and that expressions of regret at having been sterilized were uncommon. Expressions of regret were more frequent in women who had had psychiatric disorder preoperatively.

The second study was carried out in Nottingham by Bledin et al. (1984). As in the Oxford study, standardized interview methods were used before sterilization and at defined intervals afterwards (6 weeks and 6 months). However, this study differed from the Oxford study in three main ways: it was deliberately restricted to women who were free from either physical or mental ill-health preoperatively; it included post-partum as well as interval sterilization; and it included two non-sterilized comparison groups drawn from family planning clinics and maternity wards. There were 65–70 women in each of these four groups.

The main findings were: there was no evidence that mental health as measured by the PSE was significantly affected by sterilization; more sterilization subjects than non-sterilized subjects reported subjectively experienced impediments in sexual satisfaction at the later follow-up; regrets and wish for reversal were rare, and were associated with higher PSE scores initially.

From these two studies, it appears that elective sterilization, as practised at two teaching centres in the UK, has no significant adverse psychological sequelae in healthy women in the first 6–18 months after the operation. It is not certain that the same would apply to women in countries with different cultures.

In the past, it was often held that age, parity and marital disharmony were determinants of psychiatric outcome after sterilization. Recent studies do not support any such associations, at least in Western cultures. It now appears that the main determinants of adverse sequelae such as psychiatric disturbance or feelings of regret after sterilization, are preoperative psychiatric disorder, previous history of psychiatric contact, and neuroticism – although all these are much less common among sterilization patients than among hysterectomy patients.

Psychiatric aspects of bilateral oophorectomy

There have been few reports of the psychiatric effects of bilateral oophorectomy, and it is difficult to draw any firm conclusions from them. There are two reasons for this difficulty. First, bilateral oophorectomy is usually performed together with other procedures, such as hysterectomy; hence it is difficult to identify any adverse effects specifically associated with removal of the ovaries. Secondly, most psychiatric studies of oophorectomy have been retrospective and based on small and unrepresentative samples, and have used variable time intervals of assessment.

Research has been concerned with two possible sequelae of oophorectomy – psychiatric disorder and psychosexual dysfunction. The four main studies of psychiatric disorder have compared psychiatric morbidity after hysterectomy with and without oophorectomy. Two of these studies were retrospective and two prospective. Both retrospective studies found that the psychiatric outcome was no worse when hysterectomy was combined with bilateral oophorectomy (Barker, 1968; Richards, 1973). In the prospective study in St Louis, oophorectomy was found to have no special association with psychiatric morbidity, but a significant association with complaints of headaches, fatigue and menopausal symptoms (Martin, Roberts and Clayton, 1980). Among the 156 women undergoing hysterectomy in the Oxford prospective study, 30 (19.2%) had bilateral oophorectomies (Gath et al., 1981). Among these bilaterally oophorectomized women, there was no evidence of an excess of psychiatric morbidity (compared with non-oophorectomized women), and no evidence of any difference in psychiatric outcome between the 18 women who received a hormone implant and the 12 who did not. From these four studies, it seems likely that the psychiatric outcome is no worse after hysterectomy combined with oophorectomy, than after oophorectomy alone.

From the clinical literature little is known about sexual dysfunction after bilateral oophorectomy alone. Four studies have examined psychosexual functioning after bilateral oophorectomy combined with hysterectomy (Huffman, 1950; Dodds *et al.*, 1961; Munday and Cox, 1967; Utian, 1975). Because all four studies were retrospective, any inference must be tentative, but the consensus finding appears to be that the risk of psychosexual dysfunction is no greater after hysterectomy with removal of both ovaries than after hysterectomy with ovarian conservation.

These studies and others concerned with psychiatric aspects of oophorectomy have been reviewed by Osborn and Gath (1983).

So far the findings on psychiatric and psychosexual complications of bilateral oophorectomy are rather inconclusive. In order to obtain more firmly based answers, it will be necessary to use prospective research designs, standardized methods of assessment, and large and representative samples.

Psychiatric aspects of surgery in general

The first part of this chapter has discussed research on psychiatric aspects of specific gynaecological operations, namely hysterectomy, sterilization and bilateral oophorectomy. This second part will deal with practical issues in the assessment and management of gynaecological patients who present actual or potential psychiatric problems. These psychiatric issues are not confined to gynaecological surgery, but may arise in any kind of surgery.

Well-conducted surveys, using strict assessment criteria, have shown that 15–25% of patients in surgical wards have psychiatric disorders, which are largely emotional disorders. It is also established that about half of these patients with psychiatric disorder are not recognized as such by the ward staff. Generally, patients with psychiatric disorder are recognized only if they show outward signs such as weeping, agitation or obtrusive behaviour, but not if they are quiet and inconspicuous.

Is it important that patients with psychiatric disorder should be detected in gynaecological and other surgical wards? The answer is affirmative for two reasons. First, the patient's psychiatric state may influence her response to management, and particularly her postoperative course and rehabilitation. Secondly, the patient may need psychiatric treatment to relieve distress, to prevent deterioration, or to guard against self-harm.

For these reasons it is desirable that the gynaecologist should be able to recognize psychiatric disorder, even when it is inconspicuous. Of course, the busy gynaecologist cannot be expected to have the time or expertise to make a detailed psychiatric examination of every gynaecological patient. However, it should be feasible for him to make a quick but reasonably reliable assessment whenever appropriate, as explained below.

The rest of this chapter is in four sections: the detection of psychiatric disorder; the assessment of psychiatric disorder; some basic principles of psychiatric management; examples of psychiatric syndromes likely to be met in gynaecological surgery.

Detection of psychiatric disorder

Two groups of patients will be discussed under this heading – those who are currently psychiatrically well but vulnerable to becoming unwell; and those who are currently psychiatrically unwell.

DETECTION OF PATIENTS WHO ARE PSYCHIATRICALLY WELL BUT VULNERABLE

It is desirable that patients in this group should be detected at an early stage in the process of selection for surgery, so that the indications for surgery and the timing of the operation can be assessed in relation to the degree of vulnerability.

Vulnerability to psychiatric disorder is determined by many factors, including family psychiatric history, patient's psychiatric history, personality, social circumstances and physical health. A psychiatrist would try to assess all these factors, but the gynaecologist would need to limit his enquiry to one or two criteria. For this purpose, the patient's previous psychiatric history would probably be the best guideline. If a patient has had a psychiatric illness at any time previously in her life, then she has a considerably increased risk of breaking down psychiatrically under the stress of gynaecological illness, admission to hospital, surgery and postoperative experiences. The risk is not absolute; many people have a single episode of psychiatric illness and then meet subsequent stressful circumstances without recurrence of the illness. Nevertheless, previous psychiatric illness is a good indicator of increased vulnerability. This was well shown in the Oxford study of hysterectomy (Gath et al., 1981), in which a highly significant association was found between a poor psychiatric outcome after hysterectomy and a history of psychiatric consultation at any time in the patient's life before the operation.

It is useful to enquire first whether the patient has ever been referred to a psychiatrist or nerve specialist, because of emotional, psychiatric or nervous problems (the choice of words will depend on the type of patient). If the answer is yes, enquiry should be made about dates, inpatient or outpatient care, nature of problem, treatment, response to treatment, and outcome. Similar enquiries should be made about psychiatric contacts with the GP, not involving psychiatric referral.

It is worthwhile obtaining information in this detail, because it gives some indication of what might happen in any future relapse. Generally, although not always, subsequent psychiatric disorders resemble previous psychiatric disorders in individual patients.

DETECTION OF PATIENTS WHO ARE CURRENTLY PSYCHIATRICALLY UNWELL

As mentioned above, some patients with psychiatric disorder can be recognized because of their disturbed behaviour, while others show little or no outward sign of disturbance.

When the gynaecologist takes the history, he may observe abnormalities in the patient's appearance, general behaviour and attitudes, talk, mood and intellectual functioning. Thus the patient may be retarded in movement, speech and thought (suggesting depression); sad and miserable-looking (depression); agitated and jumpy (anxiety disorder or agitated depression); excited and overactive (manic disorder); suspicious and guarded (paranoid state); or forgetful and muddled (organic brain disorder or emotional disorder). Further details of such signs are given in the section on psychiatric syndromes.

When there is little or no outward sign of disturbance, the detection of psychiatric disorder may be more difficult. However, it is usually feasible to ask a few simple screening questions to select patients who need further assessment. For example, the gynaecologist can ask whether the patient has been sad, miserable, tense, worried or frightened; sleeping as well as usual; energetic; or keeping up usual interests and activities. Of course, the answers to some of these questions may be influenced by the patient's gynaecological condition. Some patients may give evasive answers through diffidence or stoicism. But at least some patients will take the opportunity to reveal a psychiatric problem.

Assessment of psychiatric disorder

Once he has detected a psychiatric disorder, the gynaecologist will need to assess it briefly. Four questions can usefully be considered:

1. What is the nature and severity of the psychiatric disorder?
2. Is the psychiatric disorder caused by an underlying physical disorder?
3. Is the psychiatric disorder a psychological response to the gynaecological problem, or to other factors?
4. Is the patient's personality important in aetiology?

The answers to these questions are important because they may influence management of both the psychiatric and the gynaecological problem.

In making these assessments, it is usually helpful to talk to other informants – a close relative of the patient, the general practitioner or a psychiatrist who has known the patient in the past. This is highly important because patients with psychiatric disorder often give inaccurate accounts of themselves. Such misrepresentation may occur through deliberate evasion or exaggeration, or because the patient's recollections and judgements are distorted by her psychiatric state.

What is the nature and severity of the psychiatric disorder?
The nature of the disorder can be determined only through familiarity with the various psychiatric syndromes and their constituent features. These are reviewed briefly in the later section on psychiatric syndromes.

The severity of the disorder is determined by several criteria, including the intensity of the patient's distress, the degree of impairment of normal social functioning, the presence of symptoms such as delusions and hallucinations, and the duration of the disorder. Examples of these criteria are given in the section on psychiatric syndromes.

Is the psychiatric disorder caused by an underlying physical disorder?
Psychiatric disorders may be directly induced by physical agents, including brain diseases (such as degenerations, tumours, vascular lesions), endocrine disorders (such as Cushing's disease), and drugs used in treatment (such as reserpine or laevodopa). Such causes should be excluded by history-taking, physical examination and suitable investigations.

Is the psychiatric disorder a psychological response to the gynaecological problem, or to other factors?
Many psychiatric disorders appear to be psychological reactions induced by the impact of stressful circumstances on a vulnerable personality. Among gynaecological patients, the stressful circumstances may be gynaecological, or may be coincidental factors such as marital problems, bereavement or financial difficulties.

The gynaecological problem may be psychologically stressful for several reasons. First, it may result in pain, discomfort, social embarrassment or restricted activity. Such factors are particularly likely to be stressful if they are chronic. Secondly, the experience of consultation with the GP and the gynaecologist may be psychologically stressful, particularly because of the patient's uncertainty and fear about the future. Thirdly, admission to hospital for surgery is usually very stressful. The sources of this stress have been well documented by Cartwright (1964). They include: disruption of life (separation from home, husband, children); the nature of the illness (is it cancer?); the possible outcomes of the operation (death, inability to cope with a job, sexual dysfunction); the passive role of the patient (acceptance of medical and nursing care, probably without understanding it); the presence of other patients who are aged, querulous or suffering from unsightly conditions; lack of privacy when talking to doctors or visitors.

It is important to determine whether psychiatric disorder is a response to such gynaecological factors, or to other factors, because the answer has important implications for management (see below).

Is the patient's personality important in aetiology?
The patient's personality may influence many aspects of her illness behaviour – how far she complains of symptoms or seeks medical help, whether she stays off work, how she responds to treatment, recovers from an operation, or adjusts to disability.

Personality factors also largely determine vulnerability to psychiatric disorder. Probably the main factor is the lifelong capacity to cope with adversity. Generally, patients who cope best with gynaecological illness or surgery are those who have previously coped well with life's challenges.

Certain types of people are particularly prone to psychiatric breakdown when faced with illness or surgery. For example, vulnerability to breakdown is greater in anxiety-prone patients, who have lifelong anxiety and react to every difficulty, real or imaginary, with fear; cyclothymic patients, who alternate between elation and depression to an abnormal degree; and obsessional patients whose rigidity may be disabling when they are faced by the new routine of a surgical ward.

It would not be necessary in gynaecological practice to identify these personality types accurately; the main requirement, as emphasized above, is to determine how well the patient has coped with previous adversity.

Basic principles of psychiatric management

As mentioned earlier in the chapter, psychiatric factors may influence selection for surgery when the procedure is elective – for example hysterectomy or sterilization. In addition, psychiatric factors may influence three other management issues: timing of surgery; the patient on psychotropic medication; and the patient's need for explanation.

TIMING OF SURGERY

If a patient needs a gynaecological operation but is currently psychiatrically ill, is it better to perform the operation promptly, or to postpone it? This decision depends on a number of factors, including the nature and origins of the psychiatric disorder. Sometimes there is a considerable risk that surgery will make the patient psychiatrically worse. For example, in the case of major mental illnesses such as schizophrenia or manic depressive psychosis, surgery may have detrimental effects on patients with delusions and hallucinations. Such illnesses often have a fluctuating course, and it may be better to wait for a remission before operating.

On the other hand, if a patient has emotional symptoms secondary to menorrhagia, then it is probably best to perform hysterectomy while the patient is still psychiatrically unwell. In this case it may help the patient to experience any necessary stressful events without delay, so that she can begin psychiatric recovery with all adversity behind her.

Clearly, the timing of surgery for psychiatric patients is difficult, and needs to be tailored to the individual patient's needs. In most cases it will be best to arrive at a decision after discussion with the GP or psychiatrist, and with the patient herself.

THE PATIENT ON PSYCHOTROPIC MEDICATION

Patients seen in gynaecological practice may be taking psychotropic medication. This medication may have been prescribed for a concurrent psychiatric illness, such as an emotional disorder or schizophrenia. On the other hand there may be no concurrent illness, and the drug may have been prescribed to prevent recurrence of a remitting and relapsing illness. Examples of such prophylactic medication are chlorpromazine or intramuscular fluphenazine for schizophrenia, and lithium for manic depressive psychosis. These prophylactic drugs may be taken for several years.

An important principle is that no psychotropic medication, whether for concurrent symptoms or for prophylaxis, should be stopped without consulting the patient's GP or psychiatrist. There are several reasons for this precaution; one good reason is that a highly vulnerable patient may be exposed to the stresses of hospital admission or surgery without much-needed protection against psychiatric relapse.

This warning applies even to minor tranquillizers such as diazepam. Discontinuation of such drugs before surgery may lead to resurgence of severe anxiety symptoms, or (if the drug has been taken regularly over a lengthy period) to withdrawal symptoms.

THE PATIENT'S NEED FOR EXPLANATION

Careful surveys have shown that 90% of patients in surgical wards want to be given information about their illness – what their symptoms mean, why investigations are necessary and how they will be done, when surgery will be carried out, what the operation will consist of, what the implications will be for work, sexual activity or swimming, and many other issues.

It is also known from surveys that about two-thirds of patients do not receive the information they are hoping for. Why do patients not receive adequate explanations? The reasons are complex. Understandably busy surgeons are short of time. The relationship between doctor and patient is not always conducive to explanation; patients are often diffident, while the doctor has a 'professional' attitude which protects him from close involvement with the patient.

Although these barriers to communication are understandable, there can be no doubt that most patients need to have their illness and its management explained in some detail, and that such explanation may alleviate anxiety, depression and other psychiatric symptoms.

Giving a satisfactory explanation to a patient calls for the use of simple, non-technical language which is tailored to her capacity to understand. It is important to allow the patient opportunities to ask questions, as this will indicate how full and direct the explanation needs to be.

Common psychiatric syndromes

Finally, we come to the various psychiatric syndromes that may be met in surgical practice. The main syndromes and their clinical features are listed in *Table 2.1*. This section will give an account only of the two commonest syndromes among surgical patients – emotional disorders and acute organic psychiatric syndromes. For more details the reader is referred to a standard textbook of psychiatry (for example, Gelder, Gath and Mayou, 1983).

TABLE 2.1. Some common psychiatric syndromes and their clinical features

Psychiatric disorder	Main presenting features
Emotional disorders	
Depressive disorder	Mood sad, also often anxious and irritable. Reduction in energy, interest, self-confidence, decisiveness. Concentration impaired. Thoughts gloomy. In severe cases, biological symptoms: weight loss, appetite reduction, constipation, sleep disturbance (early morning waking), reduced sexual desire. Suicidal inclinations, expressed or concealed. Recovery from surgery may be delayed
Anxiety disorder	Fearfulness out of proportion to circumstances. Tension, irritability, sleep disturbance (difficulty getting to sleep). Autonomic symptoms, e.g. palpitations, tremor, diarrhoea, urinary frequency. Sometimes panic attacks (acute fear with autonomic symptoms). Recovery from surgery may be delayed
Mania	Behaviour typically overactive, energetic, distractable and sometimes aggressive. Mood sometimes elated, but not always; sometimes distressed, irritable. Commonly grandiose ideas, extravagant overspending, and increased sexual interest. This disinhibited behaviour may cause disturbance in the ward, and interfere with treatment
Organic disorders	
Acute organic disorders	Impairment of consciousness, with impaired concentration, thinking, memory. Disorientation common. Mood fearful. Behaviour may be restless, overactive, noisy, irritable; or slow, inactive, quiet. Visual hallucinations or illusions common. Condition often worse at night
Dementia	Slowly progressive intellectual decline, with memory impairment, poor judgement, loss of abstract thinking. Mood may be euphoric, depressed, anxious or fluctuating. Behaviour often impaired, with poor self-care and lack of consideration for others. Condition often shown by vague and inconsistent history-giving; acute emotional distress doing simple mental tasks; onset of confusion and disorientation in unfamiliar surroundings, e.g. hospital
Schizophrenia	Widespread disorder of many psychological functions, and of the connections between them. Disorder of thought including vagueness, lack of connection, and delusions (false, unshakable beliefs) which may be bizarre. Hallucinatory voices characteristic. Mood may be depressed, anxious, frightened, elated or flattened. Behaviour may be withdrawn, uncommunicative, suspicious, perplexed, aggressive or sometimes normal
Paranoid states	Delusions of persecution, often with anxious and distressed mood, and suspicious and unco-operative attitude. Patient may believe that medical and nursing staff are acting against her best interests (e.g. poisoning her with injections)

TABLE 2.1. continued

Psychiatric disorder	Main presenting features
Neuroses Obsessive-compulsive neurosis	Obsessions are recurrent thoughts which patient resists and struggles against, but cannot exclude, e.g. thoughts about cancer or death, harming other people, contamination by dirt or germs, or religious themes. Often combined with extreme indecisiveness. Compulsions are ritualized patterns of behaviour, e.g. repeated hand washing. Depressed mood and anxiety often accompany
Hysterical neurosis	Impairment of bodily function which is not caused by physical disease. Numerous symptoms and signs, such as loss of sensation, limb paralysis, constricted visual field; these often correspond to patient's conception of the disorder but not to anatomy or physiology. Hysterical symptoms often occur with actual organic disorder. Psychiatric symptoms include memory loss and visual hallucinations, often with a mood of depression or anxiety, although patient sometimes shows 'la belle indifférence'. Hysterical symptoms lead to a lowering of anxiety (the 'primary gain') by avoiding contact with the stressor. They may also confer other advantages (the 'secondary gains')
Personality disorder	Lifelong abnormalities of behaviour which cause suffering to the patient or other people. Patients may be demanding, manipulative and attention-seeking; shy, aloof and solitary; prone to frequent mood swings between elation and depression; aggressive, irresponsible and antisocial, etc. Patient often has a lifelong history of difficult relationships with other people and a poor work record
Alcohol and drug dependency	Most likely presentation in surgery is onset of withdrawal syndrome within 48 h of admission. Features include tremor, anxiety, and features of acute organic syndrome described above (*delirium tremens*). Dependency often not admitted, but suggested by job (e.g. publican), related physical disorders (e.g. liver disease), or demands for analgesics. Dependency often damages family and social relationships, work, finances and physical health

EMOTIONAL DISORDERS

By far the most common psychiatric syndromes in surgical practice are depressive disorders and anxiety disorders. Often the two occur together, but it is convenient to describe them separately.

In *depressive disorders*, the common symptoms are a mood of sadness, often combined with some irritability. Concentration is impaired, and thoughts may be gloomy, self-reproachful and pessimistic. There may be 'loss' symptoms, such as reduction of energy, interest, self-confidence and decisiveness. There may also be 'biological' symptoms, such as poor appetite, weight loss, constipation, sleep disturbance (particularly early morning waking), reduced sexual desire, impotence or amenorrhoea. Towards the evening the depressed mood may lift, but if there is also marked anxiety it may worsen. The onset of a depressive disorder may evoke other psychiatric symptoms, such as obsessive-compulsive or phobic symptoms.

Depressive disorder may be suggested by the patient's appearance – facial expression of sadness, bowed stance and heavy gait. When the disorder is severe, there may be paucity and slowing of speech and movement. In agitated depression the opposite picture may be seen – restlessness, hand-wringing and over-talkativeness.

In *anxiety disorders*, there are feelings usually described as tension, edginess or nervousness. The patient is afraid for no apparent reason, and sees threats in every situation. Here, too, there is often marked irritability. Sleep is disturbed by frightening dreams and there is often difficulty in getting off to sleep. In severe disorders, the patient may experience uncontrollable panic attacks. Some patients complain of bodily symptoms such as palpitations, diarrhoea and frequency of micturition.

On examination, the patient may seem jumpy and distractable. Irritability may manifest itself as frank rudeness or aggression (which is best disregarded by the interviewer). There may be signs of autonomic overactivity such as paleness, sweating, dilated pupils, and rapid pulse and respiration.

The *detection* of an emotional disorder should be reasonably easy if the patient complains of the typical symptoms listed above, or shows the typical signs. In the absence of such features, emotional disorder may be revealed if the gynaecologist asks the screening questions listed in the earlier section on detection of psychiatric disorder. If these screening questions are positive, it is obviously important to seek confirmatory evidence of emotional disorder by enquiring directly about other symptoms, such as depressive thought content, biological features of depression, panic attacks and bodily symptoms of anxiety.

On the combination of symptoms and signs present, it is usually possible to make a fairly confident *diagnosis* of depressive disorder or anxiety disorder. Mistakes can be made, however, because patients with other disorders such as schizophrenia may present with features apparently typical of an emotional disorder. An anxiety disorder may need to be differentiated from thyrotoxicosis; the latter may be recognized by intolerance of heat, raised sleeping pulse, exophthalmos and lid lag, and biochemical tests.

An assessment of the *severity* of an emotional disorder requires considerable experience of seeing other patients with similar disorders. However, most clinicians can make a reliable assessment of the intensity of distress and impairment of functioning experienced by the patient. In depressive disorders, the presence of the biological features described above, or of psychotic features such as delusions or hallucinations, certainly points to a severe disorder. It should be remembered that anxiety is a very common symptom in surgical patients. It usually starts before the operation, seems to reach a peak 4 days before surgery, and continues for several days afterwards (Johnston, 1980). Anxiety is more frequent and severe in surgical patients than in medical patients, even when their illnesses are less severe (Volicier and Burns, 1977).

The *aetiology* of emotional disorders should be assessed along the lines described in the earlier section on aetiology.

The *treatment* of emotional disorders (as of all psychiatric disorders) falls under three headings – psychological, physical (medication or ECT) and social. No attempt will be made here to review treatment in detail; for this the interested reader is referred to a textbook of psychiatry (see also Chapter 5). Two points need to be stressed. First, many patients with emotional disorders can be helped by psychiatric referral. Secondly, many emotional disorders in surgical patients can be considerably alleviated by explanation and reassurance provided by the gynaecologist, as explained in the earlier section on the patient's needs for explanation.

ACUTE ORGANIC PSYCHIATRIC SYNDROMES

Organic psychiatric syndromes are disorders that arise either from demonstrable structural disease of the brain (such as brain tumours, injuries or degenerations), or from brain dysfunction which is caused by disease outside the brain (such as myxoedema or heart failure). These disorders are well described in the textbook on organic psychiatry by Lishman (1978). These syndromes may be divided into an acute syndrome, sometimes called delirium or confusional state, which is described below; and a chronic syndrome, otherwise known as dementia, which is summarized in *Table 2.1*.

The acute organic psychiatric syndrome is described here because it is common in surgical practice. It occurs in 5–15% of patients in general medical or surgical wards, and about 20–30% of patients in surgical intensive care units (Lipowski, 1980).

The most important clinical feature is impairment of consciousness or awareness, sometimes referred to as 'clouding'. This impairment varies in intensity during the day, and is usually worst at night. The patient is disorientated in time and place, and shows impairment of concentration, thinking and remembering. The patient's behaviour may be restless, overactive, noisy and irritable; or else it may be slow, inactive and quiet. Visual distortions may occur as illusions or hallucinations. The mood is often fearful. The early signs of the acute brain syndrome are slight drowsiness, a tendency to make silly mistakes and some bewilderment. Often these early signs are missed and the diagnosis is not made until the onset of florid behavioural disturbance.

When the acute brain syndrome is diagnosed, the next step is to search for the cause. The main causes include: drug intoxication or withdrawal, e.g. delirium tremens; metabolic, endocrine and nutritional disorders; systemic infections; and brain lesions, including tumours, injuries and infections.

The search for causes requires a thorough physical examination. Basic investigations usually include haemoglobin and blood count, ESR, blood urea and electrolytes, urinary sugar and protein, and bacterial cultures. Chest X-ray and skull X-ray will almost certainly be required. Judgement is required about the indications for more intensive investigations such as CAT scan, EEG and lumbar puncture. The advice of a psychiatrist or neurologist may be helpful in relation to these investigations.

The treatment of the acute organic psychiatric syndrome is first and foremost to treat the underlying physical cause, if possible. The most important general measures are to reduce the patient's anxiety, and to avoid sensory over- or under-stimulation. The patient should be nursed in a quiet, well-lit side room. At night there should be enough light to allow the patient to see where she is. Nursing should be provided by a small number of nurses, whom the patient can recognize as familiar. The nurses should be tactful and gentle, and should give the patient repeated explanations of her condition.

The principles of drug treatment should be to give as few drugs as feasible, and to avoid any drugs that may further impair consciousness. By day it may be necessary to calm the patient without inducing drowsiness, For this purpose a suitable preparation is haloperidol; a commonly used alternative is chlorpromazine. Haloperidol has the advantage of causing less hypotension and cardiac side effects. By night, the patient may need help to sleep; for this purpose a sedative anxiolytic drug, such as a benzodiazepine, is suitable, although caution is needed with elderly patients.

References

BALLINGER, C. B. (1977) Psychiatric morbidity and the menopause: survey of a gynaecology out-patients clinic. *British Journal of Psychiatry*, **131**, 83–89

BARKER, M. G. (1968) Psychiatric illness after hysterectomy. *British Medical Journal*, **2**, 91–95

BLEDIN, K. D., BERAL, V. and ASHLEY, J. S. A. (1978) Recent trends in sterilization in women. *Health Trends*, **10**, 84–87

BLEDIN, K. D., COOPER, J. E., MACKENZIE, S. and BRICE, B. (1984) Psychological sequelae of female sterilisation: short term outcome in a prospective controlled study. *Psychological Medicine* **14**(2), 379–390

CARTWRIGHT, A. (1964) *Human Relations and Hospital Care*. London; Routledge and Kegan Paul

CHIMBIRA, T. H., ANDERSON, A. B. M. and TURNBULL, A. C. (1980) Relation between measured menstrual blood loss and patients' subjective assessment of loss, duration of bleeding, number of sanitary towels used, uterine weight and endometrial surface area. *British Journal of Obstetrics and Gynaecology*, **87**, 603–609

COOPER, P., GATH, D., FIELDSEND, R. and ROSE, N. (1981) Psychological and physical outcome after elective tubal sterilization. *Journal of Psychosomatic Research*, **25**, 357–360

COOPER, P., GATH, D., ROSE, N. and FIELDSEND, R. (1982) Psychological sequelae to elective sterilization in women: a prospective study. *British Medical Journal*, **82**, 461–464

DODDS, D. T., POTGEITER, C. R., TURNER, P. J. and SCHEEPERS, G. P. J. (1961) The physical and emotional results of hysterectomy. *South African Medical Journal*, Jan., 53–54

GATH, D. and COOPER, P. (1982) Psychiatric aspects of hysterectomy and female sterilisation. In *Recent Advances in Clinical Psychiatry*, (Granville-Grossman, K., Ed.). London; Churchill Livingstone

GATH, D., COOPER, P., BOND, A. and EDMONDS, G. (1981) Hysterectomy and psychiatric disorder: demographic, psychiatric and physical factors in relation to psychiatric outcome. *British Journal of Psychiatry*, **140**, 343–350

GATH, D., COOPER, P. and DAY, A. (1981) Hysterectomy and psychiatric disorder: levels of psychiatric morbidity before and after hysterectomy. *British Journal of Psychiatry*, **140**, 335–342

GELDER, M., GATH, D. and MAYOU, R. (1983) *Oxford Textbook of Psychiatry*. London; Oxford University Press.

HALLBERG, L. and NILSSON, L. (1964) Determination of menstrual blood loss. *Scandinavian Journal of Clinical Laboratory Investigation*, **16**, 244–248

HAYNES, P. J., ANDERSON, A. and TURNBULL, A. C. (1979) Patterns of menstrual blood loss in menorrhagia. *Research Clinic Forums*, **1**, 73–78

HUFFMAN, J. W. (1950) The effect of gynecological surgery on sexual reactions. *American Journal of Obstetrics and Gynecology*, **59**, 915–917

JOHNSTON, J. (1980) Anxiety in surgical patients. *Psychological Medicine*, **10**, 145–152

LINDEMANN, E. (1941) Observations on psychiatric sequelae to surgical operations in women. *American Journal of Psychiatry*, **98**, 132–137

LIPOWSKI, Z. J. (1980) Organic mental disorders: introduction and review of syndromes. In *Comprehensive Textbook of Psychiatry*, 3rd edn (Kaplan, H. I., Freedman, A. M. and Sadock, B. J., Eds). Baltimore; Williams and Wilkins

LISHMAN, W. A. (1978) *Organic Psychiatry: The Psychological Consequences of Cerebral Disorder*. London; Blackwells Scientific Publications

MARTIN, R. L., ROBERTS, W. V. and CLAYTON, P. J. (1980) Psychiatric status after hysterectomy – one-year prospective follow-up. *Journal of the American Medical Association*, **244**, 350–353

MARTIN, R. L., ROBERTS, W. V., CLAYTON, P. J. and WETZEL, R. (1977) Psychiatric illness and non-cancer hysterectomy. *Diseases of the Nervous System*, **38**, 974–980

MELODY, G. F. (1962) Depressive reactions following hysterectomy. *American Journal of Obstetrics and Gynecology*, **83**, 410–413

MUNDAY, R. N. and COX, L. W. (1967). Hysterectomy for benign lesions. *Medical Journal of Australia*, **17**, 759–763

NILSSON, L. and RYBO, G. (1971). Treatment of menorrhagia. *American Journal of Obstetrics and Gynecology*, **110**, 713–720

OSBORN, M. and GATH, D. (1983) Psychological aspects of gynaecology surgery. In *Handbook of Psychosomatic Obstetrics and Gynaecology* (Dennerstein, L. and Burrows, G. E., Eds). Amsterdam; Elsevier Biomedical Press

PATTERSON, R. M. and CRAIG, J. B. (1963) Misconceptions concerning the psychological effects of hysterectomy. *American Journal of Obstetrics and Gynecology*, **85**, 104–111

RICHARDS, D. H. (1973) Depression after hysterectomy. *Lancet*, **2**, 430–432

SCHWYHART, W. R. and KUTNER, S. J. (1973) A re-analysis of female reactions to contraceptive sterilisation. *Journal of Nervous and Mental Disease*, **156**, 354–370

UTIAN, W. H. (1975). Effect of hysterectomy, oophorectomy and oestrogen therapy on libido. *International Journal of Gynaecology and Obstetrics*, **13**, 97–100

VOLICIER, B. J. and BURNS, M. W. (1977) Pre-existing correlates of hospital stress. *Nursing Research*, **26**, 408–415

WING, J. K. (1976) A technique for studying psychiatric morbidity in in-patient and out-patient series and in general population samples. *Psychological Medicine*, **6**, 665–671

WING, J. K., COOPER, J. E. and SARTORIUS, N. (1974). *The Measurement and Classification of Psychiatric Symptoms*. London; Cambridge University Press

Chapter 3

Pelvic pain

Robert O. Pasnau, Steven Soldinger and Barbara L. Andersen

Definition and diagnosis of pelvic pain

Pelvic pain is a common complaint of women. The aetiology of the discomfort is often difficult to establish, partially due to the variability in the nature, intensity and site of the pain. Often, no cause can be found. On other occasions, the origin of the pelvic pain can be discovered through a careful study of the patient's history. With such a process, particular attention is given to variables such as the time and circumstance of pain at the onset, the nature and pattern of current pain symptoms, any associated difficulties, and the co-variation of pain symptomology with the normal activities of bodily functioning (e.g. movement, urination, defaecation, menstruation) and daily routines (e.g. sleep, eating, physical activity).

Pelvic pain may originate in the genital or in extragenital organs. The mechanisms that produce pain can include intense muscular contractions or cramps, inflammation or direct irritation of nerves, or psychological factors. Both smooth and skeletal muscles can produce pain by strong or sustained contractions, which can result from over-distension or obstruction, hypoxia of the muscle cells, or tetany. Nerves can be irritated by acute or chronic trauma, fibrosis, pressures, spillage of bowel or abscessed contents, serous exudates, or intraperitoneal blood. Psychological factors are more difficult to enumerate, but it is believed they can play both a direct role in the aetiology of pain and an indirect role in pain exacerbation. Thus, it is not surprising that pelvic pain is often regarded as an 'enigma'.

The options in the differential diagnosis of pelvic pain (Berkow, 1977) include: acute salpingitis; ectopic pregnancy; ovarian cysts or haemorrhage into cysts; uterine myoma; genital tumours; malposition of the uterus, especially when the uterus is retroflexed and there are fixed adhesions or scars binding the uterus; and endometriosis. In pregnant women, sudden pelvic pain may be due to an associated torsion of an ovarian cyst, acute degeneration of a uterine myoma, placental abruption, rupture of the uterus, or parametritis. One rare condition that can occur in pregnant women is a loosening of the pelvic joints which may cause pelvic pain with motion. Another cause of pelvic pain is *mittelschmerz*, usually experienced as a severe hypogastric pain occurring for a few hours midway through the menstrual cycle. This particular pain can be misdiagnosed as appendicitis.

49

Also found in the differential diagnosis of pelvic pain is the pelvic congestion syndrome. This is an incompletely understood condition affecting the pelvic vasculature. The syndrome is most often found in women aged 25–45. Frequent complaints include lower abdominal or back pain, dysmenorrhoea, dysuria, menorrhagia, dyspareunia, leucorrhoea, and pelvic discomfort on sitting or standing. Other frequently reported symptoms include anxiety, fatigue, headache, and insomnia.

A kind of pelvic pain localized in the genital area is dyspareunia (i.e. pain during sexual intercourse). Dyspareunia can be secondary to vaginismus. It may also be associated with other sexual difficulties such as a lack of sexual desire or arousal deficits. Such pain may occur upon penetration or with thrusting. Specific organic causes of dyspareunia include minimal lubrication due to lack of sexual excitement, acute or recurrent pelvic infections, pressure against the vaginal wall, atrophic changes of the vagina after the climacteric period, or vaginal lacerations. Dyspareunia occurring in the presence of sexual arousal is usually of organic aetiology.

Other causes of pelvic pain originate extragenitally and may be related to the urological, gastrointestinal or skeletal systems or the supporting tissues. Pain of urological origin is most commonly associated with frequency, dysuria, burning, fever, chills, haematuria, and ureteral colic. Pain of the pelvis associated with the musculoskeletal system can occur from the spine or the pelvis itself. It may be located at the point of involvement or be referred. Pain not found upon vaginal, abdominal or rectovaginal examination, but rather with leg or other bodily movement, suggests a skeletal aetiology, as does any pelvic pain which produces a change in sensation in the abdominal wall. Other causes of pelvic pain relate to the supporting tissues and may be an indication of cystocele, rectocele or uterine descensus. Pelvic tumours and threatened abortion may produce a similar discomfort. Backache is a common symptom, but it is seldom due to chronic gynaecological disease except in cases of advanced tumours. Pelvic pains which originate from the gastrointestinal tract or its appendages include: appendicitis, diverticulitis, peritonitis, and functional diseases of the bowel, including irritable or spastic colon. Porphyria and blood dyscrasias may cause pelvic pain.

Basu (1981) presented a quick review article encompassing the way to proceed with diagnostic entities that can be a source of pelvic pain. He provided a brief, yet clear, summary of all the diagnostic possibilities relating to the types of pelvic pain mentioned above in simple-to-follow tables. Also included is a table for delineating organic versus psychogenic causes of pelvic pain. He listed the following characteristics of 'organic pain':

1. It has characteristic features usually indicative of an underlying disorder.
2. It is usually well-defined.
3. It follows a definite pattern of radiation.
4. The pain is not necessarily ascribed to a specific organ by the patient.
5. There are few related or associated symptoms.
6. The pain is often exaggerated by any manipulation or exercise.
7. There is no specific trend to note in terms of social or personal history.
8. There are no specific trends present in terms of previous hospitalization.

When considering the 'psychogenic' causes of pelvic pain, Basu described:

1. The nature of the pain is generally ill-defined and felt over many areas of the body.

2. There is poor localization, the pain often shifting to other areas previously not affected.
3. The pain usually does not radiate – it may sometimes follow unpredictable pathways.
4. The patient often specifically localizes her pain.
5. There are many unrelated symptoms.
6. The aggravating factors seem to be related to emotional factors.
7. There are well-marked personal and social-type history difficulties.
8. There may be many admissions to general hospitals, rarely to psychiatric hospitals.

Treatment of pelvic pain may be symptomatic or require the treatment of the specific cause when identified. Often, however, treatment for pelvic pain is unsuccessful, with frustration for physicians and patients alike. This may lead to unwarranted pelvic surgery to eradicate the continuing painful condition. This may begin a vicious cycle of other complications (e.g., adhesions, drug addiction, multiple surgical operations, the concomitants of chronic pain problems.

Review of the literature on pelvic pain

Despite 100 years of inquiry, the medical literature on pelvic pain is not definitive. Although pelvic pain is a frequent complaint brought to primary care physicians and gynaecologists, few studies using adequate controls and measurements have been attempted. The pelvic pain literature can be divided into five categories, discussed below, which are useful for identifying and organizing the major problem areas in it.

The enigma of pelvic pain

Hyslop (1972) described pelvic pain as the '*bête noire* of gynaecology'. He noted that most gynaecologists approach the problem of pelvic pain in the classical manner, i.e. differential diagnosis dividing causes into congenital and acquired. The acquired causes are further subdivided into trauma, infection (acute or chronic), tumours (benign or malignant), and a miscellaneous group related to complications of pregnancy and endometriosis. At the bottom of the list is the psychosomatic group. In the usual course of events, each patient is subject to extensive examination and investigation to decide which of the possible causes is the problem. Usually, examinations and tests are uncomfortable and prolonged. When all tests fail to reveal any pathology, the condition is labelled 'psychosomatic'. By the time this diagnosis is made, the patient's mind may not surprisingly be firmly fixed on her pelvic organs.

Hyslop suggested that a 'new' classification be adopted, dividing causes into psychosomatic and organic, with priority to psychosomatic since he concluded that the former is 'undoubtedly a major cause of pain'. He postulated that psychosomatic conditions are stress and nervous tension. They lead to abnormal functioning of the autonomic nervous system and a state of colon spasm leading to congestion of the lower intestinal tract and pelvic organs. The spasm typically presents as lower abdominal pain with abdominal distension and tenderness. If the condition continues and progresses, the congestion leads to oedema of the connective tissue and hypertrophy of the organs. However, conservative treatment can reverse the condition in its early stages. In longstanding cases and where the 'psyche has been fixed on the pelvis for years', the patient may have already undergone some kind of pelvic surgery and the tissue changes may be permanent.

The essentials for a correct diagnosis and successful treatment of the condition as outlined by Hyslop are as follows:

1. An unhurried history, allowing the patient time to explain completely her pain.
2. A careful physical examination.
3. A specific, clearly communicated diagnosis.
4. An optimistic attitude during treatment and follow-up.

Mills (1978) noted gynaecologists' longstanding concern with pelvic pain for which there appeared to be no organic pathology. Lawson Tait (1883), a famous gynaecologist during the Victorian age, observed that the piano lessons common for women at that time involved long periods of sitting with an unsupported back. This circumstance, he hypothesized, might affect the blood flow through adolescent ovaries and thus cause ovaralgia. A more 'liberated' view was offered by French physicians, who blamed sexual dissatisfaction and contraceptive practices (i.e. coitus interruptus). The Germans ascribed the cause to chronic cervicitis. Whitehouse (1935) suggested excessive stimulation of the sympathetic nerves. Taylor (1949) described pelvic congestion. More recently, authors have blamed increased sensitivity of the pelvic nerves and the cerebral cortex, dysfunction of the large bowel, varicosities, and thrombophlebitis.

Mills (1978) believed that much pelvic pain is due to pelvic congestion and that the symptomatic pain is referred from the uterus. The ovaries may exhibit the congestive pathology. He hypothesized that stress may provoke such congestion of the pelvic organs which in turn leads to acute symptoms – a bleeding ovary or, more usually, chronic uterine congestion. For pain relief, physical exercise may help. He found the uterine congestion apparent in laparotomy often associated with pelvic varicosities. He concluded that 'after attention to possible stress factors, there will be some patients with enigmatic pelvic pain for whom hysterectomy will bring relief as satisfactory as that achieved by appropriate gastric surgery for peptic ulceration'.

The *British Medical Journal* (Editorial, 1978) discussed 'enigmatic pelvic pain'. In the year previous, over 10 000 women in Britain had diagnostic laparoscopies for lower abdominal pain. Quite often, no disease/condition could be diagnosed and, when the pain was longstanding, the likelihood of a specific diagnosis was decreased. Patients received several diagnostic labels including congestive dysmenorrhoea or pelvic sympathetic syndrome. These patients exhibited the following characteristics:

1. They were usually parous and pre-menopausal.
2. They described their pain as a dull ache in the suprapubic area or in one or both iliac fossae, which may be referred to the inner thighs.
3. Pain would be generally worse before the menstrual period.
4. They often had deep dyspareunia, which may persist after intercourse.
5. There may be associated leucorrhoea, menorrhagia, or irritability of the bladder, but bowel dysfunction was infrequent.
6. The majority of the women appeared to be anxious and to be undergoing a

current period of stress. Patients with 'enigmatic pelvic pain' were described as being significantly more neurotic and having less satisfactory sex lives than a comparable control group.

This report did not offer a specific treatment plan but suggested that it is important to give the reassurance that no specific pathology is present. Immediate psychiatric referral was not recommended since some patients may view this as a suggestion that their pain is 'in their head' and not 'in their body'. The general practitioner or gynaecologist may have established rapport with a particular patient and may be able to provide the necessary supportive care. Psychiatric referral may be appropriate at some later follow-up point.

Philipp (1978) also described the pain as an 'enigma'. Comparison was made to cardiac pain, inasmuch as the receptors involved in each have not yet been identified. In the female pelvis, the reaction to sensory stimuli both pleasant and unpleasant is 'mysterious'. He stated, 'We do not know what is the cause of pelvic pain, which nerves pick it up and take it to the brain, where in the brain it is appreciated, nor how to treat it'. Even with endometriosis it has been noted that the bigger cysts are painless unless they have leaked their chocolate contents, while patients with small 'partridge eye' lesions may have the worst dysmenorrhoea. Ischaemia of the pelvic organs during menstruation may also be the cause of dysmenorrhoea. Presumably under autonomic nervous control, these organs have immensely complex biochemical mechanisms partly controlled by the cerebral cortex, the basal ganglia, thalamus, and hypothalamus. Hormones modify both the level of nervous activity and the motor response, making the unravelling of the puzzle still more difficult.

Philipp emphasized that it is 'wrong to neglect the psychological factors which help to cause, aggravate, or augment sensation interpreted as pain by the patient'. He noted that such a perspective currently considers the influence of cerebral cortex on the neurohormonal secretion and the sympathetic and parasympathetic nervous systems' role in mediating the pelvic pain response.

Philipp also noted that individual differences among women, specifically physiological and anatomical variability, may account for the reasons why some women have pelvic pain and others do not. For instance, he noted that there are several types of receptors in the pelvis. In the vulvar skin alone there are tactile discs and at least four kinds of sensory corpuscles. The concentration of each varies markedly from woman to woman. Thus, a woman who cannot 'feel' sensation may have too few or too many of one or another type of sensory transducer. Similarly, the vagina, which is by comparison relatively insensitive to painful or pleasurable sensation with its fewer Pacinian corpuscles, does, however, have nerve fibres returning to it (and thus a pathway for pain) so that it can distend and react physiologically.

While he acknowledged the research of the electrophysiologists in stimulation of larger fibres in order to block other fibres – the gate-control theory of pain – Philipp stated that in dysmenorrhoea and pelvic pain 'we must still depend mainly on the pharmacologist'. He noted the need to continue the search for pain receptors in the pelvis and elsewhere in the lower abdomen.

Pelvic congestion syndrome

Duncan and Taylor (1952) presented the first descriptive information on pelvic pain patients. They interviewed 36 patients, 10 from private sources and the remaining

26 from a New York City gynaecology service. On the basis of their interviews Duncan and Taylor concluded that the sample could be described as 'psychologically ill'. The patients were seen as having experienced an insecure childhood period, particularly lacking a suitable mother or mother substitute. In addition, they were seen as 'inadequate' as women in terms of their sexual or maternal functioning. Finally, this initial report linked pelvic congestion to stressful life situations. While this first report suggested a number of useful hypotheses for further investigation, its limitations should be noted. Most obvious is the small sample size, lack of comparison group, and the subjective nature of the data reported.

Taylor (1954) summarized the psychiatric status of another 100 cases of pelvic pain patients. He viewed these patients to be similar to those in the previous report. Factors specifically noted included previous psychiatric treatment and current sexual difficulties. Despite the larger sample size, the methodological limitations are still applicable.

Edlundh and Jansson (1966) surveyed 21 Swedish gynaecology patients reporting pelvic pain. Sixteen of the sample were found to have pelvic varicosities when examined by a roentgenological technique, and the remaining five showed no vascular disturbance. Psychiatric evaluations were conducted for all subjects. Since the number of subjects in each subgroup was small, the findings were reported for the entire sample. They found their 'typical patient' to be 'fairly intelligent, tense, and a striver'. They did not, however, find such factors as lack of harmony in childhood and youth, disturbed mother relationships, early marriage, deficient sexual education, sexual dysfunction, or pregnancy fear as characteristic of their sample. However, they did report 'previous psychiatric vulnerability' (i.e. previous outpatient psychiatric treatment) for 8 of 21 patients. While some of the patients were depressed, such mood problems did not characterize the sample. In concluding, Edlundh and Jansson suggested that many factors may be influential. They hypothesized that psychological vulnerability may co-vary with other factors, and cases of 'pure' psychiatric aetiology were probably few.

Jeffcoate (1975) described what he called 'congestive dysmenorrhoea', often in the form of a diffuse dull ache in the pelvis and/or back. This was seen as the result of increasing tension in the pelvic tissues associated with premenstrual engorgement. Pain typically peaked during the 2–3 days preceding menstruation. He hypothesized that there is sometimes an organic cause for this syndrome, but for many the congestion is probably 'functional', and possibly due to such factors as emotional distress, marital and sexual distress, or even a sedentary life-style. Without a specific aetiology, surgery is unwarranted. He proposed that such procedures as dilatation of the cervix, excision of veins, or of an appendage for broad ligament varicocele are of little value. The best approach may be one focused on life changes or alleviation of emotional distress.

Hobbs (1976) reviewed the history of pelvic pain study. He listed the various causes for chronic pelvic pain in women that have been suggested over the years. Before 1915, physicians were likely to ascribe 'inflammatory causes'. After 1915, the suggestion of a hormonal aetiology was popular. This theory postulated pelvic congestion and fibrosis similar to chronic mastitis. The review by Taylor (1949) of the history of chronic pelvic pain, and conclusion that pelvic pain was a vascular condition, was viewed by Hobbs as a turning point. This paper supported a psychosomatic concept in that the abnormal vascular state was the result of a disordered function of the autonomic nervous system; the 'abnormal' mental state was not secondary to a pain syndrome. In his paper, Hobbs stressed the need for careful examination of the vulvar area and the pelvis for pelvic congestion. Diagnosis is confirmed by vulvar venography, which demonstrates pelvic varicosities and their communications. He proposed that treatment might range from supportive care to surgery (i.e. hysterectomy). Left untreated, symptoms might resolve after the menopause.

Psychological parameters of pelvic pain

Gidro-Frank, Gordon and Taylor (1960) surveyed 'emotional factors' in 40 pelvic pain patients. All were referred from a gynaecological pain clinic and several had undergone prior treatment for their complaints. While the investigators were aware of those patients who did or did not have demonstrable gynaecological pathology, they were unable to differentiate the groups on the basis of their findings. Subjects were interviewed by the investigators on a number of occasions. Partial comparison data were also presented for a sample of pregnant patients. Psychiatric disturbances were seen frequently among the pain patients. Sexual, menstrual and gestational performances were regarded as 'disturbed'. Once again, the hypothesis was proposed that 'patients with pelvic pain were unable to establish and preserve that sense of feminine identity which permits the execution of feminine functions'.

Frederick (1976) examined the psychological aspects of chronic pelvic pain and described the 'typical' pelvic pain patient. Many of the women with pelvic pain tend to be in their reproductive years, 20–40 years old. Often, symptoms start during or following a first pregnancy. When onset is in the post-partum period, Frederick suggested that it may be a coping mechanism for crisis management. Somatic complaints can also be viewed from a psychoanalytic framework and be conceptualized as conversion reactions – symbolic body representations of forbidden psychological wishes or fantasies. The conversion symptom may be an attempt to form a relationship with another person based on multiple past experiences. It expresses the forbidden wish, the defence against the wish, or both. It can condense many different themes from the past.

In some patients, Frederick found that the pain is accompanied by guilt. For example, women from rejecting families often marry rejecting husbands. Many women with pelvic pain report disturbed childhoods. They have early memories of abandonment or threat of injury or rejection, or they actually have lost a parent. Often, their parents' marriages were troubled. The women are described as immature, dependent and longing for a peaceful marriage or seeking a home life which they had never experienced. They often repeat the past and their marriages and families are often troubled by many of the same difficulties. Pain can be a familiar experience. When they cannot have forbidden angry feelings, they may develop pain as a way of coping.

Some patients who have pelvic pain with such psychological concomitants may also have organic changes (e.g. chronic pelvic congestion). Frederick suggested that there may be a predisposition to automatic nerve discharge in the pelvic region in response to stressful situations. Laparoscopic examination reveals that there are some patients without pathology and others with minor pathology but severe pain. Frederick noted that, at this time, there is no 'correct' way of handling many of these patients. He suggested that open-ended questions and taking time to gather a complete social and psychological history might facilitate the establishment of a therapeutic relationship between physician and patient. The importance of answering 'why the pain now?' is emphasized. It should be explained to the patient that pelvic pain is a difficult problem and diagnostic examinations and historical data gathering are time consuming, but specific treatment recommendations will be made as soon as possible. Frederick concluded that physicians should utilize their interpersonal and medical expertise in caring for pelvic pain patients.

Another short recent review and analysis of the psychological factors in the management and treatment of pelvic pain was given by Reading (1982–83). He reported a number of patients who had no actual physiologically definable reason for their pelvic pain. He suggested courses of treatment and evaluation which have, as their main guide, a strengthening of the alliance between doctor and patient towards achieving the desired results of alleviating the patient's complaints. He proposed methods for this in the form of 'relaxation, distraction, hypnosis, stress management, and operant methods whereby reinforcement contingencies are changed'.

In another review, Nadelson, Notman and Ellis (1983) concurred with Reading regarding the psychosomatic aspects of pelvic pain. They stated that 'patients with chronic pelvic pain tend to resist accepting the psychological aspects of their illness'. They agreed with Reading as to the usefulness of a behavioural approach to treatment.

Physical diagnostic considerations in the evaluation of pelvic pain

McFayden (1981) provided a comprehensive review suggesting how the family practitioner or gynaecologist should approach patients with pain in the lower abdomen. She paid careful attention to the combined physical and psychological aspects of the pain, focusing specifically on the physical problems that need to be considered more carefully, as well as on the details in the history that may lead to a diagnosis. She stated that 'clinical examination starts from the time the patient is first seen until her illness is resolved'. She expected the integration of the physical and psychological in the physician's attitude towards the patient throughout the examination.

The term 'functional' pelvic pain is used differently by physicians in different countries and with differing medical specialities. For instance, Thalheim (1975), in an article written for a German orthopaedics and traumatology journal, reviewed 100 patients who were diagnosed as having 'functional disturbances in the pelvis area, all complaining of pelvic pain'. In this series, 30 patients had 'coxalgia', 41 'ileosacral blockage', and 29 'pelvic ringing'. The three groups were separated, based on physical findings and diagnostic tests. In all of the cases in this survey, the pain could be attributed to physical causes.

While this paper described conditions that seem to bear little resemblance to pelvic pain in women, it is also important to remember that orthopaedic conditions must be ruled out before ascribing a psychological diagnosis (e.g. psychosomatic pelvic pain). Thalheim pointed out that pelvic pain, associated with 'pelvic ringing', can be common in women due to the loosening of the ring during pregnancy and delivery. It was particularly encountered in younger patients. In most of these cases the patient also complained of low back pain accompanied by occasional radiation of pain into the legs.

A syndrome reported by Sinaki, Merritt and Stillwell (1977) involved what they termed 'tension myalgia of the pelvic floor'. They described this as 'a form of tension myalgia involving the musculature of the pelvic floor and causing pain in these muscles or in their areas of attachment, such as the sacrum, coccyx, ischial tuberosity, and pubic ramae'. These symptoms associated with pelvic myalgia are often vague, and they are frequently difficult for the patient to describe or localize accurately. Such patients usually complain of an aching discomfort in the rectum, pelvis or lower back; indeed, a number of these patients were initially treated fruitlessly for low back pain, lumbar disc syndrome or degenerative joint disease of the lumbar spine.

In their review of the literature, Sinaki and colleagues noted that a number of different authors have described pelvic pain problems. The origin of the particular pelvic pain they described is in one of several muscles of the pelvic floor or in the areas of attachment on neighbouring bony structures. This syndrome should be differentiated from urinary tract infections, various rectal diseases and trauma. The clinical features of this syndrome were described from the case histories of 94 patients, 78 women and 16 men. The women in their study often described the pain they were having as pelvic pain, although the most frequent complaint of pain in this particular study was rectal pain. They found that the majority of their patients had high scores, on the Minnesota Multiphasic Personality Inventory (MMPI), in hysteria and hypochondriasis. They found that high depression scores were absent. These findings are consistent with other studies of chronic pain patients described later.

DeValera and Raftery (1976) studied cases of lower abdominal and pelvic pain with two common organic causes: nerve entrapment in the abdominal wall and internal pelvic ligamentous strains. Both of these pains were worse premenstrually, during pregnancy and in the puerperium. They found that two factors contributed to these entities. These included fluid retention with tissue oedema (possibly due to prolactin secretion) and relaxation of the pelvic joints and ligaments by the action of hormones secreted by the corpus luteum or placenta.

The nerve entrapment occurs by the nipping of the thoracic and upper lumbar nerves as they emerge through the rectus sheath. The pain is chiefly abdominal, but it may radiate through the posterior division of the nerve causing some backache which is usually not severe. This diagnosis should be considered whenever there is chronic lower abdominal pain and discomfort. By putting the rectus muscle into a position of tension and then pressing upon it, the pain is generally exacerbated. Treatment of these patients by injection of less than 0.5 ml of 6% aqueous phenol was described.

Intrapelvic ligamentous strain was diagnosed by vaginal examination. The pelvic side walls in the sacroiliac joints were carefully palpated, as were the sacrospinous ligaments. Often a sharply localized trigger area was found. Pressure on the particular area evoked the characteristic pain of which the patient had been complaining. Treatment consisted of injecting the trigger area with a small amount of local anaesthetic with corticosteroids. Recurrence rate in this syndrome was high, and repeated injections were often required. When the strain was located anteriorly, 6% aqueous phenol injection produced better results. One complication after intrapelvic injection with a local anaesthetic (bupivacaine) involved numbness of the legs, but this disappeared after several days. With the phenol they found that numbness was more persistent, and in one of their cases a foot drop developed which lasted for a week. They also found some vaginal bleeding following the injections. In one patient, an ischiorectal abscess developed.

Pelvic pain has often been associated with the use of an intrauterine device (IUD), according to Trobough (1978). He stated that insertion pain is one of the causes of pelvic pain associated with the IUD. He reported that 21% of 1121 removals of IUD were for pain and an additional 18% were for pain and bleeding. The cause of pelvic pain in patients wearing IUDs is unknown. One hypothesis is for myometrial irritability secondary to endometrial prostaglandin release triggered by the presence of a foreign body. Another hypothesis is that perhaps the physical characteristics of the device may play a role in pain production. He wrote that another problem with IUDs and pelvic pain is most often caused by infection of the pelvis, and that pelvic infection can be separated into three basic categories which have distinctive pathology, pathogenesis and microbial aetiology. He described: (a) infections that occur post-D and C, post-partum and post-abortal following intrauterine trauma; (b) postoperative infections most usually from organisms which are introduced from the skin or vagina during the operation; and (c) pelvic inflammatory disease (PID) which is a bacterial pelvic infection occurring in the non-pregnant patient without a history of prior surgical entry. In this situation, the primary pathology is an endosalpingitis, usually caused by gonococcus bacteria.

Trobough described the aetiology, diagnosis and treatment of acute pelvic inflammatory disease, but noted that chronic pelvic infections may be caused by *Mycobacterium tuberculosis*, parasites or fungus. However, these are almost never encountered in developed countries. They cautioned that the so-called 'chronic' bacterial salpingitis is usually either an indolent infection in patients who have received inappropriate or suboptimal antibiotic therapy or recurrent salpingitis. Even though recurrent bacterial salpingitis or recurrent PID is a very commonly occurring clinical event, the timing of recurrence suggests that most are attributable to new infection rather than chronicity or a relapse.

Between 10% and 17% of all women with gonorrhoea develop PID, accounting for approximately 20% of all gynaecological admissions to Bellevue Hospital from 1935 to 1951, 10% of all gynaecological admissions to King's County Hospital in New York from 1951 to 1959 and approximately 5% of all gynaecological patients at the University of Washington Hospital in Seattle between 1968 and 1972. There is some mystery as to how the micro-organisms obtain entry into the fallopian tubes. The cervix of a healthy woman normally contains all of the opportunistic pathogenic bacteria that are involved in infection and it must be remembered that most women who develop gonorrhoea do not develop PID.

The factors responsible for the failure of local defence mechanisms in the minority of patients who do develop PID require further study. It appears that menstruation may be important, in that 66% of patients with gonococcal salpingitis develop symptoms during or within 7 days of onset of menstruation. The IUD also apparently reduces the efficiency of local barriers to the spread of gonococcal and other organisms into the upper genital tract. It may be that menstrual blood may be refluxed through the fallopian tubes, since blood is often detected in the peritoneal dialysis returns in menstruating women with chronic renal failure. It is also conceivable that spermatozoa could carry the organism into the tubes, as the gonococci are capable of attachment to spermatozoa.

Acute PID is not an easy diagnosis to make but usually includes findings of a mass, fever and elevated peripheral white blood count and erythrocyte sedimentation rate. Physical examination nearly always shows pelvic tenderness which is maximal in the adnexal areas. Cervical tenderness with movement is usually found but is a non-specific sign which may be present in any pelvic inflammatory condition. It must be recognized that not all features will be found in each patient, and care must be taken in diagnosis to rule out acute pelvic inflammatory disease when a patient complains of pelvic pain.

Trobough noted that over one-third of his patients with salpingitis developed recurrent pain and adnexal tenderness following at least one normal pelvic examination after completion of therapy. Since all the patients had experienced a symptom-free interval, these occurrences were not considered to represent chronic infections, but rather recurrent infection. Such patients could be confused with patients with chronic pelvic pain syndromes.

Lundberg, Wall and Mathers (1973) also found poor correlations between pain, physical findings and pathology in a study of 95 patients with pelvic pain. Twenty-four of 47 patients who had normal pelvic examinations were found to have organic pathology on laparoscopy, while 16 of 46 patients with abnormal pelvic examinations were found to have no pathology on laparoscopy. Although the purpose of this paper was to emphasize the importance of performing laparoscopy in the evaluation of pelvic pain patients with normal pelvic examinations, the findings support the observations of others that one-third or more of all patients with pelvic pain fall into a category of no demonstrable pathology to account for the symptoms. Obviously, laparoscopy should be used first before subjecting patients with pelvic pain to laparotomy.

Chatman (1981) reviewed a cause of pelvic pain associated with the Allen–Masters syndrome, 'laceration(s) of uterine supports with resultant defect(s) in the broad and/or uterosacral ligaments'. This article pointed to the importance of laparoscopic examination and that the pelvic peritoneal defects may be related to endometriosis, thus delineating quite a specific cause of pelvic pain that is physical in nature.

Empirical investigations

Castelnuovo-Tedesco and Krout (1970) compared three groups of pelvic pain patients. Group 1 included 40 women with chronic pelvic pain, ranging in age from 28 to 64; 25 women had demonstrable organic pathology and 15 did not. Group 2 included 27 women within the same age range with pelvic pathology, but without report of chronic pain. Group 3 included 25 chronic pain patients ranging in age from 21 to 48. However, it is unknown how many of the sample exhibited pelvic pathology. Extensive data were gathered from group 1, including two psychiatric interviews by the investigators, MMPI, Sentence Completion, Thematic Appercep-tion Test (TAT) and Rorschach. Groups 2 and 3 completed only a life-history questionnaire and the MMPI.

Demographic and medical history differences between the groups were noted. With regards to employment status, 3 patients in group 1, 7 patients in group 2, and 20 women in group 3 were employed. The educational level for groups 1 and 2 patients was comparable (i.e. tenth grade), whereas the group 3 average number of grades completed was slightly over 12. In terms of parity, for group 1, only 1 patient had never been pregnant, the average number of pregnancies was 5.7 and the average number of children was 3.6. In group 2, all of the patients had been pregnant once, with the average number of pregnancies being 6.5 and the average number of children 4.7. In group 3, 5 of the patients had never been pregnant and the average number of pregnancies was 2.5, with an average of 2.2 children per patient.

Castelnuovo-Tedesco and Krout described the psychological characteristics of their pelvic pain patients as a group rather than differentiating subgroups (e.g. organic vs. non-organic, reporters vs. non-reporters). As in previous reports, 'A striking degree of psychopathology and social disorganization was characteristic'. For instance, of the 40 women in group 1, only three were seen as 'normal'. They were seen as having deficits in interpersonal relations in that they appeared bland, detached and depressed. Sexual relations were reportedly unsatisfactory and disappointing. The mean MMPI profiles of the three groups were compared. Those with pelvic pain, groups 1 and 3, showed greater elevations on almost all scales in comparison to group 2, the group with pelvic pathology but without pain. Groups 1 and 3 also had higher scores on hypochondriasis and hysteria scales. Groups 1 and 3 also showed substantially greater evidence of paranoia, psychasthenia and schizoid responses than group 2. Group 3 had a little less depression and somatization than group 1. Overall, the MMPI profiles of the patients in groups 1 and 3 were viewed as comparable. Organic pathology was found in 25 of the 40 patients in group 1. There was no apparent relationship between the organic findings and psychiatric findings.

Sixteen of the patients underwent surgery; 13 no longer had pain, although in 1 patient the pain returned. Twenty-one patients underwent culdoscopy, 6 of these patients became completely pain free, and 3 of them partially pain free. Those patients who experienced pain relief had all been treated surgically. Psychiatric follow-up of 17 of these latter patients was undertaken. Five of the patients were noted as having experienced some improvement; pain for the remaining 12 patients was unchanged, worse or in other body locations.

Castelnuovo-Tedesco and Krout concluded that 'substantial psychopathology is characteristic of chronic pelvic pain patients, regardless of the presence or absence of pelvic pathology'. The pain appeared to be more closely related to psychiatric disturbance than to any organic pathology. Their principal conclusions were:

1. The psychiatric characteristics did not differentiate between patients with organic pelvic pathology and those without.
2. Pelvic pain patients, regardless of presence or absence of organic pelvic pathology, showed considerable psychopathology, especially mixed character disorders with predominant schizoid features. The majority of those who received hysterectomy became pain free, but in a minority, other symptoms appeared.
3. The patients without pelvic pain had a more normal composite MMPI profile than those with pain.
4. Among patients with pelvic pain, social class had little apparent bearing on the degree of psychopathology.

This investigation is important in that it surveyed different groups of gynaecology patients in an attempt to equate for pain reports. In such a study it is important that care be taken to equate comparison groups on any variable that can co-vary with outcome (e.g. demographic variables, gynaecological history). The authors reported that MMPI profiles of groups 1 and 3 were slightly elevated relative to the mean profile of group 2. However, statistical analyses were not performed to determine whether or not the differences were statistically significant. In addition, subsequent research (Sternbach, 1974) has noted that the profiles of these patients are typical ones for *pain* patients (i.e. the 'conversion V profile') and are probably not configurations unique to pelvic pain patients.

An investigation by Beard *et al.* (1977) was the first to present a clear comparison between pelvic pain patients with and without demonstrable pathology. Eighteen women with pain and negative laparoscopy findings were compared with 17 women with similar complaints and positive findings. Of those with diagnosed conditions, 6 had chronic infection with adhesions, 3 had endometriosis, 1 had a recent infection, 4 had tubal-ovarian masses, 2 had chronic tubular ectopics, and 1 had had a previous tube operation. The remaining 18 were not found to have any pathology on laparoscopy and were considered the laparoscopy negative group. In addition, a control group of women with no gynaecological complaints was evaluated.

For each patient a clinical history, pelvic examination, cervical smear and blood counts were obtained. A urinalysis was done with culture and, when indicated, an intravenous pyelogram was obtained. All of the above tests were normal for all patients. Within a month, the patients were admitted for laparoscopy. Prior to laparoscopic examination, the patients completed the Eysenck Personality Inventory (EPI) – a general screening test for neuroticism and extroversion; the Middlesex Hospital Questionnaire (MHQ) – an instrument used to measure anxiety, obsessional traits, somatic aspects of anxiety, depression and hysterical symptoms; and a Semantic Differential – an attitude measure. Also, a psychosocial questionnaire was given to the patients to provide information about parental relationships, childhood influences, sexual activities and relationship with husband/partner. All of the patients were reviewed 6 weeks and 3 months after laparoscopy. Successful treatment was indicated by the patients' self-report of improvement. The patients who did not experience any improvement 3 months after their laparoscopy were referred to a psychiatrist.

The neuroticism subscore of the EPI was significantly higher for the laparoscopy negative women than that of the control. The score for the laparoscopy positive group fell midway between the other two (and was not significantly different from either). The semantic differential scores from the MHQ also revealed a similar pattern in that women with negative laparoscopy were significantly less positive in their attitudes toward themselves and their partners than were those in the control group. These women described themselves as less pleasing, less sexually attractive and more anxious. Also, it is particularly noteworthy that both groups of pain patients reported experiencing significantly fewer orgasms during sexual activity than those women in the control sample. There was some indication that the laparoscopy negative group had more family problems than the laparoscopy positive group or the control group.

The incidence of associated symptoms was higher in the laparoscopy positive group, with the exception of dyspareunia which was high in both the laparoscopy positive and the laparoscopy negative groups. Interestingly enough, the laparoscopy negative group reported pain which was different from the laparoscopy positive patients. The laparoscopy negative group more often described their pain as dull in character, whereas the laparoscopy positive patients more often described their pain as colicky. Movement of the cervix elicited pain in only one of the laparoscopy negative patients as compared with 5 of 16 of the laparoscopy positive patients. They also noted that the laparoscopy negative group complained of exacerbation of their pain by movement or exercise. In other respects the clinical characteristics of the two groups were similar. Seven women in each group found no way to relieve their pain. About half of the patients in each group said that the site of their pain was variable.

A comparison of their menstrual histories, obstetric histories and other illnesses showed no significant difference between the two groups. In the laparoscopy negative group reassurance was enough to help 5 of the patients, while the other 13 received no improvement. Nine of these 13 patients agreed to see a psychiatrist. In 3, symptoms remained unchanged after relaxation therapy or sexual counselling over three months postoperatively. With the group of 14 who showed improvement, 8 were cured and 3 showed marked improvement.

Beard *et al.* (1977) noted that it is difficult, if not impossible, to distinguish patients in whom organic conditions are detected from those in whom no condition is found. They suggested that the psychological aspect of pelvic pain may arise from a woman's difficulty in externalizing her feelings when distressed. They concluded that psychosomatic disturbance should be considered a *bona fide* cause of pelvic pain and one which gynaecologists and family practitioners should be prepared to treat.

This investigation provided the first objective data suggesting that women with pelvic pain but no demonstrable pathology may differ as a group from other gynaecology patients with pain and diagnosed pathology conditions. While patients with positive laparoscopy findings may have similar difficulties, the data at present are insufficient to make this conclusion. These findings were strengthened by the inclusion of comparison groups and the equation of groups on variables which potentially co-vary with outcome.

Renaer *et al.* (1979) presented data from a comparison investigation. Three groups were contrasted: group 1, 15 patients with chronic pelvic pain without obvious organic cause; group 2, 22 endometriosis patients with pelvic pain; and group 3, 23 gynaecology patients being treated for benign, non-painful conditions. Numerous measures were used to describe the groups and all data were subjected to statistical analyses.

Data from the MMPI indicated that mean profiles for the two pain groups were similar and each was significantly different from the control; however, they did not differ from each other. In fact, the profiles were similar to those presented by Castelnuovo-Tedesco and Krout (1970), resembling the patterns provided by chronic pain patients. Groups were also compared on the Interpersonal Relations Questionnaire which examined male–female relationships. Analyses indicated that patients from group 1, in comparison with those from group 3, described themselves as significantly more suspicious, detached and unfriendly toward their husbands. Again, the pain patients as a group did not differ from one another.

Henker (1979) reported on the psychological characteristics of 20 consecutive patients with chronic pelvic pain referred to the Psychiatry Consultation Team of the University of Arkansas Medical Center. He reported that the majority of women at his facility with pelvic pain complaints responded to definitive treatment or symptomatic measures, while a small number presented with no significant physical abnormality, but continued to have pain. When these latter patients underwent laparoscopy, the following results were reported: 45% had some type of pelvic infection, 15% had endometriosis, 7% had other diseases and 33% showed no disease entity. This paper discussed 20 consecutive patients with chronic pelvic pain who were referred to psychiatrists during a 2-year period from 1976 to 1978. The sample was predominantly white, with low to middle socioeconomic status, and married.

Henker described the characteristics of pelvic pain among this sample. For the majority, the pain varied from constant and dull to intermittent and stabbing. The most common kind was a dull, continuous pain. Location of this pain was retropubic in 4 cases, right iliac fossa in 4, left iliac fossa in 3 and deep pelvic or rectal in 2. Some of the patients described non-localized pelvic discomfort. Four of the women characterized their pain as sharp; 2 located their pain within the vagina. One described a deep retropubic pain radiating down her right leg, and 1 had pain in the left iliac fossa associated with and often inhibiting her ability to urinate or have a bowel movement. One reported a colicky-type pain. Fourteen patients reported some dysmenorrhoea. Eight had problems with sexual intercourse, 6 experiencing moderate pain on penetration. One patient was able to enjoy intercourse, but often felt severe sharp pain afterwards. The duration of the pain varied. All had been symptomatic for over a year. The longest was 36 years. There was organic disease present within the majority of these patients, but specific evaluation or treatment failed to bring any relief. Ten of the patients had hysterectomy, with or without a bilateral oophorectomy.

In terms of psychiatric diagnosis, the author reported that the symptoms were sufficiently varied for all patients such that no trend appeared obvious; however, 8 of the 20 patients were seen as 'histrionic'. Psychophysiological disorders (i.e. tension/migraine headaches, GI disturbances, asthma) were frequent. Two of the women did have some mild organic brain syndrome findings. Five showed mild depression.

On the basis of this survey, Henker identified three classes of patients. The first was composed of 11 patients who had had an operation in the past, but in whom the pain continued postoperatively. The second group consisted of 6 patients, 3 with gynaecological disease and 3 with post-traumatic abnormalities in whom the existing disease did not seem to be sufficient to explain the magnitude of the pain. The final group comprised 3 patients in whom there was no demonstrable disease. When offered relaxation training or psychotherapy, patients were resistant. Six patients rejected the suggestion, and 6 rapidly terminated therapy shortly after beginning. Henker recommended that extensive psychiatric interviews be conducted for patients with complaints of continuing pelvic pain, but that supportive psychotherapy is best provided by the primary physician.

Case histories

The preceding review of the pertinent medical and psychiatric literature demonstrates the confusing state of knowledge and treatment approaches to patients suffering from a most common gynaecological complaint. Many patients with organic problems have concomitant emotional problems which may or may not complicate their painful illness. Many patients have no physical pathology at all, and some do not have enough to 'justify' their pain in the view of competent medical authority. Some patients who have had pain for a long time, regardless of aetiology, have developed personality disorders which have been described as 'chronic pain personalities' (Sternbach, 1974).

The authors have recently evaluated several patients who seem to represent the diversity of the clinical problems encountered. The cases which follow suggest a taxonomy for categorizing pelvic pain patients with implications for management or treatment.

Case 1
This patient represents an example of a patient with clear-cut painful pelvic disease who experienced some emotional problems during the course of treatment.

The patient was a 20-year-old female admitted to a community hospital with a complaint of pelvic pain. The pain was experienced in the pelvis, more or less continually throughout the month, but more intensely during the menstrual period. Investigation as an outpatient failed to reveal any significant pathology. The patient was admitted for a laparoscopy examination to rule out endometriosis. The laparoscopy revealed extensive endometriosis through the pelvis. Initially, the patient was relieved to discover the cause for the pelvic pain, inasmuch as in the past she had been told that her pains were 'psychosomatic' and she had some doubts as to whether there was any organic pathology. However, she did experience some psychological difficulties, including a transient depression, before she was able to adjust to the demands of taking medication over a prolonged period and accepting the fact that she had developed a chronic physical ailment at such a young age. These difficulties were felt to represent a normal reaction to a painful illness, however, and not the manifestation of psychiatric disorder.

Case 2

This is an example of a case in which there is demonstrable organic pathology which does not totally account for the patient's reaction to the pain.

The patient was a 21-year-old female, admitted to the gynaecology service through the Emergency Medical Department of a large university hospital. The patient had two previous admissions to the gynaecology service with a history of tubal-ovarian abscesses and recurrent salpingitis. During each of these, she had seen a psychiatric consultant because of 'management problems'. The patient's white blood count was elevated and her temperature was raised. It was the physician's opinion that her reaction to the pain was out of proportion to the physical findings. Nevertheless, he felt obliged to begin another course of antibiotics in the hospital. During the course of hospitalization, the patient became increasingly unco-operative and demanding. She was accusatory towards the staff, she berated the other patients on the ward, and she was unco-operative with her treatment regimen. The staff found her to be an extremely difficult patient and her physician again requested help from the psychiatric department to assess in managing the patient.

The past social history, which was elicited by the psychiatrist, revealed a childhood and adolescence filled with significant losses, including an alcoholic mother, an absent father, multiple foster home placements, social isolation, lack of close interpersonal relationships, truancy, and many legal difficulties including drug abuse and assault. The patient was facing a jail sentence upon her release from the hospital.

Although rapport with the patient was difficult to develop due to her suspicion and resistance, gradually she began to respond to the interpersonal efforts of the consultant and a boyfriend whose help was enlisted. The consultant listened patiently to her many complaints and was able to provide some help for the staff in setting limits for the patient. The pain gradually resolved, and the patient left the hospital.

Case 3

This illustrates a case of a possible physical condition which could contribute to the pelvic pain, but one in which there is some controversy as to the validity of the physical syndrome.

The patient was a 35-year-old female who came to the walk-in clinic of a large community hospital with a complaint of pelvic pain for the prior 3 months. She had seen her family physician 1 month earlier. He had diagnosed a 'muscle strain' and had given her some pain pills. However, the pain persisted and the patient came seeking another opinion. She reported that the pain, which occurred primarily in the left lower quadrant of her abdomen, was aggravated by work and lifting her children. The pelvic examination was within normal limits as was an examination of her abdomen. The positive finding occurred when the patient was instructed to tense her abdominal wall. She experienced pain when pressed in the left lower quadrant. Presumptive diagnosis of nerve entrapment in the abdominal wall or myofascial pain syndrome was made. The patient was reassured and returned to her family doctor for follow-up treatment. The patient accepted this without further question.

Case 4

This exemplifies one of the less commonly encountered cases in which there is no demonstrable organic cause for the patient's pelvic pain.

The patient was a 22-year-old married college student who consulted a private gynaecologist with the complaint of chronic pelvic pain and dyspareunia. A presumptive diagnosis of endometriosis had been made, but laparoscopic examination failed to reveal any demonstrable cause for the pain problem. Notable history events included separation from her parents during childhood, early assumption of responsibility for a large number of younger children in a foster family, poor relationships during adolescence and academic over-achievement in high school and college. The patient was a pre-law student, as was her husband. The couple claimed to have no interest in having children. The patient was convinced that if her uterus were removed, her pain problems would disappear. Psychological testing was consistent with the diagnosis of a 'pain-prone personality', and a recommendation was made that the patient enter psychotherapy. The couple were resistant to this idea, and they convinced the surgeon that an operation would be appropriate. Following hysterectomy, the patient had no further pain complaints and remained free of significant emotional problems or chronic pain behaviour.

Case 5

This illustrates a case of psychologically experienced pain, probably an hysterical conversion phenomenon.

The patient was a 27-year-old female who presented to the Emergency Medicine Department of a small community hospital with a complaint of acute pelvic pain. Pelvic examination revealed some adnexal tenderness on the right side, and the presumptive diagnosis of tubal ectopic pregnancy was entertained. However, the patient refused culdocentesis or laparoscopy. Before she was permitted to leave the hospital against medical advice, she was seen by a psychiatrist. He allowed the patient and her husband to express some of their fears of surgery and hospitalization. Following this brief interaction, the patient agreed to admission to the hospital. After admission, it was learned that her father was on another floor of the hospital dying of advanced cancer of the colon. The patient spent the evening visiting her father, and in the morning she had no further complaint of pain. She was discharged without further pelvic problem and referred for psychiatric consultation as an outpatient.

Conclusions

Even though complaints of pelvic pain are frequent among gynaecology patients, the medical literature for this perplexing problem is not extensive. Only a few conceptualizations have been proposed. Each postulates psychological and physical factors; however they differ in the role each is believed to play. For the purpose of identifying and organizing the major problem areas, the literature has been divided into five categories.

The first section includes those investigations that describe pelvic pain as an *enigma*. Hyslop (1972) urged that rather than considering psychological factors as secondary, they may be causally related to the pain for some women. Mills (1978) hypothesized that the pain may result from pelvic congestion, referred from the uterus. The *British Medical Journal* (Editorial, 1978) urged physicians to provide continuing support to patients even when they could find no physical cause to the pain. Philipp (1978) emphasized that 'psychological factors' were to be considered. However, such an analysis needs to include more than just a simplistic inquiry into sexual experience of early youth. Instead, inquiry needs to be directed into the processes by which cerebral cortical activity influences neurohormonal secretion and autonomic nervous system activity.

The second section presents descriptive studies of patients whose pain was believed to originate from pelvic congestion. Duncan and Taylor (1952) and Taylor (1954) were the first to present interview data from pelvic pain patients. They viewed their patients as 'psychologically ill' in terms of having unpleasant childhood experiences, current difficulties with sexual or maternal functioning, and ongoing life stresses. In contrast, Edlundh and Jansson (1966) found Swedish pelvic pain patients to be typically intelligent, tense and striving. Jeffcoate (1975) described 'congestive dysmenorrhoea' as pain associated with premenstrual engorgement but also due to pervasive anxiety or current life stresses. Most recently, Hobbs (1976) has supported a psychosomatic concept of pelvic pain, i.e. the abnormal vascular state was the result of a discordant functioning of the autonomic nervous system and that an abnormal mental state was not secondary to the pain syndrome.

The third section summarizes reports of the psychological observations of pelvic pain patients. Gidro-Frank, Gordon and Taylor (1960) described their pelvic pain patients as unable to establish and maintain female functions, i.e. sexual, menstrual and gestational performance. Frederick (1976) discussed the psychological responses to pelvic pain that may be conversion reactions. As others noted, Frederick also urged primary care physicians to establish a therapeutic alliance with their patients.

The fourth section discusses physical diagnostic considerations in the evaluation of pelvic pain. Authors emphasized different origins of pain. These included: tension myalgia of the pelvic floor (Sinaki, Merritt and Stillwell, 1977); nerve entrapment or internal pelvic ligament strain (DeValera and Raftery, 1976); insertion or containment pain from an IUD (Trobough, 1978); and pelvic pain from acute or recurrent pelvic infection (Eschenbach and Holmes, 1975). Also, in the evaluation of all of these cases, Lundberg, Wall and Mathers (1973) recommended routine use of the laparoscopy, in view of the low correlation often found between pain reports, physical findings and pathology.

The few empirical investigations of pelvic pain patients are included in the fifth section. A large-scale descriptive investigation was reported by Castelnuovo-Tedesco and Krout (1970). Utilizing psychiatric interviews and psychological test profiles, they concluded that substantial psychopathology is characteristic of chronic pelvic pain patients, regardless of the presence or absence of pelvic pathology. In addition, the pain was regarded as more closely related to psychiatric disturbance than to organic pathology. An investigation by Beard *et al*. (1977) was the first to present a clear comparison between pelvic pain patients with and without demonstrable pathology. These findings were the first objective data indicating that pelvic pain patients, with or without pathology, represent a population different from that of typical gynaecology patients. Data from the Renaer *et al*. (1979) investigation corroborated these findings. The report by Henker (1979) on the psychological characteristics of 20 chronic pelvic pain patients suggested that supportive psychotherapy be provided by the primary care physician.

To study adequately this difficult and perplexing problem, particular care must be taken in future research efforts. At the initial stage all physical causes must be ruled out or defined so that clear comparisons of relevant pain patients can be made (i.e. pain reporters with specific organic causes vs. pain reporters without organic cause; pelvic pain reporters without pathology vs. other body site chronic pain patients, etc.). Next, groups must be equated on variables which could potentially co-vary with outcome, such as age, parity, sexual responsiveness, etc. Structured interviews must be supplemented by data from more objective sources such as psychological tests, behavioural samples, and information from significant others. Only clear comparisons made between diagnostically 'pure' groups equated on potentially relevant variables will lead to the discovery of the factors unique to pelvic pain.

Making a diagnosis of the aetiology of pelvic pain does not necessarily lead to adequate or appropriate treatment. In the section on case histories, it is suggested that pelvic pain patients can be divided into the five categories shown below.

1. Patients who have pelvic pathology which explains the pain
These are patients with positive physical and laparoscopy examinations in which findings in the opinion of competent medical authority, provide a physical explanation of the painful symptoms. It is important to realize, however, that a patient in this category may develop a chronic pain problem or personality. Over time it may not be clear whether the patient remains in this category or overlaps into another category. Also, some patients in this category may require psychiatric treatment or emotional support. However, for most of these patients, the supportive therapy should be provided by the primary care physician.

2. Patients who have pelvic pathology which does not explain the pain
In this category, patients may have a number of physical findings which in the opinion of competent medical authority do not totally explain the painful symptoms. Such patients are often observed to be more neurotic or have significantly more emotional problems than those in the first category. For such patients, it is essential that the primary care physician takes on the role of providing supportive therapy as well as diagnostic work-up. In these patients, correcting the underlying medical problem often does not affect the pelvic pain problem to a significant degree.

3. Patients who have questionable pelvic or extra-pelvic pathology, which may or may not explain the pelvic pain
These questionable pathological states have been described as the pelvic congestion syndrome, myofascial or musculoskeletal pain syndromes, changes in pelvic blood

flow, difficulties in sexual arousal, vulvar varicosities, and pelvic sympathetic syndrome. This group blends into the one described above, with the same implications for treatment and therapy. As with the former group, it is essential that while the work-up continues and the physical symptoms are treated the primary care physicians use themselves as therapists offering emotional support and establishing therapeutic relationships.

4. Patients who have no discernible pelvic pathology to explain the pelvic pain
When this situation occurs, such patients are best described as suffering from conversion disorders in which the pelvic pain bears a symbolic relation to an underlying psychological problem. Occasionally, in either a depressed or otherwise psychotic patient, the painful symptomatology represents a somatic delusion. Most of the time, the underlying pelvic or extrapelvic pathology has not yet been discovered. It is important to continue the evaluation, establishing a positive alliance with the patient and avoiding premature psychiatric referral until the work-up is complete.

5. Chronic pain patients
These patients have been described by Sternbach and others as suffering from the psychological consequences of chronic pain over a prolonged period of time. These patients are emotionally disturbed; the form of the disturbance is neurotic. The characteristic types of this neurosis are hypochondriasis and depression. The patients state that they are preoccupied with their symptoms to the exclusion of almost everything else, and they feel quite hopeless about their situation. The evidence is clear that their reaction to chronic pain is not imaginary, but is measurable and seems consistent from patient to patient. It is not useful to differentiate 'psychogenic' pain from 'real' pain for these patients because the emotional consequences of pain appear to be independent of aetiology. When the chronic pain personality stage has been reached, most physicians are unable to provide the necessary treatment. Instead they often become involved in a series of difficult interactions with the patient which may lead to physician frustration and patient despair. Sometimes the physician is unaware that the patient has passed from one of the other categories into the chronic pain stage, and a 'pain game' interaction develops. Such patients require a multidisciplinary pain treatment approach at an outpatient or an inpatient behaviour change treatment programme. Specialists in pain management should evaluate and treat these patients to employ interventions to interrupt the pain reinforcement and assist the patient in psychological and physical rehabilitation. A large number of chronic pelvic pain patients in our university pain clinic have benefited greatly from this kind of interdisciplinary approach, using nerve blocks, group psychotherapy, medication, self-hypnosis and relaxation techniques.

Categories 2, 3 and 4 represent the 'enigmatic pelvic pain' group. Even though there is considerable overlap between these three groups, it is helpful to conceptualize a theoretical taxonomy of pelvic pain to increase flexibility in the diagnostic and therapeutic considerations. Hopefully, these categories will lead to the ability to develop earlier detection, better treatment and enhanced physician education.

References

BASU, H. K. (1981) Major problems of pelvic pain. *British Journal of Hospital Medicine,* **26,** 150–159

BEARD, R. W., BELSEY, E. M., LIEBERMAN, B. A. and WILKINSON, J. C. M. (1977) Pelvic pain in women. *American Journal of Obstetrics and Gynecology,* **128,** 566–570

BERKOW, R. (Ed.) (1977) *Merck Manual of Diagnosis and Therapy,* 13th edn, Raleigh, New Jersey; Merck, Sharpe and Dohme Research Laboratories

CASTELNUOVO-TEDESCO, P. and KROUT, B. M. (1970) Psychosomatic aspects of chronic pelvic pain. *Psychiatry in Medicine,* **1,** 109–126

CHATMAN, D. L. (1981) Pelvic peritoneal defects and endometriosis: Allen–Masters syndrome revisited. *Fertility and Sterility,* **36,** 751–756

DeVALERA, E. and RAFTERY, H. (1976) Lower abdominal and pelvic pain in women. In *Advances in Pain Research and Therapy,* Vol. 1, pp. 933–937 (Bonica, J. J. and Albe-Fessard, D., Eds.) New York; Raven Press

DUNCAN, C. H. and TAYLOR, H. C. (1952) A psychosomatic study of pelvic congestion. *American Journal of Obstetrics and Gynecology,* **64,** 1–12

EDITORIAL (1978) Enigmatic pelvic pain. *British Medical Journal,* **2,** 1041–1042

EDLUNDH, K. O. and JANSSON, B. (1966) Pelvic congestion syndrome – preliminary psychiatric report. *Journal of Psychosomatic Research,* **10,** 221–229

ESCHENBACH, D. A. and HOLMES, K. K. (1975) Acute pelvic inflammatory disease: current concepts of pathogenesis, etiology and management. *Clinical Obstetrics and Gynecology,* **18,** 35–56

FREDERICK, M. A. (1976) Psychological aspects of chronic pelvic pain. *Clinical Obstetrics and Gynecology,* **19,** 399–406

GIDRO-FRANK, I., GORDON, T. and TAYLOR, H. C. (1960) Pelvic pain and female identity. *American Journal of Obstetrics and Gynecology,* **79,** 1184–1202

HENKER, F. O. (1979) Diagnosis and treatment of non-organic pelvic pain. *Southern Medical Journal,* **72,** 1132–1134

HOBBS, J. T. (1976) The pelvic congestion syndrome. *The Practitioner,* **216,** 529–540

HYSLOP, R. S. (1972) Some thoughts on pelvic pain. *New Zealand Journal of Obstetrics and Gynecology,* **12,** 40–42

JEFFCOATE, T. N. A. (1975) *Principles of Gynaecology,* 4th edn. London; Butterworths

LUNDBERG, W. I., WALL, J. E. and MATHERS, J. E. (1973) Laparoscopy in evaluation of pelvic pain. *American Journal of Obstetrics and Gynecology,* **42,** 872–876

McFAYDEN, I. R. (1981) Gynecological pain in the lower abdomen. *Clinics in Obstetrics and Gynecology,* **8,** 33–47

MILLS, W. G. (1978) The enigma of pelvic pain. *Journal of the Royal Society of Medicine,* **71,** 257–260

NADELSON, C. C., NOTMAN, M. T. and ELLIS, E. A. (1983) Psychosomatic aspects of obstetrics and gynecology. *Psychosomatics,* **24,** 871–884

PHILIPP, E. (1978) Pelvic pain. *Journal of the Royal Society of Medicine,* **71,** 244–246

READING, A. (1982–83) Critical analysis of psychological factors in the management and treatment of chronic pelvic pain. *International Journal of Psychiatry and Medicine,* **12,** 129–139

RENAER, M., VERTOMMEN, H., NIJS, P., WAGEMANS, L. and VAN HEMELRIJCK, T. (1979) Psychological aspects of chronic pelvic pain in women. *American Journal of Obstetrics and Gynecology,* **134,** 75–80

SINAKI, M., MERRITT, J. L. and STILLWELL, G. K. (1977) Tension myalgia of the pelvic floor. *Proceedings of the Mayo Clinic,* **52,** 717–722

STERNBACH, R. A. (1974) *Pain Patients: Traits and Treatment.* New York; Academic Press

TAIT, L. (1883) *Pathology and Treatment of Diseases of the Ovaries.* Birmingham, UK; Cornish

TAYLOR, H. C. (1949) Vascular congestion and hyperemia. *American Journal of Obstetrics and Gynecology,* **57,** 211

TAYLOR, H. C. (1954) Pelvic pain based on a vascular and autonomic nervous system disorder. *American Journal of Obstetrics and Gynecology,* **67,** 1177–1196

THALHEIM, W. (1975) Differential diagnosis of important functional disturbances in the pelvic area. *Beitrage zur Orthopedie und Traumatologie,* **22,** 430–434

TROBOUGH, G. E. (1978) Pelvic pain and the IUD. *Journal of Reproductive Medicine,* **20,** 167–174

WHITEHOUSE, J. B. (1935) *Eden and Lockyer's Gynaecology,* 4th edn, p. 755. London; Churchill

Chapter 4

The premenstrual syndrome

Lynne M. Drummond and Clive M. Tonks

Introduction

At first sight, premenstrual tension is a very attractive subject for study. The timing of the symptoms is predictable. The patient can often serve as her own control because symptoms are also absent at predictable times. Alas, like so much in life, the reality is far from this simple ideal. As one tries to focus closely on the premenstrual syndrome, it assumes a mirage-like quality, tending to become blurred and indistinct. Pinning it down has similarities to picking up a globule of mercury; the moment you seem to have it, it escapes between your fingers. The superficial attractiveness as a subject for study has led to a voluminous literature, but the difficulties have made that literature confused and contradictory. As we shall see, the subject abounds in speculation and dogma but is remarkably low on fact.

Historical aspects of the premenstrual syndrome

According to Ricci (1950), physicians at the time of Hippocrates were aware that some women had symptoms prior to menstruation. He translates their work as follows: '(preceding menstruation, some women have) . . . a sense of heaviness similar to that which occurs in the eighth month of pregnancy, lumbago, chills, febrile reactions, severe headaches, ringing in the ears, heat in the spinal column and specks before the eyes.'

Ricci also translates Soranus of Ephesus (c. A.D. 100): 'The menses are about to occur when a women feels somewhat uneasy on walking, when a feeling of heaviness appears in the loins. Some develop a torpor, yawning and pandiculation, while others develop nausea and loss of appetite.'

Both these descriptions mention 'heaviness', which we equate with the bloated feelings found in present-day descriptions, but little of the rest is recognizable to modern ears.

Historically, there now appears a great gap in the record until the publication of the paper 'The hormonal causes of premenstrual tension' (Frank, 1931). Before this, apart from a mention of premenstrual pain in varicose veins (Goodman, 1878), attention had seemed confined to the phase of menstruation itself.

Certainly, according to the older literature, a host of hazards confronted the menstruating women. Sutherland (1892) cited Icard (1890) as observing the following during menstruation: 'Kleptomania, pyromania, dipsomania, suicidal mania, erotomania, nymphomania, delusions, acute mania, delirious insanity, impulsive insanity, morbid jealousy, lying, calumny, illusions, hallucinations and melancholia.' One can only conclude that the later nineteenth century must have been an exciting time in which to menstruate!

There have been religious prohibitions on menstruating women in many cultures. The medical profession have also added to and elaborated many of the myths about the baleful effects of menstruation. Macht (1943) mentions many warnings issued by doctors. It was said that meat would spoil if salted by menstruating women, and one report warned against playing stringed instruments while menstruating because the strings would fail to emit the correct note or might even snap during a performance!

Luckily, the paper by Frank (1931) turned interest toward the premenstrual phase and allowed menstruating women to get on with the business of living normally. The changes often complained of in the premenstrual phase are now know as the premenstrual syndrome.

Definition of the premenstrual syndrome

There are no generally agreed criteria for either the timing of the premenstrual phase or for the premenstrual syndrome. Indeed, after a two-day workshop on the premenstrual syndrome at the National Institute of Mental Health, USA, panellists agreed that the premenstrual syndrome existed but were unable to offer a precise definition of the disorder (Blume, 1983). Various authors have taken the premenstruum as 14 days, 7 days or 4 days before the onset of bleeding. The premenstrual week is probably the most commonly used definition.

The symptoms which have been described in this phase are legion. Dalton (1964) gave a list involving almost all organs and systems. Most authors are more restrictive, the most commonly noted being tension, irritability, depression, bloated feelings of the abdomen, swelling of the fingers, legs and breasts, and breast pain (Rees, 1953). Rarer symptoms include hypersomnia, thirst and increased appetite. Sometimes an increased liability to pre-existing conditions such as asthma or migraine is included. Rees (1953) found that the symptoms began 2–12 days before the onset of the menses and, in 85% of women, disappeared immediately with blood flow. The most common complaints were tension and irritability, present in all sufferers, depression in 80%, anxiety in 77%, swelling of fingers or legs in 74% and painful swelling of breasts in 60%. This is a fairly middle-of-the-road description of the syndrome.

Halbreich and Kas (1977) used the following criteria:

1. Symptoms recur cyclically only in the premenstrual phase.
2. There is a dramatic and complete relief with the onset of full blood flow.
3. There are no permanent symptoms, similar to or different from the symptoms of the premenstrual syndrome, during other phases of the cycle.

We would think that criterion 3 would rule out almost everyone. Certainly the use of such strict criteria would lead to much lower figures for prevalence than would the use of the broader clinical description of Rees (1953). Many workers have reported that women with premenstrual tension or depression are more likely than non-sufferers to report these symptoms in other phases of the cycle (Tonks, 1975) and all these patients would be excluded by criterion 1.

Recently, there has been increasing popularity for the idea that there may be a number of different types of premenstrual syndrome which could have differing aetiologies and responses to treatment (Clare, 1977; Moos and Leideman, 1978; Abraham, 1980; Halbreich and Endicott, 1982; Abraham, 1983). The most specific claims so far concern dysmenorrhoea and mastalgia. Coppen and Kessel (1963) found that abdominal pain was commonest on the first day of blood flow rather than premenstrually. They also found that the presence of dysmenorrhoea was not correlated with a high neuroticism score on the Eysenck Personality Inventory as were premenstrual complaints. It thus seemed they were different entities.

Stephenson, Denney and Aberger (1983), however, using the Menstrual Symptom Questionnaire, Eysenck Personality Inventory and Life Experiences Survey Questionnaire in 423 college students, found that premenstrual physical and psychological symptoms as well as menstrual pain were all positively correlated with neuroticism scores.

Preece, Mansell and Hughes (1978) gave the Middlesex Hospital Questionnaire to 317 women complaining of breast pain and to 170 controls attending hospital with varicose veins. There was no difference in mean scores between subjects and controls, and the mean scores were much lower than those obtained from psychiatric outpatients. They also divided the mastalgia patients into a clearly organic group, with periductal mastitis and patients with pain related to the menstrual cycle. The mean scores of the two groups were not significantly different and they claimed that cyclical pronounced mastalgia is not psychoneurotic. The condition is usually bilateral with diffuse pain in the breast, and is worst premenstrually and during the first few days of bleeding (Preece et al., 1976).

Clare (1983) performed a large study on 521 women in the fertile period of life, selected from GP practices, and 170 women who were attending a gynaecological clinic for premenstrual complaints. He administered the General Health Questionnaire (GHQ) and a modified version of the Moos Menstrual Distress Questionnaire to both groups. In his sample from GP practices he found that 74.8% of women reported at least one symptom on the Menstrual Distress Questionnaire. Analyses of his total sample showed that women who had a score on the GHQ suggestive of psychiatric morbidity, were more likely to report premenstrual symptoms of a psychological or behavioural type, but no difference was found in their reporting rate of physical symptoms.

Recent work has tended to show that symptoms are much less time restricted than originally claimed. Silbergeld, Brast and Noble (1971) studied 8 female students intensively over 4 cycles and found that some psychological and physical complaints were more common both premenstrually and menstrually. Beumont, Richards and Gelder (1975) studied 25 volunteers throughout a complete cycle. Daily records were made on a mood self-rating scale for depression, a psychological symptom checklist and a physical symptom checklist. They found that scores on all scales were significantly higher in the premenstrual and menstrual weeks. It is interesting to note that a small group of hysterectomized women with functioning ovaries showed the same trends. The cycle phase was determined endocrinologically. The trends were not statistically significant, possibly because there were only 7 subjects.

Bäckström, Boyle and Baird (1981) recorded daily symptom ratings on complaints of premenstrual symptoms for 1 month prior to and up to 2 months after hysterectomy. Ovarian activity was monitored by twice weekly measurement of urinary hormones. They found that cyclical changes in mood persisted following hysterectomy, with the most physical and psychological symptoms being complained of in the late luteal phase of the cycle. The also found a marked decrease in ratings of activity and vigour which started in the late luteal phase and persisted through the time of menstruation. Most of the women showed a small but significant improvement in symptoms after hysterectomy. Theoretically, this group is important because their ratings would not be biased by knowledge of their cycle phase, as menstruation had been abolished.

In another careful study, Beumont et al. (1978) demonstrated a rise in complaints about mood through the 4 premenstrual days to a maximum on the second day of menstruation, followed by a fall on day three. Physical complaints were at a maximum on the first day of menstruation. A study using daily recording on a 17-item self-rating scale also showed that high scores in the premenstrual phase ran on into menstruation (Taylor, 1979b). Perhaps we are edging forward to the idea of a paramenstrual rather than a premenstrual syndrome.

There are, of course, negative findings such as a study of 28 women over 2 cycles which found that anxiety, hostility and depression scores did not correlate with the phase of the cycle (Friedman and Meares, 1978).

Sampson and Jenner (1977) used a novel statistical technique, which has subsequently been used by other workers, to overcome technical objections to the usual methods of allowing for the different lengths of cycles. Nineteen volunteer student health visitors filled in a Menstrual Distress Questionnaire daily. This gave scores on 8 aspects of the syndrome every day throughout one cycle. A sine wave was then fitted to each of these scores over the full cycle by a least squares method. They found that the peak value of these curves for pain, poor concentration and behavioural change occurred about 1 day prior to the start of menstruation. The peak for water retention was 2 days before and for negative affect it was the day following the onset of bleeding.

Overall, despite the lack of agreed criteria, there does appear to be a tendency for certain symptoms to cluster premenstrually and menstrually.

Prevalence of the premenstrual syndrome

The prevalence of the premenstrual syndrome varies greatly according to the criteria for selection and the sample taken. Studies reporting questionnaire data or straightforward verbal complaints of premenstrual symptoms tend to give much higher prevalence rates than those obtained by the analysis of daily records of mood state (Tonks, 1975; Sampson and Prescott, 1981; Endicott and Halbreich, 1982).

In a study where postal questionnaires were sent to 500 women, 22% complained of moderate or severe premenstrual headache, 32% complained of moderate or severe premenstrual irritability and 23% complained of moderate or severe premenstrual depression or anxiety. No less than 72% of the sample reported some premenstrual swelling (Coppen and Kessel, 1963).

In a Scandinavian study, questionnaires were sent to 1083 randomly selected women. Between 50% and 70% of the women, dependent on age group, complained of some premenstrual symptoms. The most frequently reported symptoms were irritability, swelling of the abdomen or swelling of the breasts premenstrually and these occurred whether the women were taking oral contraceptives or not. Oral contraceptives had the effect of apparently reducing the reported severity of symptoms (Andersch and Hahn, 1981). This finding is contrary to the claims of Dalton (1982) that oral contraceptives increase the frequency and severity of premenstrual complaints.

Rees (1953) interviewed 61 normal women and 84 patients attending psychiatric, psychosomatic or allergy outpatient clinics. Severe premenstrual symptoms were reported by 5% of the normals and 32% of the outpatient group. Moderate premenstrual symptoms were reported by a further 16% of the normals and 30% of the outpatients. The total prevalence in his normal group was therefore 21% and in the clinic attenders was 62%.

Gynaecological patients ($n = 1395$) who were not on hormonal treatment were given a Menstrual Symptom Questionnaire and 50% reported some premenstrual symptoms, with a peak incidence of 60% between the ages of 30 and 40 years (Hargrove and Abraham, 1983). Sheldrake and Cormack (1976), using a questionnaire with first-year university students, found complaints of premenstrual irritability in 32.5% and premenstrual depression in 31% of those who responded and were not taking oral contraceptives.

In two separate studies using a modified Menstrual Distress Questionnaire, Clare (1977, 1983) found that three-quarters of women visiting general practitioners for other reasons complained of at least one premenstrual symptom. This is probably high because of the broad criteria and possibly because the sample were already attending a general practitioner.

All these prevalence figures are at variance with those found by McCance, Luff and Widdowson (1937). These workers asked 167 women to fill in daily records about their symptoms. They found a great discrepancy between complaints made about premenstrual symptoms and the actual analysis of the daily records. Only 3 subjects showed clearly recurrent cycles of premenstrual depression, and clearly recurrent cycles of premenstrual irritability were hard to find. Combining records for the whole cohort, a process tending to reduce the random variation, showed that complaints of depression and irritability were more common premenstrually. This study is supported by that of Wilcoxon, Schrader and Sherif (1976) who also used daily reports with 92 volunteers. In addition, these workers gathered data about life events. They found that reported stressful events accounted for more of the variance in 'negative' mood than did the phase of the menstrual cycle.

Probably there is an underlying rhythmicity of mood related to the menstrual cycle but it seems to be easily swamped by the random variation in environmental stress. It is also clear that a substantial number of women will complain that they have premenstrual or paramenstrual symptoms, although the prevalence varies. Indeed, the prevalence clearly varies with the sample as shown when clinical attenders are compared with normals (Rees, 1953). Coppen (1965) found that premenstrual complaints were commoner in women with a neurotic illness, intermediate in those with affective disorders and least in women with schizophrenic illnesses.

Physiological correlates of the menstrual cycle

Here we intend to look at some of the reported changes other than those of the sex hormones themselves. A large number of such changes have been reported, the best known being the temperature change occurring at ovulation and forming the basis of the rhythm method of contraception.

A number of changes could affect water and salt metabolism. It has been reported that fasting, supine plasma aldosterone levels in women tended to be higher in the luteal and late luteal phases of the menstrual cycle. Plasma renin activity did not demonstrate such periodicity (Katz and Romfh, 1972). Total solute excretion in urine was higher during the second half of the cycle due to a mild natriuresis. This extra excretion of sodium was particularly seen in the urine secreted during the night. Indeed, in the late luteal phase, some women showed a decrease in the daytime excretion of sodium and an increase in nocturnal sodium excretion. This led to there being no overall change in the 24-hour sodium excretion (Parboosingh, Doig and Michie, 1973). A diurnal variation in sodium excretion of this kind might explain some of the failures to demonstrate premenstrual water retention. These studies are usually performed by repeat weighings in the early morning *after* voiding urine. Any daytime water retention would have been lost by the increased sodium excretion overnight.

Theoretically, alterations in circulating progesterone throughout the menstrual cycle may be thought to affect fluid balance. Progesterone acts as a partial agonist of aldosterone and has been thought to induce a temporary natriuresis followed by compensatory increases in the renin–angiotensin–aldosterone axis (Reid and Yen, 1983). However, as these authors point out, the finding that the conversion of progesterone to the mineralocorticoid deoxycorticosterone is enhanced during the luteal phase (Parker et al., 1981) leaves the overall effect of progesterone unresolved.

An increased capillary permeability to plasma protein in the second half of the menstrual cycle has been demonstrated using a sphygmomanometer venous occlusion method on the arm. This could certainly account for complaints of swelling but, in their subjects, the changes did not correlate with such complaints (Jones et al., 1966).

Breast changes have been reported. Breast volume has been shown to increase in the luteal phase of the cycle, using a water displacement measurement technique (Milligan, Drife and Short, 1975). Increased breast volume in the second half of the cycle was also found using plaster casts as a measurement of volume. Heat flow from the breast was also measured and was found to be higher in the second half of the cycle. The authors postulated that these changes could be due in part to increased blood flow in the breasts at this time (Nassar and Smith, 1975). It has also been claimed (Robinson and Short, 1977) that breast sensitivity, as judged by two-point discrimination, shows peaks at ovulation and around the beginning of menstruation. Skin pain threshold for the breast did not show any relationship to the menstrual cycle.

Changes with a less direct relationship to the premenstrual syndrome are also often reported. Alveolar carbon dioxide tension has been measured throughout the cycle and found to fall after ovulation until the time of menstruation (Goodland and Pommerenke, 1952). Later workers also reported that carbon dioxide tension was lowest premenstrually and speculated that this might account for some premenstrual complaints. They suggested that as they found that minimal hyperventilation at this time could cause symptoms such as headache, dizziness and restlessness by reducing carbon dioxide to unacceptably low levels, this could be part of the mechanism of some premenstrual symptoms (Damas-Mora et al., 1980).

Belmaker et al. (1974) reported changes in platelet monoamine oxidase activity.

A peak at ovulation, followed by a low 5–11 days later, was found. No significant relationship between platelet monoamine oxidase activity and a global scale of menstrual mood variation in their subjects was shown. A problem here is that platelets have an estimated life of 10 days or so and therefore any hormonal effects on the parent megakaryocytes would have taken place some days earlier. Cerebral monoamine oxidase is thought to play a part in mood, and indeed monoamine oxidase inhibiting drugs are widely used to treat pathological depression.

Many other cyclic changes have been reported, for example in eosinophil count and bile lipids. They probably have no relationship to the premenstrual syndrome.

Behavioural and psychological correlates of the menstrual cycle

Many changes have been reported and they are not confined to those women who actually complain of premenstrual tension. Dalton has been an indefatigable investigator in this field. She has claimed increases in aggressive behaviour as well as a decline in performance in women in the paramenstrual period (Dalton, 1964).

There have been cases brought to court where women charged with violent crime have made pleas of mitigating circumstances or diminished responsibility due to premenstrual syndrome. This tended to increase media coverage and public interest in premenstrual symptomatology. It has been suggested that such extensive publicity, together with the lack of agreed diagnostic criteria, has led to an extremely confused public attitude towards premenstrual complaints and may well cause women to attribute any negative affect, incautious behaviour or physical symptoms as due to the premenstrual syndrome (Rose and Abplanalp, 1983).

An editorial in the *Lancet* drew attention to the problem of attributing abnormal behaviour to the premenstrual syndrome. It suggested that, although there had been claims of increased crime, epileptic seizures and depression in the premenstrual phase, the data could as easily have been interpreted as lowered crime, fewer epileptic seizures and increased self-esteem in the mid-cycle phase (Editorial, 1981).

Aggressive behaviour in female psychotic patients has been reported as more common premenstrually (Gregory, 1957). However, in a study of 29 subnormal females over 3 months, analysis of ratings made by the nursing staff failed to show that specific mood changes, overactivity, aggression or attention-seeking behaviour were correlated with the premenstrual or menstrual phases. It was concluded that menstruation was not a significant factor causing behavioural change in mentally handicapped females (Sampson, 1980).

There have been reports of correlations between the premenstrual or menstrual phases of the cycle and commission of violent crime but, as concluded by Clare (1983), most of these have major methodological flaws. Two studies, however, have attempted to overcome the problems by not relying on data collected retrospectively or obtained by self-report.

In one study, 45 inmates of the North Carolina Correctional Center for Women were studied. Their menstrual activity and details of physical or verbal attacks on staff or other inmates were recorded by staff. The results showed that the greatest number of aggressive outbursts occurred during the premenstrual and early menstrual phases. The women who reported feeling more irritable during these phases were found to be no more likely to be aggressive than women who did not report these symptoms (Ellis and Austin, 1971). The other study followed 50 females remanded to prison for offences of violence against persons or property. Information was obtained about their menstrual cycles and the day of the offence was estimated as a particular day of an ideal 28-day cycle. Days 25–28 were regarded as premenstrual and days 1–4 as menstrual. Both together were regarded as paramenstrual. They found that an excessive but not statistically significant number of offences had been committed in the premenstruum. The excess committed in the menstrual phase was statistically significant. There was also a statistically significant lack of offences committed in the ovulatory and post-ovulatory phase. Complaints of premenstrual tension were not correlated with the offence taking place premenstrually. The authors point out that these findings, if reliable, do not mean that all women are more likely to be violent paramenstrually. It may merely mean that women with a propensity for violence find it more difficult to control themselves in the paramenstruum (d'Orban and Dalton, 1980).

A behaviour extensively studied in relation to the menstrual cycle has been attempted suicide. A significant excess of suicide attempts has been reported in the premenstrual week (Tonks, Rack and Rose, 1968). Wetzel and McClure (1972) reviewed the literature and, although they found the results confusing, concluded that there was an excess of attempted suicide in the premenstrual and menstrual phases. Since then two studies of women attempting suicide failed to find a statistically significant excess during menstruation or the premenstrual phase (Holding and Minkoff, 1973; Birtchnell and Floyd, 1974). It is difficult to explain these discrepant findings and the question of some relationship remains open.

There have also been reports of less dramatic behavioural changes being associated with the paramenstruum. For example, 45% of women factory workers reporting sick were found to be between 1 and 3 days premenstrual or were menstruating (Dalton, 1964). She also stated that half of the acute female admissions to hospital were in this phase as were approximately half the acute female admissions to psychiatric beds.

It has been found that women in the paramenstrual phase were more likely to bring their children to a paediatric clinic than they were at other times. The paediatrician (blind to the mothers' menstrual phase) rated the children of mothers in the paramenstrual phase as less sick than the children of mothers in other phases (Tuch, 1975). Like so many other studies, this shows some methodological weakness in coping with cycles of varying length.

There have also been claims that both physical performance and cognitive performance (as in examinations) might vary throughout the cycle. The evidence for changes in physical performance is virtually non-existent and much doubt has been cast upon any evidence for cognitive changes. In a study where psychological tests were given through the cycle, no change was demonstrated in cognitive performance (Sommer, 1972). A review of the literature also reached an essentially negative conclusion (Sommer, 1973).

Clare (1983) has also found little evidence to support the idea that women are more accident-prone premenstrually. He suggests that, even if it can be shown that women have more road accidents around menstruation, the rate of accidents is still less than that for men and that the accidents in which women are involved are generally less serious.

The disparate findings reviewed here lend support to Parlee (1973) in her swingeing attack on most of the work reporting correlations between cycle phase and behaviour. She found most such work to be methodologically unsound and of doubtful reliability. Sommer (1973) also reached a similar negative conclusion after reviewing the literature. She wrote: 'Behaviours related to the female menstrual cycle have been the stuff of mythology, a basis of vocational and social discrimination and an apparently inexhaustible source of speculation and observation.'

Attempts have been made to demonstrate mood changes during the cycle in women who do not necessarily complain of premenstrual symptoms. Some of this work has been mentioned earlier, in the section looking at definitions of the syndrome. Some studies using daily records did demonstrate higher scores for psychiatric and somatic complaints premenstrually and menstrually (Beumont, Richards and Gelder, 1975; Beumont et al., 1978, Taylor, 1979b).

Not all studies agree however. Friedman and Meares (1978) failed to find correlations between cycle phase and scores of negative mood. In a study when many variables were measured during the menstrual cycle, it was found that there was more day-to-day variability in scores in the premenstrual and menstrual phases (Moos et al., 1969). This would suggest that lability and unpredictability characterized these phases.

Much of the work attempting to correlate behavioural change and the menstrual cycle is contradictory. One is forced to conclude that such correlations are probable rather than certain. The methodological problems produced by the variability of cycle length have not been solved. Bias also stems from subjects knowing the purpose of the study and yet knowing when the next bleed is likely to occur.

Aetiology of the premenstrual syndrome

There have been many speculations as to the cause or causes of premenstrual tension. Extensive review of the subject has shown that there is little evidence to support any of them (Tonks, 1975). Some of the main theories are listed and discussed below; readers will note that there are overlaps.

1. Abnormalities of sex hormones:
   (a) high blood levels of oestrogen;
   (b) high ratio of oestrogen to progesterone in blood;
   (c) allergic sensitivity to endogenous oestrogen;
   (d) direct pharmacological effect of progesterone;
   (e) allergic sensitivity to endogenous progesterone;
   (f) increased secretion of prolactin.
2. Water and sodium retention due to the following:
   (a) salt-retaining effects of sex hormones;
   (b) increased production of antidiuretic hormone;
   (c) increased aldosterone production;
   (d) some hypothalamic malfunction;
   (e) increased capillary permeability to protein.
3. Miscellaneous physical theories:
   (a) a specific menotoxin produced in the endometrium;
   (b) changes in monoamine oxidase activity;
   (c) lowered alveolar carbon dioxide tension;
   (d) oestrogen increasing serotonin-receptor sensitivity;
   (e) endogenous opioid peptides;
   (f) prostaglandin-induced symptoms.

4. Psychological theories:
   (a) it is a 'neurotic' disorder;
   (b) it stems from early experience about menstruation.

Abnormalities of sex hormones

The theories implicating female sex hormones have been extensively studied. The most popular has been the suggestion that there might be a premenstrual deficiency in progesterone leading to a high ratio of oestrogen to progesterone premenstrually. Some oestrogen would thus not be 'antagonized' by progesterone and cause symptoms (Israel, 1938). Recent work on this possibility has been conflicting.

Plasma levels of progesterone and oestradiol were measured by radioimmunoassay in 20 women with premenstrual complaints and compared with the results in blood from 10 normal volunteers. It was found that the pooled progesterone values from patients were significantly lower than control values from the 9th to the 5th days premenstrually. Oestradiol levels were higher in subjects than controls over the last 4 days of the cycle (Munday, Brush and Taylor, 1981). In another study, plasma oestrogen and progesterone levels in the 6 days preceding menstruation were measured in 12 women with premenstrual syndrome and 8 controls. Plasma oestrogen levels were higher for subjects than for controls from the 5th to the 2nd premenstrual days. Plasma progesterone levels were lower in subjects than in controls from the 6th to the 4th day premenstrually. The oestrogen/progesterone ratio was higher for subjects than controls from the 6th to the 3rd premenstrual days (Bäckström and Cartensen, 1974). Shader and Harmatz (1982) studied 18 women with either 'minimal' or 'maximal' premenstrual symptoms. It was found that the women with the more severe symptoms had lower urinary pregnanediol levels and higher urinary oestrogens in the early luteal phase.

The results of these studies tend to support the theory, except that the time relationship to blood flow differs from that reported for symptoms, and the criteria for the diagnosis of premenstrual syndrome were not clearly stated.

Most other studies fail to support the idea. Kerr (1977) found that 65 out of 70 patients with premenstrual complaint had no abnormality of progesterone. Andersch et al. (1978) studied 19 patients and 20 controls and found no differences in the blood levels of oestradiol-17β or progesterone premenstrually. O'Brien et al. (1979) and O'Brien, Selby and Symonds (1980) studied 18 women with premenstrual syndrome and 10 symptomless controls. They reported that mean serum progesterone levels in the post-ovulatory phase were actually higher for subjects than for controls. However, rather idiosyncratic criteria were used to define the presence of premenstrual symptoms in their work. No difference in plasma progesterone or oestradiol-17β was found by Taylor (1979a) when studying volunteers which he divided into high and low premenstrual complaint groups. Clare (1983) found no difference in serum progesterone or prolactin among 42 women with and without premenstrual complaints. The use of oral contraceptives did not appear to alter the frequency of premenstrual symptoms in this study.

On balance, it seems unlikely that abnormalities of progesterone or oestrogen levels can be implicated for most women with premenstrual symptoms. The idea of high levels of oestrogen unopposed by progesterone being causative is inherently unlikely when one considers normal hormonal variations through the cycle. There is a high pre-ovulatory peak of oestrogen and its precursors in the presence of low values of progesterone. Oestrogenic activity rapidly falls and then, after ovulation, there is a slow rise both in oestrogen and progesterone. There is a sharp fall in both just before blood flow. By far the highest level of unopposed oestrogenic activity occurs around ovulation (Short, 1972). If also the recent findings suggesting that symptoms are paramenstrual rather than premenstrual are correct, it would be difficult to invoke this theory.

Recently, it has been suggested that sex hormone binding globulin (SHBG) might be implicated in premenstrual complaints. When SHBG binding capacity was measured in 50 women with 'severe' premenstrual syndrome and 50 age-matched controls, it was found to be significantly lower in the subjects (Dalton, 1981). The selection criteria used for inclusion in this study were, however, unusual as they were defined by psychiatric hospital admission, suicidal attempts, criminal offences, violence, epilepsy, alcoholism or asthma premenstrually, with at least 7 clear days post-menstrually. The author suggests that the SHBG binding capacity may be useful in the diagnosis of premenstrual syndrome and also postulates that lowered capacity may lead to an increase in free oestradiol at tissue level which she relates to the aetiology of the syndrome. In another study, however, when women were defined as suffering from premenstrual syndrome by the use of anxiety rating scales, the 15 subjects were found to have significantly higher plasma SHBG than the 15 controls (Bäckström and Aakvaag, 1981).

The possible role of prolactin has attracted some attention in recent years. Halbreich et al. (1976) studied 28 women with premenstrual syndrome and 21 controls. Serum prolactin levels were estimated in the 2nd, 3rd and 4th week of a menstrual cycle. They reported that the mean serum prolactin levels for women with the syndrome was higher than for controls throughout the cycle. It is difficult to equate this with the phasic nature of the condition. However, Jeske et al. (1980) found that when they measured serum prolactin in 21 women with premenstrual syndrome and 12 controls, subjects had slightly higher levels of prolactin throughout the cycle, but significant differences were only noted in the premenstrual week. This study also reported that the stimulation of prolactin with metoclopramide was much greater in subjects than controls.

Other studies have failed to find differences in serum prolactin between sufferers and controls in the luteal phase of the cycle (Andersch, Andersson and Isaksson, 1978), or throughout the course of the cycle (O'Brien and Symonds, 1982).

The literature on prolactin studies in premenstrual tension appears conflicting, and some workers have concluded that abnormal prolactin levels could not be implicated. Horrobin (1983), however, has suggested that the finding that most women with premenstrual symptoms have normal prolactin levels could be explained by women with the syndrome being abnormally sensitive to normal levels of prolactin. He claims that there is evidence that in the absence of prostaglandin E_1, prolactin has exaggerated effects and he therefore postulates a deficiency of prostaglandin E_1 as the cause of premenstrual symptoms. What this fails to explain, however, is that symptoms of hyperprolactinaemia are not at all like those of the premenstrual syndrome. Even those studies reporting high levels of prolactin agree that the high levels might be a concomitant of the syndrome rather than a cause, since stress itself is known to raise prolactin levels (Franz, Kleinberger and Noel, 1972).

The other listed sex hormone abnormalities such as allergic sensitivity or a direct pharmacological action of progesterone are now of historical interest only (Tonks, 1975).

Water and sodium retention

Salt and water retention premenstrually still remains a popular belief despite much evidence against it. The origin is presumably that many women complain of swelling of the ankles, fingers, breasts and abdomen premenstrually.

Water retention should show itself by weight gain, and careful weighing each morning after voiding urine has been a favourite method of investigation. In a small group of subjects, there was found to be an average weight gain of 1.25 lb (0.56 kg) 5 days premenstrually. This gain did not, however, correlate with the presence or absence of premenstrual symptoms (Reeves, Garvin and McElin, 1971). Nassar and Smith (1975) failed to find evidence of luteal phase weight gain in 13 women and also showed that breast volume increases premenstrually were not accompanied by measurable changes in body weight. Statistical differences in follicular and luteal weights were not shown by Elsner *et al.* (1980) in 24 women who complained of long-standing symptoms of bloating, swelling and premenstrual weight gain.

Body weight and total body water using tritiated water was measured in 39 patients with cyclical pronounced mastalgia and 17 controls by Preece *et al.* (1975). Measurements were taken on the 5th and 25th days of the cycle. No significant difference in the ratio of total body water/total body weight between the two measurement days or between the two groups was demonstrated. A similar lack of increase in total body water or body weight between the follicular and luteal phase of women with premenstrual syndrome or control subjects has also been reported by Andersch, Andersson and Isaksson (1978). In a very careful study of psychiatric patients with and without premenstrual exacerbations of symptoms, Bruce and Russell (1962) could not demonstrate premenstrual weight gain. Also, in careful metabolic balance studies they could not demonstrate premenstrual water and sodium retention. Indeed, the tendency was for water retention to take place preferentially at ovulation when oestrogen, a weak salt-retaining hormone, was at its highest level. Reflecting on this research and other evidence, Russell (1972) was led to state: 'the retention of salt and water in the body before the onset of menstrual flow . . . [is] . . . one of the medical myths which seem to have captivated the minds of examination candidates and authors of standard textbooks of psychiatry. . . . It still holds the field in popular mythology.'

Such studies do not really rule out shifts of water between intracellular and extracellular spaces, as have been postulated in affective disorders. Nor do they rule out localized water retention in breasts or fingers. Indeed, as Nassar and Smith (1975) reported, premenstrual breast volume increases were not accompanied by detectable increases in body weight. The work of Parboosingh, Doig and Michie (1973) reporting nocturnal sodium loss and diurnal retention, mentioned earlier, should make us look again at the subject with a critical eye. The question remains unsettled, but as Russell (1972) points out, water retention around ovulation does not provoke symptoms similar to those found in the premenstrual syndrome. The possibility therefore that it is a major causative factor is remote.

If good evidence for salt and water retention is lacking, looking for the causes of that retention is unlikely to be fruitful. However, there are cyclic physiological changes during the menstrual cycle, in addition to the changes in sex hormones. Some of these could be associated with water retention. Aldosterone levels have been shown to increase significantly in the premenstrual phase, but the rise was unrelated to the presence or severity of premenstrual symptoms (O'Brien *et al.*,

1979). Failure to find significant differences in aldosterone levels in women with or without premenstrual complaints has been reported by Munday, Brush and Taylor (1981). There is a report of increased capillary permeability to protein premenstrually, but again it was unrelated to the presence of symptoms, even those of swelling and bloating (Jones et al., 1966).

Miscellaneous physical theories

We can now move on to the miscellaneous physical causes which have been raised. One of the most enduring was the idea of a specific menotoxin elaborated in the aging endometrium. This menotoxin could be absorbed into the general circulation and cause symptoms. The shedding of the endometrium with menstruation would cause relief of the symptoms. The literature was replete with the dire consequences of injecting menstrual blood into experimental animals. The idea lost favour following reports that the dire consequences to experimental animals failed to materialize if good asepsis was practised (Tonks, 1975).

Monoamine oxidase activity has long been thought to play a role in the control of mood. Belmaker et al. (1974) reported cyclic variations in platelet monoamine oxidase activity without being able to demonstrate any relationship between those levels and mood.

A recent speculation was based on reports of lowered levels of carbon dioxide in expired air premenstrually and menstrually. In parallel with this, the time taken to provoke delta activity on an EEG by hyperventilation was found to be minimal in these phases. The hyperventilation produced symptoms of dizziness, restlessness, headache and so on. It was suggested that this increased sensitivity to hyperventilation might be part of the cause of premenstrual symptoms (Damas-Mora et al., 1980). Clearly, these findings need corroboration and further investigation.

Other theories have involved central mechanisms. Fluctuations of serotonin, gamma-aminobutyric acid (GABA) and interrelated neuroendocrine processes have been postulated. Evidence for this was claimed from the effectiveness of Danazol, an anti-oestrogen drug, in reducing premenstrual symptoms in a small uncontrolled trial (Labrum, 1983). He suggested that oestrogen might increase serotonin receptors in the brain and that serotonin stimulates the secretion of prolactin. He, therefore, suggests that breast symptoms would be expected in women with relatively high oestrogen and that this would decrease before menstruation.

Another proposal is that premenstrual symptoms are a result of cyclic gonadal-steroid induced change in opioid peptide activity. Studies on the use of naloxone have indirectly suggested that oestrogen and progesterone acting alone or in combination could increase central opioid peptide activity. It has been suggested that all the symptoms of the premenstrual syndrome may be a result of either excess opioid activity in the luteal phase or be caused by opioid withdrawal following the onset of menstruation (Reid and Yen, 1983; Reid 1983).

Other theories have suggested that premenstrual symptoms may be caused by metabolic products of prostaglandins (Wood and Jakubowicz, 1980), by excess prostaglandins themselves (Budoff, 1983) or by a deficiency of prostaglandin E_1 (Horrobin, 1983). The evidence for these theories has mainly come from the alleged efficacy of antiprostaglandin drugs or precursors of prostaglandin E_1 in combating premenstrual symptoms.

Psychological theories

Psychological theories of aetiology have also been advanced. Many studies have shown a correlation between the presence of premenstrual complaints and measures of 'neuroticism'. Frequently, women with premenstrual complaints are reported as having an increased incidence of similar complaints in other phases of the cycle (Moos et al., 1969; Tonks, 1975). Sampson and Jenner (1977), reporting on 19 volunteer student health visitors, failed to find any significant relationship between the neuroticism score on the Eysenck Personality Inventory and the presence of premenstrual complaints. One must remember that the group was small. Clare (1977) reported that a high score on the General Health Questionnaire (designed to screen psychiatric disorder) was a good predictor of the presence of premenstrual complaints, but that the presence of premenstrual complaint did not predict a high score on the questionnaire. A later study, however, showed that a high score on this questionnaire was predictive only of complaints of premenstrual psychological or behavioural symptoms and had no relationship to physical complaints (Clare, 1983).

Taylor (1979c) reported a significant positive correlation between neuroticism scores on the Eysenck Personality Inventory and high scores on the affect subscale of his measure of premenstrual distress. He found no correlation between 'neuroticism' and the presence of physical symptoms premenstrually.

In general, it seems that 'neuroticism', which is often regarded as a tendency to complain, does correlate with the presence of premenstrual symptoms. It is clear, however, that this correlation is unlikely to be the whole explanation of the syndrome.

Many more specific 'psychogenic' theories have been propounded but have not been extensively researched. It had been reported that women with premenstrual tension often said that they had been informed about menstruation during childhood in a very disparaging manner (Fortin, Wittkower and Kalz, 1958). A recent study of 179 women which examined the relationship between the memory of their menarche, adult attitudes toward menstruation and current experiences of paramenstrual symptoms failed to support this assertion. It was found that negative recollections of the first menstrual bleed had little affect on current menstrual attitudes and that, indeed, positive recollections of the menarche were more associated with current paramenstrual negative effect and impaired performance. Current menstrual symptoms were more strongly associated with current menstrual attitudes that any other factor (Woods, Dery and Most, 1982). Friedman et al. (1982), in a study of 28 psychiatric patients with what they described as 'premenstrual affective syndrome', reported that 16 (57%) of the patients had abnormal sexual histories compared with only 1 in 17 patients who had no premenstrual affective changes. The authors suggest that 'premenstrual affective syndrome may signify unresolved sexual conflicts in subgroups of psychiatric inpatients'. However, the patients included in this study suffered from a wide range of severe psychiatric disorders and this, together with the retrospective nature of the study, must shed some doubt on their claims.

One must conclude that the aetiology of the premenstrual syndrome is still obscure and, indeed, that many widely held beliefs are untrue.

Treatment of the premenstrual syndrome

Many different forms of treatment have been advocated over the years. The proponents of the approach usually base it on one or more of the aetiological ideas which have been discussed. Unfortunately, evaluation of the results of treatment by trials of sound methodology have been sparse. Many of the approaches have been reviewed in detail (Tonks, 1975; Clare, 1979). Here, only some of the more popular treatments will be discussed.

Early workers, brave or foolhardy according to taste, suggested radium therapy to the ovaries (Frank, 1931) or low dosage radiation to the pituitary (Israel, 1938), to lower the amount of circulating oestrogen. Rather less drastic treatments are now in vogue.

Hormone treatments

The hypothesis that a relative deficiency of progesterone premenstrually causes the syndrome has led to treatment with progesterone or synthetic progestogens. Dalton (1977) has been, over many years, the leading proponent for the efficacy of progesterone given in the premenstrual phase. It has been suggested that oral progesterone is ineffective, although this has been questioned by Whitehead et al. (1980), so treatment has meant daily injections of 50 mg or 100 mg of progesterone or the use of suppositories or pessaries in doses of 200–400 mg twice daily for the 14 days prior to the onset of menstruation. This is often not really acceptable to patients. Sampson (1979) reported a methodologically sound double-blind controlled trial of progesterone given by suppository or pessary against a placebo for the 12 premenstrual days; she failed to find any significant difference between placebo or progesterone 200 mg twice daily or progesterone 400 mg twice daily. As is so frequently reported in this disorder, the placebo response rate was high. At the present time, proof of the efficacy of progesterone is lacking.

Synthetic progestogens such as are used in oral contraceptive preparations have also had their advocates. A double-blind controlled trial of norethisterone 7.5 mg daily from the 16th to the 25th day of the cycle against diuretic and placebo showed norethisterone to be significantly better at relieving complaints of swelling and bloating, but unhelpful at relieving psychological symptoms (Coppen et al., 1969). There have been reports that women on oral contraceptives had significantly less premenstrual depression and irritability than women using other forms of contraception, but that complaints about swelling did not differ between the groups (Herzberg and Coppen, 1970). These two reports are at variance. Another placebo-controlled double-blind study measured the effects of norethisterone against bromocriptine in 36 women and found that norethisterone alleviated breast tenderness whereas bromocriptine decreased the total score of both physical and psychological premenstrual symptoms (Ylöstalo et al., 1982). There have also been reports of the beneficial effect of oral contraceptives in all premenstrual symptoms (Andersch and Hahn, 1981). On reviewing the literature, Clare (1979) found the evidence for the efficacy of the 'pill' to be conflicting. In his study he found no significant increase or decrease in the frequency of premenstrual symptoms in pill users (Clare, 1983).

When the effects of different oral contraceptives on premenstrual complaints were examined in 191 women, it was found that premenstrual depression and bloating were more commonly found in women taking preparations containing lynoestrol, which has only a weak progesterone effect, as opposed to those taking preparations containing the stronger progestogen, norgestrol (Andersch, 1982).

A new progestogen, dydrogesterone, has been marketed as a treatment for premenstrual syndrome. Taylor (1977) reported an open trial of this drug, given in a dosage of 10 mg twice daily from the 12th to the 26th day of the cycle. He reported that 32% of the patients were cured and 40% improved. The best results were with complaints of swelling and bloating. In a condition with a high placebo response rate, this evidence is far from compelling. Another placebo-controlled, although not double-blind, trial on this drug reported a 43% placebo response and 72% improvement with dydrogesterone compared with the pretreatment measures. Breast symptoms were reported not to respond well to the treatment. Although 67 patients completed the trial, 36 patients dropped out at an early stage (Kerr *et al.*, 1980).

The supposed role of raised prolactin levels in causing the syndrome has led to the use of bromocriptine which lowers serum prolactin levels. The results have been variable. Harrison and Letchworth (1976) in a double-blind controlled trial against placebo failed to demonstrate significant differences. In a multicentre double-blind study on 24 women described as having moderate to severe premenstrual symptoms, bromocriptine resulted in statistically signficant improvement in daily ratings of breast tenderness, bloating and depression (Elsner *et al.*, 1980). When bromocriptine 2.5 mg twice daily during the luteal phase of the cycle was assessed against placebo by Andersen *et al.* (1977), only complaints of breast pain were significantly more relieved by bromocriptine. In an open trial of bromocriptine in 16 women with severe premenstrual mastalgia, 13 women responded to a dose of 2.5 mg of bromocriptine per day (Palmer and Monteiro, 1977). Blichert-Toft *et al.* (1979) reported a double-blind, cross-over trial of bromocriptine vs. placebo in 10 patients with severe mastalgia and fibrocystic disease of the breasts. Dosage used was 2.5 mg bromocriptine daily for the first week of the cycle and 2.5 mg twice daily for the rest of the cycle. Pain was significantly more relieved by bromocriptine. Given the pathology of the subjects, it is difficult to evaluate the relevance of this report. In a double-blind trial of bromocriptine 1.25 mg daily from the 19th day of the cycle onwards, against 1 mg daily of the diuretic bumetanide, bromocriptine was significantly better at relieving psychiatric symptoms, whereas the diuretic was better at relieving complaints of swelling (Andersch *et al.*, 1978). This finding conflicts with that of Andersen *et al.* (1977) discussed previously. On balance it would seem that bromocriptine is of minimal benefit. It might be worth trying if breast pain is a major symptom.

Robinson, Huntington and Wallace (1977) treated 32 patients with Bellergal (which contained belladonna alkaloids, ergotamine tartate and phenobarbitone). Ergotamine is said to depress serum prolactin levels (Andersen and Larsen, 1979). They used one tablet of bellergal three times daily for the last 10 days of the cycle. Bellergal was found to be significantly better than placebo both for psychiatric symptoms and breast tenderness. This is an isolated report and the statistical treatment accorded to scores from visual analogue scales was suspect.

Treatment with diuretics

Failure to demonstrate premenstrual water retention has not prevented the use of a wide variety of diuretic drugs in treatment.

Conflicting reports can be found both in open trials and in the few double-blind controlled trials reported (Tonks, 1975). Further publications have done little to clarify the matter. Mattsson and Schoultz (1974) compared chlorthalidone with lithium carbonate and placebo. The dose of chlorthalidone used was 25 mg daily from the 14th to the 21st day and then 25 mg twice daily from the 21st to the 28th day. They found placebo to be superior to chlorthalidone or lithium. Metolazone has been compared with a placebo in a dose of 1 mg or 2.5 mg daily for the 7 premenstrual days and throughout menstruation by Werch and Kane (1976). They reported that metolazone was significantly better than placebo for both psychiatric symptoms and complaints of swelling. It is interesting that they only included women who were at least 3 lb (1.36 kg) heavier premenstrually than they were 6 days postmenstrually.

Andersch et al. (1978) compared bromocriptine with bumetanide 1 mg daily given from the 19th day onwards. A placebo was not used in the trial but both drugs gave lower scores for complaints than were seen in untreated cycles. Bumetanide was found superior to bromocriptine in relieving swelling. Carstairs and Talbot (1981) reported on women who were entered into a cross-over study with a commercial combination of bendrofluazide 3 mg and meprobamate 200 mg (Tenavoid) and either placebo, bendrofluazide 2.5 mg or meprobamate 200 mg, all given 3 times daily. Relief of symptoms was reported in 66% of patients receiving the combination drug, 48% on placebo, 42% on meprobamate and 36% on bendrofluazide. In a double-blind trial of spironolactone 25 mg 4 times daily from the 18th to the 26th day of the cycle, against placebo, spironolactone significantly reduced the premenstrual symptoms (O'Brien et al., 1979). The measure of symptoms used in this trial, however, is not known to be a reliable or valid measure. Interestingly, spironolactone owes its diuretic properties to its aldosterone antagonism and, as we have seen, increased aldosterone production has been suggested as a cause of the premenstrual syndrome.

On reviewing the literature on the use of diuretics, we must still conclude that their efficacy is open to question.

Other treatments

On the basis that the major symptoms of the premenstrual syndrome are 'affective', the use of lithium has been advocated. In one double-blind trial it was found to be ineffective, even when serum lithium levels were kept within the therapeutic range (Singer, Cheng and Schou, 1974). Another study, using 24 mmol of lithium carbonate daily for the 14 premenstrual days, found it less effective than placebo (Mattsson and Schoultz, 1974). However, in view of the dangers of lithium, its use seems scarcely justifiable.

Reports that the depression encountered with oral contraceptive use was sometimes responsive to pyridoxine have led to trials assessing its use in the premenstrual syndrome. In an open trial, doses of 40–100 mg were used from 3 days before symptoms were expected until the beginning of bleeding. Improvement was reported in between 50% and 60% of patients (Kerr, 1977). This would not be much in excess of placebo response in this condition. Abraham and Hargrove (1980) reported a double-blind cross-over study performed over 3 cycles on 25 women using pyridoxine 50 mg or placebo. Pyridoxine was found to have beneficial effects in measures of anxiety, irritability and tension in both follicular and luteal phases.

Minor tranquillizers have also been used to combat the psychiatric symptoms encountered. A study of 13 women reported that diazepam was superior to placebo in reducing premenstrual high anxiety levels (Shader and Harmatz, 1982). This finding does not seem surprising in view of the pharmacological effects of diazepam. Minor tranquillizers probably do have immediately beneficial effect with some patients but, as the condition is a very chronic one, the physician should carefully weigh any immediate advantage against the ever present risk of addiction and misuse.

Recently, the use of oil of evening primrose has been heralded as a cure for premenstrual tension. Its advocates suggest that premenstrual symptoms may be cause by prolactin having exaggerated effects in the absence of prostaglandin E_1. Oil of evening primrose contains gamma-linolenic acid which is the essential fatty acid precursor of prostaglandin E_1. Horrobin (1983) reported 3 double-blind placebo-controlled studies, one large open study on women who had failed to improve on other kinds of therapy and one open study on new patients. He claimed that, in all these studies, oil of evening primrose was shown to be a highly effective treatment for premenstrual depression, irritability, breast pain and tenderness and fluid retention. However, the paper gives few details on the methods used in these studies to obtain subjects or to assess outcome.

Other workers who believe that premenstrual symptoms are caused by excess prostaglandins have suggested measures to reduce these levels, including the use of prostaglandin inhibitors (Budoff, 1983). Wood and Jakubowicz (1980), in a double-blind cross-over study of 37 patients, assessed mefenamic acid, a prostaglandin inhibitor, against placebo. Mefenamic acid was given in a dose of 500 mg 3 times daily during the luteal phase of the cycle. Medication was found to improve significantly premenstrual symptoms of tension, irritability, depression, pain and headache, but to be ineffective for breast symptoms.

Thiomucase-H, a mucopolysaccharide, has been claimed to be effective in several exclusively French studies for premenstrual symptoms which were deemed secondary to water retention (Hauser, 1983). The anti-oestrogen drug danazol has also been claimed to be effective in a small uncontrolled trial by Labrum (1983). Atton-Chamla et al. (1980) examined the relationship between atopy and premenstrual symptoms in 138 women. It was reported that there was a high incidence of personal or family history of allergy in these patients compared with normal controls. A double-blind trial using a course of gammaglobulin-histamine complex injected subcutaneously vs. placebo injections was performed on 86 women. A significantly higher proportion of subjects on active treatment reported symptomatic relief.

A whole panoply of other drugs have been used, ranging from testosterone to vitamin A and epsilonaminocaproic acid. None of them has stood the test of time and they have, for one reason or another, fallen into disfavour.

There have been claims that psychotherapy might be of value. This is even more contentious a subject than the efficacy of drugs. The assessment of the value of psychotherapy in any condition has proved very difficult and we do not know its value in the premenstrual syndrome. There would seem, however, to be a prima facie case for thinking that many sufferers are helped by being able to discuss their problems and symptoms openly with their doctor, i.e. psychotherapy in its broadest sense.

One must agree with the Editorial (1979) in the British Medical Journal which stated: 'What we need is a more precise definition of the syndrome with well-planned, carefully controlled trials of various treatments – including simple reassurance, mild sedation or tranquillizers.'

One should not let this essentially negative review of available treatments force one to take a nihilistic view of the possibilities. Very many trials have shown a high placebo response rate (Clare, 1979) and any attempts at treatment are likely to be of help to a number of sufferers. Probably the act of taking a history and showing understanding of the problem is in itself therapeutic. The prescription of some harmless medicament such as pyridoxine may also be of great benefit. Should this approach prove unrewarding, one finds that a number of patients need contraceptive advice and the provision of one or other oral contraceptive may help both problems. For patients who are convinced they retain fluid, then small quantities of a safe diuretic in the premenstrual phase may be crowned with success. One should not cavil at such an essentially pragmatic approach. Much of medicine is still a practical art rather than a hard science.

Conclusions

In February 1980, and again in November 1982, premenstrual syndrome was accepted, in the USA, as being a 'disease of the mind' within the meaning of section 2 of the Homicide Act 1957 and had the result that charges of murder against two women were commuted to manslaughter by reason of diminished responsibility (Brahams, 1983). In the UK there have also been cases in the Courts where women have successfully pleaded diminished responsibility or mitigation due to premenstrual syndrome in crimes of arson and assault (Dalton, 1980). In France, premenstrual syndrome has long been recognized as a cause of temporary insanity (Oleck, 1953). Whether it can be considered justifiable to accept a plea of diminished responsibility on the grounds of a condition which, as we have seen, is a subject of wide controversy, must remain an open question.

Parlee (1973) published a very critical review of previous work on behavioural changes correlated with the menstrual cycle and on premenstrual tension. She concluded that 'as a scientific hypothesis, the existence of the premenstrual syndrome has little other than face validity'. This would seem to be an extreme view.

On balance, there seems to be evidence for minor psychological and physiological changes to be connected with the menstrual cycle. These changes, particularly the psychological ones, are probably easily swamped by variations stemming from random environmental events. Some women, especially those with high levels of 'neuroticism' or 'complainingness', recognize the underlying rhythmicity, note the changes and complain of them, despite the huge variations in severity between cycles. Once the underlying rhythmicity is perceived, if a woman is premenstrual when she feels depressed or tense, the expectation that it is only premenstrual tension may be actually helpful because it carries the hope of relief when menstruation is established. To paraphrase Voltaire, 'if the premenstrual syndrome did not exist, it would be necessary to invent it'.

As clinicians, we share the view of many of our colleagues that there are a small number of women only, perhaps the tail end of a distribution curve, who do have regularly recurring distressing and severe premenstrual symptoms. It is a task for the future to distinguish these from the generality of women who think they have premenstrual complaints and concentrate our research on them.

References

ABRAHAM, G. E. (1980) Premenstrual tension. In *Current Problems in Obstetrics and Gynecology*, pp. 1–48 (Leventhal, M., Ed.). Chicago; Year Book Medical Publishers

ABRAHAM, G. E. (1983) Nutritional factors in the etiology of the premenstrual tension syndromes. *Journal of Reproductive Medicine*, **28**, 446–464

ABRAHAM, G. E. and HARGROVE, J. T. (1980) Effects of Vitamin B on premenstrual symptomatology in women with premenstrual syndrome: a double-blind crossover study. *Infertility*, **3**, 155–165

ANDERSCH, B. (1982) The effect of various oral contraceptive combinations on premenstrual symptoms. *International Journal of Gynaecology and Obstetrics*, **20**, 463–469

ANDERSCH, B., ANDERSSON, M. and ISAKSSON, B. (1978) Body water and weight in patients with premenstrual tension. *British Journal of Obstetrics and Gynaecology*, **85**, 546–550

ANDERSCH, B. and HAHN, L. (1981) Premenstrual complaints. II. Influence of oral contraceptives. *Acta Obstetricia Gynecologica Scandinavica*, **60**, 579–583

ANDERSCH, B., HAHN, L., WENDESTAM, C., OHMAN, R. and ABRAHAMSSON, L. (1978) Treatment of P.M.T. syndrome with bromocriptine. *Acta Endocrinologica* (Kopenhavn) **88**, Suppl. 216, 165–174

ANDERSEN, A. N. and LARSEN, J. F. (1979) Bromocriptine in the treatment of the premenstrual syndrome. *Drugs*, **17**, 383–388

ANDERSEN, A. N., LARSEN, J. F., STEENSTRUP, O. R., SVENDSTRUP, B. and NIELSEN, J. (1977) Effect of bromocriptine on the premenstrual syndrome. A double-blind clinical trial. *British Journal of Obstetrics and Gynaecology*, **84**, 370–374

ATTON-CHAMLA, A., FAVRE, G., GOUDARD, J.-R., MILLER, G., ROCCA SERRA, J.-P., TEITELBAUM, M., VALLETTE, C. and CHARPIN, J. (1980) Premenstrual syndrome and atopy: a double-blind clinical evaluation of treatment with a gamma-globulin/histamine complex. *Pharmatherapeutica*, **2**, 481–486

BÄCKSTRÖM, T. and AAKVAAG, A. (1981) Plasma prolactin and testosterone during the luteal phase in women with premenstrual tension syndrome. *Psychoneuroendocrinology*, **6**, 245–251

BÄCKSTRÖM, C. T., BOYLE, H. and BAIRD, D. T. (1981) Persistence of symptoms of premenstrual tension in hysterectomized women. *British Journal of Obstetrics and Gynaecology*, **88**, 530–536

BÄCKSTRÖM, T. and CARTENSEN, H. (1974) Estrogen and progesterone in plasma in relation to premenstrual tension. *Journal of Steroid Biochemistry*, **5**, 257–260

BELMAKER, R. H., MURPHY, D. L., WYATT, R. J. and LORIAUX, D. L. (1974) Human platelet monoamine oxidase changes during the menstrual cycle. *Archives of General Psychiatry*, **31**, 553–556

BEUMONT, P. J. V., ABRAHAM, S. F., ARGALL, W. J. and SIMSON, K. G. (1978) A prospective study of premenstrual symptoms in healthy young Australians. *Australian and New Zealand Journal of Psychiatry*, **12**, 241–244

BEUMONT, P. J. V., RICHARDS, D. H. and GELDER, M. G. (1975) A study of minor psychiatric and physical symptoms during the menstrual cycle. *British Journal of Psychiatry*, **126**, 431–434

BIRTCHNELL, J. and FLOYD, S. (1974) Attempted suicide and the menstrual cycle – a negative conclusion. *Journal of Psychosomatic Research*, **18**, 361–369

BLICHERT–TOFT, M., ANDERSEN, A. N., HENRICKSEN, O. B. and MYGIND, T. (1979) Treatment of mastalgia with bromocriptine: a double-blind crossover study. *British Medical Journal*, **1**, 237

BLUME, E. (1983) Premenstrual syndromes, depression linked. *Journal of the American Medical Association*, **249**, 2864–2865

BRAHAMS, D. (1983) Premenstrual tension and criminal responsibility. *Practitioner*, **227**, 807–813

BRUCE, J. and RUSSELL, G. F. M. (1962) Premenstrual tension. A study of weight changes and balances of water, sodium and potassium. *Lancet*, **2**, 267–271

BUDOFF, P. W. (1983) The use of prostaglandin inhibitors for the premenstrual syndrome. *Journal of Reproductive Medicine*, **28**, 469–478

CARSTAIRS, M. W. and TALBOT, D. J. (1981) A placebo controlled trial of 'Tenavoid' in the management of the premenstrual syndrome. *British Journal of Clinical Practice*, **35**, 403–409

CLARE, A. W. (1977) Psychological profiles of women complaining of premenstrual symptoms. *Current Medical Research and Opinion*, **4**, Suppl. 4, 23–28

CLARE, A. W. (1979) The treatment of premenstrual symptoms. *British Journal of Psychiatry*, **135**, 576–579

CLARE, A. W. (1983) Psychiatric and social aspects of premenstrual complaint. *Psychological Medicine*, monograph suppl. 4, 1–58

COPPEN, A. (1965) The prevalence of menstrual disorders in psychiatric patients. *British Journal of Psychiatry*, **111**, 155–167

COPPEN, A. and KESSEL, N. (1963) Menstruation and personality. *British Journal of Psychiatry*, **109**, 711–721

COPPEN, A., MILNE, H. B., OUTRAM, D. H. and WEBER, J. C. P. (1969). Dytide, norethisterone and a placebo in the premenstrual syndrome. *Clinical Trials Journal*, **6**, 33–36

DALTON, K. (1964) *The Premenstrual Syndrome*. London; Heinemann

DALTON, K. (1977) *The Premenstrual Syndrome and Progesterone Therapy*. London: Heinemann

DALTON, K. (1980) Cyclical criminal acts in premenstrual syndrome. *Lancet*, **2**, 1070–1071

DALTON, K. (1982) What is P.M.S.? *Journal of the Royal College of General Practitioners*, **32**, 717–723

DALTON, M. E. (1981) Sex hormone-binding globulin concentrations in women with severe premenstrual syndrome. *Postgraduate Medical Journal*, **57**, 560–561

DAMAS-MORA, J., DAVIES, L., TAYLOR, W. and JENNER, F. A. (1980) Menstrual respiratory changes and symptoms. *British Journal of Psychiatry*, **136**, 492–497

d'ORBAN, P. T. and DALTON, J. (1980) Violent crime and the menstrual cycle. *Psychological Medicine*, **10**, 353–359

EDITORIAL (1979) Premenstrual tension syndrome. *British Medical Journal*, **1**, 212

EDITORIAL (1981) Premenstrual syndrome. *Lancet*, **2**, 1393–1394

ELLIS, D. P. and AUSTIN, P. (1971) Menstruation and aggressive behaviour in a correction centre for women. *Journal of Criminal Law, Criminology and Police Science*, **62**, 388–395

ELSNER, C. W., BUSTER, J. E., SCHINDLER, R. A., NESSIM, S. A. and ABRAHAM, G. E. (1980). *Obstetrics and Gynaecology*, **56**, 723–726

ENDICOTT, J. and HALBREICH, U. (1982) Retrospective report of premenstrual depressive changes: factors affecting confirmation by daily ratings. *Psychopharmacology Bulletin*, **18**, 109–112

FORTIN, J. N., WITTKOWER, E. O. and KALZ, F. (1958) A psychosomatic approach to the premenstrual tension syndrome: a preliminary report. *Canadian Medical Association Journal*, **79**, 978–981

FRANK, R. T. (1931) The hormonal causes of premenstrual tension. *Archives of Neurology and Psychiatry* (Chicago), **26**, 1053–1057

FRANZ, A. G., KLEINBERGER, D. L. and NOEL, G. L. (1972) Studies on prolactin in man. *Recent Progress in Hormone Research*, **28**, 527–573

FRIEDMAN, J. and MEARES, R. A. (1978) Comparison of spontaneous and contraceptive menstrual cycles on a visual discrimination task. *Australian and New Zealand Journal of Psychiatry*, **12**, 233–239

FRIEDMAN, R. C., HURT, S. W., CLARKIN, J., CORN, R. and ARONOFF, M. S. (1982) Sexual histories and premenstrual affective syndrome in psychiatric in-patients. *American Journal of Psychiatry*, **139**, 1484–1486

GOODLAND, R. L. and POMMERENKE, W. T. (1952) Cyclic fluctuations of alveolar carbon dioxide tension during the normal menstrual cycle. *Fertility and Sterility*, **3**, 394–401

GOODMAN, J. (1878) The cyclic theory of menstruation. *American Journal of Obstetrics and Diseases of Women and Children*, **11**, 673–694

GREGORY, B. A. J. C. (1957) The menstrual cycle and its disorders in psychiatric patients. II. Clinical studies. *Journal of Psychosomatic Research*, **2**, 199–224

HALBREICH, U., ASSAEL, M., BEN-DAVID, M. and BORNSTEIN, R. (1976) Serum prolactin in women with premenstrual syndrome. *Lancet*, **2**, 654–656

HALBREICH, U. and ENDICOTT, J. (1982) Future directions in the study of premenstrual changes. *Psychopharmacology Bulletin*, **18**, 121–123

HALBREICH, U. and KAS, D. (1977) Variations in the Taylor M.A.S. of women with premenstrual syndrome. *Journal of Psychosomatic Research*, **21**, 391–393

HARGROVE, J. T. and ABRAHAM, G. E. (1983) The incidence of premenstrual tension in a gynaecologic clinic. *Journal of Reproductive Medicine*, **27**, 721–724

HARRISON, P. and LETCHWORTH, A. T. (1976) Bromocriptine in the treatment of premenstrual tension syndrome. In *Pharmacological and Clinical Aspects of Bromocriptine (Parlodel)*, pp. 103–105 (Bayliss, R. I. S., Turner, P. and Maclay, W. P., Eds). Tunbridge Wells, UK; M.C.S. Consultants

HAUSER, G. A. (1983) Therapy of the premenstrual syndrome with thiomucase-H. *Therapeutische Umschau*, **40**, 610–614

HERZBERG, B. N. and COPPEN, A. J. (1970). Changes in psychological symptoms in women taking oral contraceptives. *British Journal of Psychiatry*, **116**, 161–164

HOLDING, T. A. and MINKOFF, K. (1973). Parasuicide and the menstrual cycle. *Journal of Psychosomatic Research*, **17**, 365–368

HORROBIN, D. F. (1983). The role of essential fatty acids and prostaglandins in the premenstrual syndrome. *Journal of Reproductive Medicine*, **28**, 465–468

ICARD, S. (1890) *La Femme Pendant la Période Menstruelle*. Paris; Alcan

ISRAEL, S. L. (1938). Premenstrual tension. *Journal of the American Medical Association*, **110**, 1721–1723

JESKE, W., KLOS, J., PERKOWICZ, J. and STOPINSKA, V. (1980). Serum prolactin in women with premenstrual syndrome. *Materia Medica Polona*, **12**, 44–46

JONES, E. M., FOX, R. H., VEROW, P. W. and ASSCHER, A. W. (1966). Variations in capillary permeability to plasma proteins during the menstrual cycle. *Journal of Obstetrics and Gynaecology of the British Commonwealth*, **73**, 666–669

KATZ, F. H. and ROMFH, P. (1972) Plasma aldosterone and renin activity during the menstrual cycle. *Clinical Endocrinology*, **34**, 819–821

KERR, G. D. (1977) The management of the premenstrual syndrome. *Current Medical Research and Opinion*, **4**, suppl. 4, 29–34

KERR, G. D., DAY, J. B., MUNDAY, M. R., BRUSH, M. G., WATSON, M. and TAYLOR, R. W. (1980) Dydrogesterone in the treatment of the premenstrual syndrome. *Practitioner*, **224**, 852–855

LABRUM, A. H. (1983) Hypothalamic, pineal and pituitary factors in the premenstrual syndrome. *Journal of Reproductive Medicine*, **28**, 438–445

MACHT, D. I. (1943) Further historical and experimental studies on menstrual toxin. *American Journal of Medical Science*, **206**, 281–305

MATTSSON, B. and SCHOULTZ, B. V. (1974) A comparison between lithium, placebo and diuretic in premenstrual tension. *Acta Psychiatrica Scandinavica*, suppl. 225, 75–84

McCANCE, R. A., LUFF, M. C. and WIDDOWSON, E. E. (1937) Physical and emotional periodicity in women. *Journal of Hygiene*, **37**, 571–611

MILLIGAN, D., DRIFE, J. O. and SHORT, R. V. (1975) Changes in breast volume during normal menstrual cycles and after oral contraceptives. *British Medical Journal*, **4**, 494–496

MOOS, R. H., KOPPELL, B. S., MELGES, F. T., YALOM, I. D., LUNDE, D. T., CLAYTON, R. B. and HAMBURG, D. A. (1969) Fluctuations in symptoms and moods during the menstrual cycle. *Journal of Psychosomatic Research*, **13**, 37–44

MOOS, R. H. and LEIDEMAN, D. B. (1978) Towards a menstrual cycle symptom typology. *Journal of Psychosomatic Research*, **22**, 31–40

MUNDAY, M. R., BRUSH, M. G. and TAYLOR, R. W. (1981) Correlations between progesterone, oestradiol and aldosterone levels in the premenstrual syndrome. *Clinical Endocrinology*, **14**, 1–9

NASSAR, A. M. and SMITH, R. E. (1975) Menstrual variations in thermal properties of the human breast. *Journal of Applied Physiology*, **39**, 806–811

O'BRIEN, P. M. S., CRAVEN, D., SELBY, C. and SYMONDS, E. M. (1979) Treatment of premenstrual syndrome by spironolactone. *British Journal of Obstetrics and Gynaecology*, **86**, 142–147

O'BRIEN, P. M. S., SELBY, C. and SYMONDS, E. M. (1980) Progesterone, fluid and electrolytes in premenstrual syndrome. *British Medical Journal*, **280**, 1161–1163

O'BRIEN, P. M. S. and SYMONDS, E. M. (1982) Prolactin levels in the premenstrual syndrome. *British Journal of Obstetrics and Gynaecology*, **89**, 306–308

OLECK, H. L. (1953) Legal aspects of premenstrual tension. *International Record of Medicine and General Practice Clinics*, **166**, 492–501

PALMER, V. B. and MONTEIRO, J. C. M. P. (1977) Bromocriptine for severe mastalgia. *British Medical Journal*, **1**, 1083

PARBOOSINGH, J., DOIG, A. and MICHIE, E. A. (1973). Renal excretion of water and solutes during the normal menstrual cycle. *Journal of Obstetrics and Gynaecology of the British Commonwealth*, **80**, 733–738

PARKER, C. R., WINKEN, C. A., RUSH, A. J., PORTER, J. C., MACDONALD, P. C. (1981) Plasma concentration of 11 deoxycorticosterone in women during the menstrual cycle. *Obstetrics and Gynaecology*, **58**, 26–30

PARLEE, M. B. (1973) The premenstrual syndrome. *Psychological Bulletin*, **80**, suppl. 6, 454–465

PREECE, P. E., HUGHES, L. E., MANSELL, R. E., BAUM, M., BOLTON, P. M. and GRAVELLE, I. H. (1976) Clinical syndromes of mastalgia. *Lancet*, **2**, 670–673

PREECE, P. E., MANSELL, R. E. and HUGHES, L. E. (1978) Mastalgia: psychoneurosis or organic disease? *British Medical Journal*, **1**, 29–30

PREECE, P. E., RICHARDS, A. R., OWEN, G. M. and HUGHES, L. E. (1975). Mastalgia and total body water. *British Medical Journal*, **4**, 498–500

REES, L. (1953). Premenstrual tension syndrome. *Journal of Mental Science*, **99**, 62–73

REEVES, B. D., GARVIN, J. E. and McELIN, T. W. (1971) Premenstrual tension: symptoms and weight changes related to potassium therapy. *American Journal of Obstetrics and Gynecology*, **109**, 1036–1041

REID, R. L. (1983) Endogenous opioid activity and the premenstrual syndrome. *Lancet*, **2**, 786

REID, R. L. and YEN, S. S. C. (1983) The premenstrual syndrome. *Clinical Obstetrics and Gynecology*, **26**, 710–718

RICCI, J. V. (1950). *The Genealogy of Gynecology*, 2nd edn. Philadelphia; Blakiston

ROBINSON, J. E. and SHORT, R. V. (1977) Changes in breast sensitivity at puberty, during the menstrual cycle and at parturition. *British Medical Journal*, **1**, 1188–1191

ROBINSON, K., HUNTINGTON, K. M. and WALLACE, M. G. (1977) Treatment of the premenstrual syndrome. *British Journal of Obstetrics and Gynaecology*, **84**, 784–788

ROSE, R. M. and ABPLANALP, J. M. (1983) The premenstrual syndrome. *Hospital Practice*, **18**, 129–141

RUSSELL, G. F. M. (1972). Premenstrual tension and 'psychogenic' amenorrhoea: psychophysical interactions. *Journal of Psychosomatic Research*, **16**, 279–287

SAMPSON, G. A. (1979) Premenstrual syndrome: a double-blind controlled trial of progesterone and placebo. *British Journal of Psychiatry*, **135**, 209–215

SAMPSON, G. A. (1980) Menstruation, mood and mental handicap. *British Journal of Psychiatry*, **136**, 410

SAMPSON, G. A. and JENNER, F. A. (1977) Studies of daily recordings from the Moos Menstrual Distress. Questionnaire. *British Journal of Psychiatry*, **130**, 265–271

SAMPSON, G. A. and PRESCOTT, P. (1981) The assessment of the symptoms of premenstrual syndrome and their response to therapy. *British Journal of Psychiatry*, **138**, 399–405

SHADER, R. I. and HARMATZ, J. S. (1982) Premenstrual tension in biochemical and psychotropic drug assessment. *Psychopharmacology Bulletin*, **18**, 113–121

SHELDRAKE, P. and CORMACK, M. (1976) Variations in menstrual cycle symptom reporting. *Journal of Psychosomatic Research*, **20**, 169–177

SHORT, R. V. (1972) The control of menstruation. *British Journal of Hospital Medicine*, **7**, 552–555

SILBERGELD, S., BRAST, N. and NOBLE, E. D. (1971) The menstrual cycle: a double-blind study of symptoms, mood and behaviour, and biochemical variables using enovid and placebo. *Psychosomatic Medicine*, **33**, 411–428

SINGER, K., CHENG, R. and SCHOU, M. (1974) A controlled evaluation of lithium in the premenstrual tension syndrome. *British Journal of Psychiatry*, **124**, 50–51

SOMMER, B. (1972) Menstrual cycle changes and intellectual performance. *Psychosomatic Medicine*, **34**, 263–269

SOMMER, B. (1973) The effect of menstruation on cognitive and perceptual motor behaviour: a review. *Psychosomatic Medicine*, **35**, 515–534

STEPHENSON, L. A., DENNEY, D. R. and ABERGER, E. W. (1983) Factor structure of the menstrual symptom questionnaire: relationship to oral contraceptives, neuroticism and life stress. *Behavioural Research and Therapy*, **21**, 129–135

SUTHERLAND, H. (1892) *A Dictionary of Psychological Medicine* (Tuke, D. H., Ed.). London; Churchill

TAYLOR, J. W. (1979a) Plasma progesterone, oestradiol-17-beta and premenstrual symptoms. *Acta Psychiatrica Scandinavica*, **60**, 76–86

TAYLOR, J. W. (1979b) The timing of menstruation-related symptoms assessed by a daily symptom rating scale. *Acta Psychiatrica Scandinavica*, **60**, 87–105

TAYLOR, J. W. (1979c) Psychological factors in the aetiology of premenstrual symptoms. *Australian and New Zealand Journal of Psychiatry*, **13**, 35–41

TAYLOR, R. W. (1977) The treatment of premenstrual tension with dydrogesterone ('Duphaston'). *Current Medical Research and Opinion*, **4**, suppl. 4, 35–40

TONKS, C. M. (1975) *Premenstrual Tension In Contemporary Psychiatry, British Journal of Psychiatry*, Special Publication No. 9, pp. 399–408 (Silverstone, T. and Barraclough, B., Eds.). Ashford, UK; Headley Bros.

TONKS, C. M., RACK, P. H. and ROSE, M. J. (1968) Attempted suicide and the menstrual cycle. *Journal of Psychosomatic Research*, **11**, 319–323

TUCH, R. H. (1975) The relationship between a mother's menstrual status and her response to illness in her child. *Psychosomatic Medicine*, **37**, 388–394

WERCH, A. and KANE, R. E. (1976) Treatment of premenstrual tension with metolazone: a double-blind evaluation of a new diuretic. *Current Therapeutic Research*, **19**, 565–572

WETZEL, R. D. and McCLURE, J. N. (1972) Suicide and the menstrual cycle: a review. *Comprehensive Psychiatry*, **13**, 369–374

WHITEHEAD, M. I., TOWNSEND, P. T., GILL, D. K., COLLINS, W. P. and CAMPBELL, S. (1980) Absorption and metabolism of oral progesterone. *British Medical Journal*, **280**, 825–827

WILCOXON, L. A., SCHRADER, S. L. and SHERIF, C. W. (1976) Daily self reports on activities, life events, moods and somatic changes during the menstrual cycle. *Psychosomatic Medicine*, **38**, 399–417

WOOD, C. and JAKUBOWICZ, D. (1980) The treatment of premenstrual symptoms with mefenamic acid. *British Journal of Obstetrics and Gynaecology*, **87**, 627–630

WOODS, N. F., DERY, G. K. and MOST, A. D. (1982) Recollections of menarche, current menstrual attitudes and perimenstrual symptoms. *Psychosomatic Medicine*, **44**, 285–293

YLÖSTALO, P., KAUPPILA, A., PUOLAKKA, J., RÖNNBERG, L. and JÄNNE, O. (1982) Bromocriptine and norethisterone in the treatment of premenstrual syndrome. *Obstetrics and Gynaecology*, **59**, 292–298

Chapter 5

Psychological disorders in pregnancy

Gisela B. Oppenheim

Incidence of psychiatric disturbances in pregnancy

Does pregnancy, as has often been said, serve to protect the future mother from mental illness? Perhaps the combination of physiological change and the stress of twentieth century Western culture produces the very opposite effect. Paffenbarger (1964) studied first-admission rates to American mental hospitals from a geographically defined area, during pregnancy and 6 months post-partum. He reported that the onset of a first mental illness during pregnancy occurred in 5 per 10 000 live births. A steep rise post-partum to 19 per 10 000 was noted. The ratio of psychosis to neurosis in pregnancy for these inpatients was 1:2. This ratio was reversed in the post-partum groups.

A similar survey by Pugh et al. (1963) found fewer admissions than anticipated for all groups of mental illness during pregnancy, but a greater number than might be expected postnatally.

Both these studies support the view that pregnancy may have a protective function, preventing serious mental illness.

The epidemiological survey carried out by Kendell et al. (1976) approached the problem differently. They located all women from a defined area giving birth in 1970, and identified from the Camberwell Case Register those mothers coming to psychiatric attention. A retrospective analysis was made of the health of these women. The findings of Kendell et al. (1976, 1981) do not support the view that pregnancy reduces the occurrence of new episodes of serious psychiatric illness throughout the trimesters. Kendell et al. (1976) also noted the prominent peak of psychiatric illness in the three-month period after delivery.

These surveys are subject to certain limitations. They were retrospective and relied on the accuracy of psychiatric records. Patients were identified by contact with psychiatrists or psychiatric services or through hospital records. This approach must result in a bias towards the more severely ill. Milder neurotic disturbances, which do not lead to impairment of daily performance, frequently do not come to medical attention, or at best are only reported to the family doctor. They are thus excluded from all three studies.

Kumar and Robson (1978), working in an ante-natal clinic, carried out a prospective study which included minor neurotic disturbances in their survey of 119 primigravidae attending a London Teaching Hospital. The authors accept that their sample is slanted towards the healthier end of the social scale, and hence is not representative of all women. Kumar and Robson found an overall prevalence of neurotic illness in 21% of their mothers-to-be. They also demonstrated a clear peak in post-natal psychiatric illness.

Tod (1964) studied 700 consecutive pregnant patients in his London practice. He reported a relationship between pathological anxiety during pregnancy and puerperal depression.

Dalton (1971), in a prospective study of 500 pregnant women, reported that 37% experienced some depression during pregnancy. However, the degree of incapacity caused is not discussed.

Nilsson and Almgren (1970), in a survey of 152 pregnant women, noted a slight increase in psychiatric symptoms compared with the patients' pre-pregnancy status.

Wolkind and Zajicek (1981), in a prospective study of working class women having their first baby, showed that psychiatric illness predating pregnancy increased the prevalence of problems during the pregnancy and in the puerperium. They reported a prevalence of 14% in unselected married women at the beginning of the third trimester. Surprisingly, single mothers did not fare any worse.

Epidemiological surveys of the prevalence of mental illness in pregnancy, like the above examples, have not yet yielded completely convincing results. The concept of freedom from mental illness during pregnancy appears to be oversimplified, but there is general agreement that, post-natally, women are at high risk of developing a psychiatric illness. Welner (1982) in a review of 108 papers on childbirth-related psychiatric illness, concurs with this view (see also Chapter 6).

Emotional reactions

Many pregnant women feel perfectly content and do not report any evidence of distress. Women who are regularly plagued by severe premenstrual tension may regard the whole of their pregnancy as a kind of happy interlude. Others, by contrast, find the first three months rather stressful. Many women show considerable *emotional lability* in the pregnant state. Restlessness, irritability and touchiness, anxiety and mild depression may all be puzzling experiences. By the 16th week most mothers-to-be have regained their equilibrium.

Clinical experience, judged by psychiatric referral rates, suggests that the second trimester is the least stressful. Fava et al. (1982), studying the effect of amniocentesis on women's anxieties, lend support to this view. Thus, following amniocentesis carried out in the second trimester, workers found the expected decrease in anxiety but observed a parallel decrease in their control group. They postulate that a decrease in psychological distress is normal in the second trimester. However, looking at specific symptoms, Little et al. (1982) found no significant differences in anxiety ratings throughout pregnancy. Inspection of the data of Kumar and Robson (1978) lends support to the view that the second trimester of pregnancy is less stressful than the first, but they found little difference between the incidence of new episodes of depression or anxiety in the second and third trimesters.

Common anxieties

In a first pregnancy, natural apprehension may be compounded by ignorance. The immature teenager may have little knowledge of pregnancy and childbirth and is especially at risk. She may have an unstable relationship, lack parental support and be afraid of anyone in authority. The young mother-to-be may be frightened of hospital, physical examination and especially injections. Not infrequently the youngster is preoccupied with her loss of sexual attractiveness. The older, married and experienced woman may be in a state of conflict about the pregnancy, especially if the baby was not planned.

An unplanned pregnancy gives rise to specific problems, particularly poignant in a single girl. In theory this situation should be a rare event, as advice on family planning is readily available. In practice, this is not so, There are many reasons – personal, religious and cultural, the desire to satisfy unconscious needs or to bring pressure on a reluctant boyfriend to 'make it legal'. Even today the option to marry is backed by considerable social pressure, and 'shotgun' weddings still occur. At best, a genuine commitment existed between the young people before the undesired pregnancy was discovered.

In both groups an unhappy past experience may trigger specific fears. A previous therapeutic termination, especially if the event was hidden from the husband, repeated spontaneous abortions or a previous unexplained stillbirth may all play a part in raising the patient's anxiety level.

Fears about fetal abnormality are common and may be enhanced in women exposed to infection or drugs during the first trimester. Women who know of a hereditary risk, or who have already borne an abnormal infant, may be particularly concerned. Astbury and Walters (1979) have shown that in the last groups amniocentesis allayed maternal apprehension. Their work lends support to the view that dread of the unknown enhances the anxieties engendered by pregnancy.

Cox, Connor and Kendell (1982) found that anxiety often centres on the delivery and the health of the unborn child. Many patients dread the pains of labour and doubt their ability to cope. A fear of death in childbirth is not uncommon.

A father-to-be may have his own problems. He may either dislike his wife's changing contour or feel proud of the joint achievement. He may be anxious on his partner's behalf, but not aware of how he can be of help.

Inadequate housing is a frequent source of anxiety. Financial difficulties may arise when both parents have been working and suddenly the family income is reduced. Thus, a lower living standard may be forced on to the couple and sometimes even a change in social status.

The decision on whether to stay at home with baby in preference to a return to remunerative employment has to be faced by many mothers. Expectations, generated by the media and women's magazines, and conflicting values in our changing society make this choice difficult and may produce feelings of anxiety and guilt. This conflict of priorities is particularly worrying for the professional woman. What can be done to lessen the impact of these common symptoms?

Ante-natal psychological care should synchronize with routine physical supervision. Both these aspects of well-being lend themselves to simultaneous monitoring. Ideally, any serious problems should be discussed prior to conception.

The pre-conception clinic

It is not only past obstetric problems which require elucidation. Couples can be advised how to achieve optimum physical and mental health in the ideal setting of a pre-conception clinic.

The importance of nutrition should be emphasized. Some figure-conscious girls on the verge of anorexia nervosa (see page 100) may require guidance towards better eating habits and need to appreciate that low maternal weight may influence the birth weight of their baby. Perhaps more frequently one meets the overweight patient who had difficulty in conceiving and who runs the risk of hypertension, diabetes mellitus and a particularly large baby.

Many women do not appreciate the deleterious effects of both alcohol and tobacco on their unborn child. Discussion is aimed at modifying any faulty habits.

A mother with a history of post-natal depression, attending a pre-conception clinic, may wish to know how likely she would be to suffer a recurrence. Although a clear answer cannot yet be given, current knowledge can be discussed and placed in perspective.

Treatment of pre-existing psychiatric illness should be completed prior to conception, in case the stress of pregnancy aggravates current problems.

General management

Most women who feel anxious about some aspect of childbirth benefit from simple reassurance from their obstetrician. Others are in need of help which can only be founded on a more detailed examination of their background.

History-taking need not be formal, nor does each point require elucidation. However, it may be convenient to undertake this assessment under a number of headings:

1. *Family history.* This should cover relationships within the family. Early separation from one or both parents is very important. Do they live in reasonable proximity and are they willing to make themselves useful?
2. *Personal history.* The personal history should encompass early experience, how the mother-to-be had coped with school or other stress, her educational achievements, her work record, sexual experience, plans for the future, details of her marriage and recent life-events. How does she see her marital role? Is it an equal partnership or does one spouse dominate the marriage? Does she feel loved? Are both partners able to assume a supportive role? Was the marriage prompted by pregnancy? Was the baby planned? In the case of the single mother-to-be, is she being emotionally and practically supported by the baby's putative father?
3. *Past history.* This should elucidate marital problems, psychiatric illness and past obstetric difficulties. In case of previous psychiatric illness, attempts should always be made to obtain the relevant hospital notes.
4. *Social history.* The housing situation should be investigated. Enquiry must be made about consumption of alcohol, smoking habits and any current medication.

During history-taking, a sound working relationship can be established with the patient, enabling the obstetrician to identify those women who need specific psychiatric help.

Psychiatric assessment

This is desirable for all pregnant women who give a history of post-natal depression, irrespective of the severity of the illness. Most women are extremely fearful of a recurrence and benefit from discussing their anxiety. The realization that psychiatric help is available may be therapeutic itself. These high-risk mothers should be seen throughout their pregnancy and followed up after delivery. This approach allows the psychiatrist to detect the illness at an early stage. Prompt treatment may forestall a critical deterioration in the woman's mental health, her marital relationship and ability to care for her infant. A final check on the mother's psychological well-being should be made routinely at her post-natal examination.

Management of neurotic reactions
The neurotic reactions are not specific to the pregnant state. The emotional disorder is experienced in terms of normal variants, worrying, sadness, gloominess and feelings of restlessness or irritability (Snaith, 1983). When symptoms occur, prompt treatment is indicated, aimed at restoring the mother's well-being before confinement. Therapy is adjusted to the patient's need and presenting symptoms. Time is usually too short for insight-orientated psychotherapy, which attempts to explore subconscious mental processes and conflicts. Supportive therapy, which deals with the 'here and now' situation, is usually more appropriate and encourages the patient to talk about her difficulties. An opportunity to verbalize her anxieties and to think about them often enables her to find her own solutions. The patient who lacks the capacity to solve her own problems requires the psychiatrist to take a more directive role. It is nearly always useful to invite the husband to join in discussions. Attempts can then be made to focus on the needs of the couple.

Ante-natal preparation

Instructions are tailored to help prospective parents to meet the varying challenges of parenthood. The ideal tutor will concentrate on group discussion, but she will not neglect her teaching role. Parents-to-be require a basic fund of factual information. They need to understand the physiological and psychological changes in pregnancy so that they can take an active part in the decision-making associated with childbirth. Not every labour proceeds normally; hence some knowledge of possible difficulties may prove helpful, and prevent a feeling of failure. They should be warned that over half the new mothers will suffer from the 'baby blues' for a few days. During discussions on infant care, breast-feeding is actively promoted. Many mothers find it a source of great contentment and establish a particularly close bond with their infants. But, if serious difficulties arise, attempts at breast-feeding should be abandoned early without engendering feelings of guilt or failure.

Classes should aim to prepare the parents for the big moment of taking their new baby home. This exciting event can, otherwise, be frightening. Suddenly all the professionals have departed and the parents are literally left holding the baby. Ante-natal preparations will have succeeded if 'graduating' parents can make confident decisions and face the many challenges of parenthood.

Future trends

Despite good ante-natal care it has been difficult to anticipate and predict the development of psychiatric problems associated with pregnancy and childbirth. Research is in progress to define psychophysiological, social and biochemical variables as predictors of post-natal depression. Little *et al.* (1982) found the Hostility and Direction of Hostility questionnaire the best predictor of post-natal depressed mood.

Cox, Connor and Kendell (1982) noted that the post-natal 'blues' are not always the mild self-limiting condition we anticipate, but in their severe form the mothers were at particularly high risk of developing persistent depressive symptoms.

Paykel *et al.* (1980) found a 20% prevalence of mild clinical post-partum depression. The strongest associated factor was the occurrence of recent stressful life-events. Other important factors were a previous history of psychiatric disorder and the absence of social support.

Braverman and Roux (1978) showed that seven simple questions had a predictive value in identifying women who are at risk of developing a post-partum emotional disorder:

1. Do you feel often that your husband (boyfriend) does not love you?
2. Can you honestly say at this time that you really do not desire to have a child?
3. Do you have marital problems?
4. Was your pregnancy unplanned (accidental)?
5. Did you become very depressed or extremely nervous in the period following the birth of your last child?
6. Are you single or separated?
7. Do you more or less regret that you are pregnant?

Meares, Grimwade and Wood (1976) postulated a relationship between anxiety in pregnancy and puerperal depression, using anxiety and personality measurements. A similar relationship was reported by Tod (1964). Jones (1978) showed that neither personality nor anxiety measures could predict complications in women of low socio-economic class. The surprise finding was negative correlation with life changes: a lower life change score indicated a greater probability of complications in labour.

Standley, Soule and Copans (1979) showed that emotional reactions in pregnancy are rooted in a woman's background and have an impact on peri-natal events and infant functioning. Frommer and O'Shea (1973) reported in a prospective study that questions about the woman's childhood, in particular early separation from one or both parents before the age of 11, can identify mothers who will have difficulty in managing their infants.

Kumar and Robson (1978) found that marital tension during pregnancy was associated with post-partum depression. Patients who had problems in the relationship with their own parents were also more likely to develop a post-partum illness. Two other predictors emerged from their studies. Women over the age of 30 and those trying to conceive for 2 or more years were also more vulnerable.

Turning to the biochemical side, Sandler (1978) described an abnormality in tyramine metabolism in depressed patients. He found a significant decrease in conjugated tyramine excretion following an oral tyramine load, not only during the illness but even after clinical recovery from depression. This observation could form the basis of a laboratory predictor test for patients at increased risk from post-natal depression. Unfortunately, methods to date (1984) are still too cumbersome and expensive. We await the possible development of a simple test for clinical application.

Pre-eclampsia

Recent advances in immunology and histoincompatibility suggest that the aetiology of toxaemia will be unravelled without the need to postulate a psychosomatic component. This subject has been very ably reviewed by MacGillivray (1983).

Vomiting in pregnancy

Four distinct types may be described, only the first being common: (a) 'normal vomiting' of pregnancy; (b) hyperemesis gravidarum; (c) 'pathological vomiting'; (d) hysterical vomiting. These are dealt with below.

'Normal vomiting' of pregnancy

Nausea and vomiting is experienced by most patients early in pregnancy. Indeed, they tend not to allude to these symptoms, which usually cease spontaneously by the twelfth to fourteenth week.

Hyperemesis gravidarum

If vomiting is so severe that it leads to dehydration, ketosis and electrolyte disturbance, the special label of hyperemesis is applied. This relatively rare condition is seen in less than 0.5% of pregnant patients. Little is known of the pathogenesis of this condition, hence the sonorous title. Evidence for a psychosomatic component is mainly anecdotal. Some psychiatrists have postulated that hyperemesis occurs in patients who are subconsciously rejecting their babies. Tylden (1968) has associated it with stress, insecurity and pre-existing gastro-intestinal problems. Harvey and Sherfey (1954), in an uncontrolled clinical study, obtained a history of a vomiting tendency in response to emotional stress, in sexual disorders and in immature personalities.

The patient is usually admitted in a poor physical condition. It ought to occasion little surprise that this may be associated with an abnormal mental state. With the correction of the fluid and electrolyte imbalance, the psychological disturbance will then disappear. Nordmeyer (1946), Coppen (1959) and Sim (1968) found no evidence to support a psychosomatic aetiology. The psychiatrist has little to offer in the management of hyperemesis gravidarum. A discussion with the ward staff may help them to understand the patient's distress and encourage sympathetic management.

'Pathological vomiting'

The vomiting may be (a) directly related to pregnancy as in hydatidiform mole or red degeneration of a fibroid, or (b) independent of the pregnancy as in cerebral tumour, labyrinthitis or an acute abdominal emergency.

Hysterical vomiting

Here, the clinical picture is quite different. The patient presents in the second or third trimester of pregnancy with the complaint of vomiting after every meal. She claims she cannot even keep down a sip of water. On examination she is likely to be calm and philosophical, but convinced of an organic explanation for her symptoms. Her history is not supported by her appearance. She looks well and there are no abnormal physical or biochemical findings. Careful enquiry does not always elicit the current emotional conflict.

Anorexia nervosa

This is a psychiatric disorder with well-defined diagnostic criteria: (a) a distorted attitude towards weight and fatness, described by Crisp as an adolescent weight phobia (Crisp, 1974); (b) significant weight loss; (c) amenorrhoea.

The woman suffering from an acute form of the illness is unlikely to become pregnant, unless ovulation has been induced artificially. This may happen if the true nature of her amenorrhoea is not appreciated. The obstetrician is more likely to see a patient in relapse or suffering from a variant of anorexia nervosa, namely bulimia nervosa, described by Russell (1979). The patient has an irresistible urge to overeat. She follows this with self-induced vomiting and purging to prevent weight gain. In pregnancy, anorexia nervosa may be reactivated as a result of an increase in the body silhouette. Vomiting and diarrhoea may be the presenting features. This trap for the unwary may lead to a diagnosis of gastroenteritis or even of hyperemesis gravidarum. In both these conditions, as well as in anorexia nervosa, dehydration and ketosis may be prominent abnormalities.

CLINICAL FEATURES

Intentional starvation, cleverly disguised, with particular avoidance of carbo-hydrates, is the rule in the patient with anorexia nervosa. A feeling of emptiness after a meal is equated with a sense of elation; a feeling of fulness tends to arouse guilt. The patient feels 'bad'. Whenever the patient loses control over her dieting, she feels desperate. She may weigh herself several times a day, consult her mirror frequently, and still misinterpret her truly slim dimensions. She sees herself as fat and considerably overestimates her size. This distorted body-image goes hand in hand with a fear of growing up and assuming adult responsibilities. Paradoxically, she likes to study cookery books and enjoys cooking. Once the quest for slimness dominates her thinking, she does not stop short of lying and dishonesty to achieve her goal. It is surprising how often the girl, conscientious and reliable before her illness, may even resort to shoplifting. It is the deceitfulness which may make the diagnosis difficult.

There may be a background of overt or hidden family conflict. The pre-pubertal period of the girl tended to be free from difficulty. She was often exemplary in behaviour and had a strong wish to please. Not infrequently she had been overweight in childhood and was teased about this at school.

MANAGEMENT

The first task in the management of anorexia nervosa is correction of the electrolyte imbalance. Once this has been achieved, transfer to a psychiatric unit is almost mandatory. These units have specially trained nurses, skilled in helping the patient to re-establish normal eating patterns and reach a pre-determined target weight. A diet containing 16–20 MJ (4000–4500 kcal) daily is required to achieve a weight gain of 1–2 kg (2.2–2.4 lb) per week. The rapid restoration of an appropriate pregnant body weight will protect the fetus, but will not mitigate against relapse. While still in hospital, some weeks before discharge, the patient is encouraged to formulate a sensible diet of her own choosing. This is a useful learning experience and will demonstrate to the patient and her physician that she can maintain her correct weight and is in no danger of losing control over her eating. Relapse is a common occurrence if physical treatment to restore body weight is not followed by psychotherapy. A variety of therapeutic methods is available to treat the underlying conflict, which is frequently based on a distorted relationship with an important person in the patient's life.

INDIVIDUAL PSYCHOTHERAPY

This technique employs analytical concepts which explore and interpret the patient's childhood experience. It is used to modify unconscious mental processes which may have given rise to the patient's abnormal attitude towards weight and fatness. This approach to treatment is time-consuming and expensive. Hence, alternative methods have been evolved.

BRIEF PSYCHOTHERAPY

This differs from the above technique in that the therapist plays a more active and optimistic role. The focus of treatment is on the specific problem causing the patient's difficulties. A time limit for treatment may be agreed between patient and therapist.

GROUP THERAPY

A number of patients, perhaps 8 or 10, meet regularly for mutual help. Mixed sex groups can be very successful. The patient realizes that her problem is not unique. She finds acceptance by the group, in contrast to the rejection she has experienced in other situations. Limits are set and agreed by the group. The meeting is supervised by a group leader, usually a professional person. Group discussion and, on occasion, overt criticism aims to encourage a change of attitude and behaviour by the participants.

FAMILY THERAPY

This approach can be very helpful in anorexic patients, particularly when family relationships are disturbed. In the case of the married patient, the changing contours in pregnancy may have reactivated her adolescent weight phobia, but the underlying problem is now different. The patient may have chosen for a spouse a man who spoils her and on whom she relies heavily for support. The husband may be equally immature: doubts about his own masculinity make him sexually undemanding. He derives pleasure from his wife's dependence on him. No meaningful relationship can develop between husband and wife at that level of functioning. They will benefit from joint interviews to learn about each other's needs. Successful treatment will not only help the maturation of both partners, but also give their offspring a better start in life.

Denial of pregnancy

Denial is a mental mechanism providing an escape from unpleasant reality. A denial of pregnancy may be used by those women who perceive their pregnant state as a complete social disaster. The phenomenon is met in the young girl as well as the older woman and at all levels of intelligence. Patients who deny their pregnancy may go to term having missed all ante-natal care. Sometimes the delivery awakens strong latent maternal feelings and bonding is successful; unfortunately, more often the outlook for the infant is poor. The mother may even abandon her baby.

CASE HISTORY

Miss J., aged 18, was an undergraduate at a Scottish University, where voluminous red gowns are traditionally worn. She was the only child in a family where disharmony and tension were the order of the day. Despite this unpromising background, Miss J. did not show many neurotic traits during childhood. While under considerable academic strain, her parents decided to separate. Distressed, she sought solace from her boyfriend and conceived. Miss J. ignored this event and began her university course already 28 weeks pregnant. On the final day of term she complained of abdominal pain. The student health doctor was summoned and within two hours she had delivered a 3 kg (6.6 lb) baby.

   This crisis in Miss J.'s life altered the family dynamics. With parental support she regained her composure; the baby was adopted. Five years later she reported academic success, a fulfilling marriage and the birth of twin daughters.

COMMENT

The case history illustrates how an intelligent girl under great social pressure can ignore her own pregnancy. Subsequent events proved this to have been just an unhappy interlude in a previously stable personality.

Pseudocyesis

This is an uncommon disorder, occurring in suggestible, nulliparous women who desire children. They become convinced that they are pregnant and develop symptoms which mimic pregnancy. Amenorrhoea, abdominal enlargement, breast changes, the report of fetal movements and weight gain are commonly reported. Symptoms usually subside following ultrasound examination, open discussion and an offer of supportive therapy.

   Pseudocyesis may be the manifestation of a hysterical conversion symptom, or occur at a conscious level when it can be regarded as malingering. Occasionally it represents a delusion in a schizophrenic illness. Sim (1968) reported 6 cases, all associated with organic disease. Four of his patients suffered from intestinal obstruction.

CASE HISTORIES

Case 1
Mrs F., aged 22, married early to escape from an unhappy childhood and overbearing histrionic mother. She showed many psychological and physical features of immaturity. Frigidity was a serious problem, which she could not even acknowledge to herself. Pseudocyesis provided the perfect excuse of refusing intercourse and mollified her spouse into the bargain. In other words, she acquired a valuable hysterical conversion symptom.

Case 2

Miss T., aged 27, experienced difficulty in persuading a reluctant consort to return to her. She reported that she had planned to steal a baby, intending to pass it off as her own. Fortunately, she realized just in time that this misdeed would never achieve its purpose. She developed a pseudocyesis instead.

It is of interest that d'Orban (1976) found three cases of pseudocyesis in his review of 24 baby stealers.

COMMENT

Case 1 demonstrates an unconscious mental mechanism. A pseudocyesis was effective in reducing the patient's emotional stress. Case 2 shows, by way of contrast, how a conscious deception may present with similar symptoms.

Anxiety states

An anxiety state is characterized by an unpleasant emotional experience involving fear and dread, which may vary from chronic apprehension to a feeling of extreme intensity. Anxiety states tend to run a fluctuating course. The anxiety may be free-floating in the absence of objective dangers, or be an exaggerated response to environmental stress. Anxiety amounting to an illness must be differentiated from the almost universal anxieties experienced by most pregnant women because it disables and prevents the patient from continuing her normal activity.

Normal anxiety

Anxiety is a normal emotional reaction experienced by everyone. The universal anxieties encountered by pregnant women have been described (see page 94) and may be seen in this context.

Anxiety is often purposive – a stimulus towards useful action. A mother-to-be may actively need to feel a little anxious to galvanize herself into attending a parenthood class. As she gains the necessary knowledge, her confidence will increase and gradually her anxiety will diminish. The regular application of her newly learned skills will act as a positive feedback mechanism, which will reinforce her belief in her own competence.

Anxiety symptoms

Anxiety is conspicuous in a large variety of psychological and physical illness. It is well recognized that, in depressive illness and other psychoses, distressing anxiety may overshadow the clinical picture (see page 121). Similarly, in hyperthyroidism, anxiety may also feature prominently. The misuse of drugs represents another important causative condition. Amphetamine, LSD and atropine can cause quite severe anxiety symptoms.

Anxiety neurosis

AETIOLOGY

Typically, the patient's family background is one of personality disorder and neurotic illness (Hamilton, 1984). Thus it is not surprising that maladaptive behaviour patterns are learned in childhood from equally anxious parents and siblings. The patient tends to develop an insecure, dependent personality. She lacks the capacity to make friends and cope with stress.

CLINICAL FEATURES

The patient will present with an anxious mood, be worried about many trivia and report that she feels so tense that she is unable to cope with her life. She makes all those around her unhappy by her irritability. These psychological symptoms are likely to be accompanied by autonomic symptoms, such as palpitation, sweating, tremor and air hunger which may lead to hyperventilation, dry mouth, a feeling of constriction in the throat or 'knots' in the stomach.

Other women present with physical complaints, which they may expect the doctor to find more acceptable. Anxiety may precipitate psychosomatic symptoms in any system. Gastrointestinal complaints are common; dyspepsia, wind or loose stools are frequent complaints. This is particularly the situation when either parent suffered from gastrointestinal problems. Some women experience symptoms related to the cardiovascular or genitourinary system.

Insomnia, with difficulty in falling asleep, is common in both groups. There is often a complaint of fitful sleep, leaving the sufferer exhausted in the morning.

Equally common are classical tension headaches which start occipitally, spread forward and are then experienced as a tight band around the head. These headaches reach their peak as the build-up of the day's stress proceeds. Behaviour is often affected by anxiety. Hyperactivity and restlessness are common. A normally fit, sensible woman may become importunate, seeking constant reassurance. She presents to the physician as a classical worrier, often convinced that she suffers from organic disorder. More often, however, excessive dependence is associated with an inadequate personality.

MANAGEMENT

Diagnosis
It is especially the woman who presents her distress in physical terms who requires a full clinical examination and relevant investigations. It is important to stress to the patient that this step is essential. Negative findings must be accepted by doctor and patient alike. Failure to do so will increase the patient's anxiety and lead to unnecessary, potentially harmful and costly investigations.

Investigation of symptoms
Simple investigation of the somatic symptoms may be very helpful, although patients who are convinced of an organic explanation may find it difficult to accept reassurance.

Anxiolytic drugs
Diazepam 2 mg or oxazepam 10 mg 3 times daily may be given in the second trimester (see page 141). Drugs should only be used as a temporary measure to tide the patient over an acute episode. If insomnia is marked, drug therapy may be justified using the above criteria. It is unwise to allow women to start their labour with the handicap of a sleep debt.

Support
Regular support by the obstetrician or the psychiatrist helps most patients.

Relaxation classes
These classes can be most valuable, especially when the patient accepts that tension can cause pain. This is easily demonstrated by asking the patient to clench her fist until she experiences discomfort. The teaching sessions can be reinforced by the regular use of teaching tapes in the patient's home.

Phobic states

A phobic state is characterized by an irrational fear, evoked by a stimulus which is not a significant source of danger. The patient's reaction is not under voluntary control. She attempts to avoid the feared situation. Phobic states should be distinguished from normal, appropriate fears and from milder phobic symptoms which accompany other psychiatric syndromes by the fact that they are disabling or prevent the patient from carrying out normal activities.

Normal fears

Fear is a natural component of human experience and has a protective function. It does not constitute a handicap in daily life. Young children often tend to have a variety of fears. They may be particularly fearful of the dark, of animals or of a closed bedroom door. As the child matures, he grows out of these fears.

Phobic symptoms

Phobic symptoms may occur in association with many other psychiatric syndromes. Agoraphobia is commonly seen in depressive illness. The symptoms are usually mild, but are occasionally prominent enough to mask the underlying depressive condition.

Phobic illness: (1) agoraphobia

Marks (1969), in a comprehensive study, has classified phobias into several groups. The obstetrician is most likely to meet patients suffering from agoraphobia and needle phobia. The first of these, agoraphobia, is the commonest phobic state experienced by women of child-bearing age. The severity of symptoms tends to fluctuate and may be associated with other fears, or with mild symptoms of anxiety and depression.

AETIOLOGY

The premorbid presonality commonly shows many neurotic traits. Stressful life-events may precipitate the fear.

CLINICAL FEATURES

Characteristically, the illness commences quite acutely, with a panic attack when the patient is in her late teens or early twenties. The episode may occur in an open space, but more commonly it first takes place in a shop, theatre or church. The symptoms then tend to change to a fear of leaving home. When this becomes more marked, she avoids leaving her home altogether, becoming house-bound. Unless accompanied, she may be unable to attend for her ante-natal examinations.

MANAGEMENT

(a) Drug therapy including both anxiolytics and antidepressants; (b) behaviour therapy; (c) counselling to support the patient and to help her to resolve interpersonal problems.

Phobic illness: (2) needle phobia

Needle phobia, the second phobic illness likely to be seen by the obstetrician, is a specific fear of injections or having a blood sample taken. This phobia tends to affect stable women free from other psychiatric problems.

AETIOLOGY

Symptoms frequently commence in early childhood. Often no specific cause is known, but sometimes the onset is associated with a traumatic event involving an injection or a hospital admission.

CLINICAL FEATURES

Some women are so needle phobic that they delay starting a family. The patient will rarely volunteer her anxiety. When told in the clinic that a blood sample is required she experiences acute fear. Terror stricken, she may scream or run out of the consulting room unable to explain her distress. The phobia does not usually vary in intensity and tends to remain discrete. Some mothers are able to tolerate the feared procedure in spite of intense anxiety, provided they have learned a coping strategy from past experience. One mother used to count aloud to twelve, during which time the blood sample had to be obtained; she was quite unable to co-operate once the critical number had been reached.

MANAGEMENT

The behavioural treatment of needle phobia involves two phases. First, the mother-to-be is taught a number of anxiety management skills, which may include breathing and relaxation exercises. Some therapists teach positive thinking or a distraction technique. The second phase of treatment involves graded exposure to needles. The patient practises reducing her anxiety when confronted by the feared situation; for example, advancing from handling the needle to being touched with it at first and finally actually to having blood taken.

Obsessional states

An obsessional state or neurosis is characterized by recurrent and persistent thoughts, phobias, ruminations or activities which are associated with a sense of compulsion. The patient tries hard to dispel the obsessional thought or resist the ritual. Her efforts are accompanied by increasing anxiety. She is fully aware that the obsession is foolish and foreign to her personality. However, the compulsion is so strong that the patient cannot respond to her own reason. This disabling condition is fortunately uncommon.

Normal obsessions

Nearly all children indulge in some ritualistic activities; for example, they avoid stepping on the lines between paving stones, or perhaps they have to put Teddy to bed before they are willing to be undressed themselves. In adulthood, for instance, an obsessional approach to life is seen in our most conscientious and reliable citizens.

Obsessional symptoms

Most adults have experienced obsessional or compulsive symptoms at some time in their lives. These may just have been in the nature of a recurring musical theme or perhaps have taken the form of repeated unproductive checking of a completed task. These symptoms are particularly likely to occur during times of personal stress or fatigue.

Obsessional symptoms are not infrequently elicited as part of a depressive illness. They may also form a part of the bizarre tapestry of a schizophrenic illness or be a symptom of organic brain disease.

Obsessional thoughts
These consist of repetitive words, images or fully formed ideas which intrude into the patient's mind. These compulsive thoughts are usually unacceptable to the woman and especially disturbing when they have a sexual connotation. Some patients develop rituals in an attempt to deal with their very unpleasant symptoms. Completion of the ritual tends to allay anxiety. Compulsive hand-scrubbing and washing for minutes on end innumerable times each day may enable the mother to pick up and tend her baby, while without her ritual she would be immobilized. Her very sore hands may be the first evidence of an obsessional illness.

Obsessional phobias
These often include a morbid attitude to dirt or germs. The patient may regard herself as being contaminated and fears that she could be transmitting infection to her baby or other members of her family.

Obsessional actions or rituals
These may occur as a primary symptom. A patient who spends hours each day checking and rechecking doors, windows, fires or gas taps may be so incapacitated that she finds it impossible to go out.

Obsessional neurosis

AETIOLOGY

The premorbid personality often shows many obsessional traits. Either psychological or physiological stress may precipitate the illness.

CLINICAL FEATURES

Characteristically, the neurosis commences in the late teens. Very gradually, symptoms start to interfere with daily life at home and at work. Marked variation in the severity of symptoms is commonly observed. Consequently, the illness may run a phasic course. Medical advice is seldom sought in a first attack because these patients feel ashamed of their symptoms and may try to conceal them. Attempts to resist the compulsion are accompanied by mounting tension and anxiety. The patient obtains relief only with completion of each ritual.

MANAGEMENT

(a) Simple reassurance proves invaluable. The patient will benefit from an explanation that her troublesome symptoms are, in fact, experienced by most people at some time in their lives and that she is certainly not going mad.

(b) Drug therapy with anxiolytics should be restricted to crisis situations or to acute exacerbations.

(c) Behaviour therapy (see page 106) may be most helpful.

CASE HISTORY

Mrs D., aged 30, had been a fastidious child. Endless rituals had accompanied meals and bedtime. Every toy had to be carefully replaced in its proper box. She was meticulous in all she undertook to do – in short, she was a perfectionist. In adolescence and again shortly after her marriage Mrs D. developed a fear of spreading infection. For a time she could open a door only if she covered the handle with a handkerchief. Gradually her symptoms subsided. Three years later, when 22 weeks pregnant, Mrs D. developed quite incapacitating symptoms.

She told her obstetrician that she was terrified that she might harm her newborn infant. Her fear increased in severity whenever she saw or used a knife. Working in the kitchen became very stressful for her. Mrs D. attempted to resist the compulsion to check that no sharp objects or pins had been mislaid in the still vacant cot. She realized that her fear was groundless and quite foolish. Her symptoms aroused considerable anxiety in the staff of the obstetric department. An urgent psychiatric assessment was requested. At the consultation, Mrs D.'s obstetrician could be assured that his patient would be most unlikely to harm her baby. If anything, this child is likely to be overprotected and enjoy better than average care.

Obsessional symptoms in the context of other diseases

Obsessional symptoms frequently present in the setting of depressive illness. The clinical picture is dominated by the mood disturbance and its associated physiological concomitants. Obsessional thoughts add to the patient's misery. No attempt is made by the woman to resist her compulsion, nor does she appreciate the folly of her obsession. Thus, devoid of insight, she may act on her misguided compulsive thoughts.

CASE HISTORY

Mrs K., aged 41, was expecting her first baby after 12 years of childless marriage. She was a religious woman who had accepted her barren state as an act of God. Over the years she had often spoken to her spiritual adviser about her infertility.

He had proposed that she would find happiness if she adopted a handicapped child. Mrs K. had brooded on the idea, but had felt unable to accept his counsel. As her pregnancy advanced, she began to ruminate on her lack of moral fibre. These thoughts became ever more intrusive, recurring with great intensity and frequency. When seen at 27 weeks she was deeply depressed. Mrs K. admitted to harbouring the intent of killing herself and her baby after delivery. The patient was immediately admitted to a psychiatric unit for observation. Antidepressant therapy was commenced (see page 123). As her depression lifted, the associated obsessional ruminations resolved.

COMMENT

Obsessional symptoms are common to both case histories. Mrs D.'s first symptoms had occurred in adolescence. She attempted to resist her obsessional thoughts and rituals, realizing their absurdity. The patient suffered from an obsessional illness. She would never have acted on an obsession that transgressed her moral code. On the other hand, Mrs K.'s obsessional symptoms occurred in the setting of a depressive illness. She did not realize that her ruminations were foolish, nor did she attempt to resist them. Mrs K. had every intention of acting on her compulsive thoughts. Her depression was recognized in time. Treatment prevented the potential tragedy of a dead mother and baby.

The difficult patient

This refers to the woman who has problems in establishing a useful working relationship with her physician. At interview, the patient's behaviour is inconsistent and unpredictable. The demeanour of some patients may be at once ingratiating and flattering, while others show undue dependence or overt hostility. Obstetricians are only too familiar with the chaos which these women can create in their departments.

AETIOLOGY

Most important is parental failure to provide a secure home. All too often the family has disintegrated or is tarnished by alcoholism, criminality or overt psychiatric illness. Lack of warmth, poor example and shifting values contribute to the child's inability to acquire socially acceptable patterns of behaviour. Some women are physically immature. This can be demonstrated by their bone age on X-ray and slower than expected rhythms in the EEG.

CLINICAL FEATURES

Frequently, the patient looks younger than her stated age. She may dress in a flamboyant, provocative manner or be quite indifferent to her appearance.

Her instinctive drives and immediate needs are freely displayed in an uninhibited way. She is unaware that her behaviour has a detrimental effect on staff and other patients. Her unreliability is shown by a tendency to give a misleading history. A stranger to discipline, she fails to co-operate in treatment. Ante-natal appointments are missed and advice not heeded. She is unable to adhere to a prescribed diet or take adequate rest. Iron supplements may be consigned to the waste paper basket.

Outside the hospital setting, she has similar difficulties. Unable to sustain a relationship, family ties are lost. Rejected, she tends to mix with others of the same kind. Frequently, there is a history of drug misuse, excessive alcohol consumption or heavy smoking. Often she is without a permanent home.

CASE HISTORY

Miss W., aged 26, was admitted to hospital complaining of abdominal pain. She was found to be 30 weeks pregnant. Her pain remained unexplained and was assumed to be of psychosomatic origin. At first, Miss W. denied all her difficulties, divulging so little information about herself that the level of suspicion was raised. After time-consuming enquiries, the following story emerged.

Miss W. had been a frequent resident in psychiatric hospitals since her childhood. One admission had extended over 4 years. She led a promiscuous life and had no real friends. Two previous pregnancies had been terminated. When seen ante-natally at another hospital, she was cohabiting with an equally irresponsible man, who was not the baby's father. He used to beat her frequently. Several times she had fled from him, only to be drawn back to the same situation. Miss W. had been an erratic attender at a psychiatric outpatient department, near her temporary home. Her attendance was usually associated with a new crisis in her life. She was well known to a social worker, who expressed grave concern about her competence to manage her baby. A case conference had been convened, where the decision was reached that the baby should be taken into care. Miss W. had not accepted this decision. Instead, she absconded and decided to seek advice in a different town, where she was unknown and in a position to suppress her past history. She had visions of being allowed to leave hospital with the newborn baby in her arms. Her daydreams failed to allow for the harsh realities of caring for a demanding infant, the hard work involved and the very real responsibility. Miss W.'s anticipatory pleasure could have been likened to that of a child about to receive a new toy.

MANAGEMENT

The previous social worker visited the patient in the ante-natal ward and succeeded in convincing her that it was in her best interest to return to the original hospital. A place in a 'mother and baby' unit would be made available, if she desired it.

COMMENT

The history shows how one difficult patient can generate a great deal of work which is unproductive. Had more care been taken at an early stage to establish a good relationship with her, much time and effort might have been saved.

Drug dependence

Drug dependence is of particular importance in pregnancy, since most drugs cross the placental barrier. The drug may be teratogenic or be capable of causing an abstinence syndrome in the mother and baby. The majority of addicts appear to make use of multiple drugs. However, this does not deter many of them from expressing a preference for a particular drug from a miscellaneous assortment.

Narcotic dependence

The obstetrician is most likely to see women dependent on diamorphine (heroin), methadone, or 'Chinese', 'Turkish', 'Persian' or 'Thai' opiates in powder form. These illegal drugs are a mixture of heroin, codeine, barbiturates and various impurities. The potency varies from one packet to another.

Pregnancy is not common in drug-dependent girls, as regular narcotic use is associated with menstrual irregularities and reduced fertility. Paradoxically, this infertility constitutes the one beneficial effect which may be said to brighten the murky scene of drug dependence.

Early diagnosis of addiction contributes substantially to a successful outcome of the pregnancy. The doctor who is looking for the caricature type of 'typical junkie' will miss the diagnosis. Difficulties frequently arise because the patients are unreliable historians. Occasionally, they help the doctor unwittingly by asking for drugs. More often they deny their involvement, largely to avoid the prospect of a moralistic lecture. More realistically, they may fear that, once their drug involvement is known, they may not be trusted to care for their baby. The obstetrician should be aware that an unrelated injury or illness may not be noticed by the patient, for her pain is masked by drugs.

CLINICAL FEATURES

The heroin addict is essentially a quiet withdrawn girl. She may be ill-looking, haggard and undernourished. Track marks along veins disfigure her hands and arms. She may be heavily tattooed, which to the initiated suggests that she may have been in close contact with law-enforcing agencies, as experience shows that patients with criminal behaviour are often tattooed. The more sophisticated addict is able to avoid these obvious stigmas. It is her life-style and her preoccupation with drugs which may give the first clues to her dependence, before the pinpoint pupils are noticed.

The drug addict's behaviour is generally irresponsible and this also applies to her ante-natal care. She may attend infrequently or not at all, presenting for the first time in labour. If seen early, she is most unlikely to accept admission to hospital, which would allow her obstetrician to make an assessment of her dependence and its effect on the fetus (Fraser, 1976). The patient's lack of co-operation in her ante-natal care is in part responsible for the many fetal complications. Stillbirths and peri-natal mortality rates are both high. Placental insufficiency, leading to fetal growth retardation, is common. Often the baby is born prematurely after a relatively rapid labour. The high fetal risks make it advisable to alert the paediatric team early in the course of the patient's confinement. The children of drug abusers are at some risk of taking inadvertent overdoses of parental drugs.

COMPLICATIONS

Medical
Infection from injection sites, such as local abscess formation, septicaemia and thrombophlebitis are common. There is also an increased susceptibility to general infections. Sharing of syringes may spread AIDS, B-positive virus hepatitis, sexually transmitted diseases and rhesus sensitization in a rhesus-negative woman. Nutritional anaemia may be severe, as iron supplements are rarely taken regularly. Poor dental hygiene is a further facet of the state of general neglect.

Withdrawal syndromes

(a) *Maternal symptoms*. These can be quite mild and include restlessness, muscle cramp and gastrointestinal discomfort in the form of nausea, vomiting and diarrhoea. The patient is anxious and usually frightened of more severe symptoms. These only last for 48–72 h, but the patient may suffer from disturbed sleep for some weeks or even months.

Management. The symptoms are quickly alleviated by the administration of oral methadone mixture 1 mg in 1 ml. 10–20 ml may be an appropriate dose and can be repeated 12-hourly as necessary.

(b) *Effect on the fetus*. Fetal distress in labour will occur if the mother's opioid level falls significantly. The baby may be observed to kick quite violently.

Management. In the interest of the infant, the mother should be given methadone in labour, even if her addiction is only suspected. Naloxone must be avoided, as this morphine antagonist can induce a potentially lethal withdrawal state in the dependent fetus (Tylden, 1973).

(c) *Effect on the neonate*. Withdrawal symptoms are common. The fetus develops the same tolerance as the mother. The time of onset of symptoms depends on the drug used by the mother. Neonates previously accustomed to high heroin levels may show symptoms 4–6 h after delivery or even earlier. Methadone protects the fetus rather longer from withdrawal symptoms which may not be evident for several days after delivery. The infant is more likely to have seizures. Symptoms include a shrill cry, irritability, tremors and respiratory distress. The infant sucks only with difficulty. Vomiting or diarrhoea may lead to dangerous dehydration in a severely ill baby. If the symptoms are undiagnosed and untreated, a fatal outcome is likely. The need for active treatment is judged by the presence and severity of these symptoms.

Management. Most neonates respond to 0.1–0.2 mg of paregoric in the form of a camphorated tincture of opium, given 6-hourly, but regular administration is not always required as the following case history demonstrates. Treatment with narcotics appears to restore normal physiology more quickly. This evidence has been obtained from studies of infant sucking performances (Kron *et al.*, 1975). Other drugs have been successful in the management of neonatal narcotic withdrawal symptoms. Chlorpromazine and diazepam have proved effective.

Chlorpromazine 2.2 mg/kg per day is given orally in four divided doses. Improvement is noted in most infants within 12 h. The duration of treatment could extend to 40 days (Stone *et al.*, 1971).

Diazepam 0.5–1.0 mg is given intramuscularly every 12 h, or more frequently if necessary. Treatment may be required for 1–9 days. In the more severely ill babies who required more than 3 days of medication, the dose to abolish symptoms may be reduced gradually to 0.25 mg of diazepam towards the end of treatment (Blinick *et al.*, 1976).

CASE HISTORY

Miss J., aged 22, was having maintenance treatment of 18 ml methadone mixture daily, at the time she went into premature labour. At first, both mother and baby were doing well; artificial feeding was instituted. Seventy-two hours post-partum the baby showed signs of drug withdrawal. Restlessness and irritability were followed by a shrill cry and feeding difficulties. Morphine 0.2 mg, given by mouth once daily for 2 days, proved effective in overcoming these moderate withdrawal signs.

COMMENT

In view of the short half-life of morphine in the adult, this satisfactory response to a single dose is surprising. The neonate's limited capacity to detoxicate drugs could provide an explanation.

BREAST-FEEDING

This may present a hazard for the baby of a drug-dependent woman. The obstetrician may feel tempted to trust the patient's assurance that she has finally foresworn the use of illegal drugs. This laudable determination may evaporate in a crisis once she has returned to her consort and drug-orientated friends. Narcotics, benzodiazepines and most other drugs of misuse enter breast milk in sufficient quantities to affect the baby. Bottle feeding is therefore much safer.

GENERAL MANAGEMENT OF NARCOTIC DEPENDENCE

In the UK, under the Misuse of Drugs Regulations 1967 and 1973, a doctor who suspects his patient to be narcotic dependent is required to notify the Medical Officer, Drugs Branch, Home Office, Queen Anne's Gate, London SW1. Notification of the addict's name(s), date of birth and other details will identify the patient and yield statistics of the prevalence of addiction. More important, from the doctor's point of view, it provides an information service. By contacting the Home Office's Addict Index, the obstetrician can ascertain if his patient is currently under treatment. This facilitates contact with the patient's psychiatrist. There is no similar arrangement in the USA or Western Europe.

Management in the first trimester
A decision on management can be made only after the careful evaluation of the patient's physical state and drug problem. The choice lies between two alternatives: pharmacological detoxification or methadone maintenance therapy. The mother's own drug history will give a guide to her degree of dependence. Where possible, it should be corroborated. A complete physical examination is followed by relevant laboratory studies. These comprise a full blood count with erythrocyte sedimentation rate, liver function tests and serology, including Australia antigen. A drug screen is carried out on successive urine samples. A positive result will tell the physician only that his patient has used a drug, but not that she is dependent. Conversely, a patient in withdrawal may show no drug or its metabolites in her urine. If the patient is found to be dependent on opioids in early pregnancy, the painful topic of a therapeutic termination may be broached. The immature, young single girl may greet the suggestion with enthusiasm. This facility is, however, not available in all countries, nor is it the wish of the majority of women presenting in this situation.

(1) *Detoxification.* Ideally, the patient accepts hospital admission and pharmacological detoxification. This is a realistic goal in the highly motivated girl.

The dose of oral methadone to suppress withdrawal symptoms is carefully established. The mother is observed after taking 20 ml of methadone mixture (1 mg in 1 ml). A drowsy patient suggests the dose is too high; if withdrawal symptoms return within 8–10 h it is too low. Over the next 2–3 weeks, methadone is gradually withdrawn. Poor sleep may be a major problem during withdrawal, a symptom which persists for some weeks. Some mothers improve their sleep by practising relaxation exercises; drugs should not be used to treat their insomnia. Emphasis must be placed on supportive therapy during drug withdrawal. Unfortunately, not all pregnant addicts consent to detoxification. Reluctantly, the psychiatrist will agree to methadone maintenance therapy, fully aware of the dangers which will face the fetus and neonate.

(2) *Methadone maintenance.* Treatment can be arranged on an outpatient basis, if the mother refuses admission. The narcotic addict who uses drugs intravenously has a genuine, if exaggerated, fear of withdrawal symptoms. She will also miss 'the needle'. In outpatients, the dose of methadone mixture required to suppress withdrawal symptoms is more difficult to gauge. The patient, who anticipates that her demands will be trimmed down, tends to exaggerate her normal requirement. Her psychiatrist, battle-hardened and with a modicum of intuition, has to make an informed guess at the patient's daily methadone dosage. Methadone mixture 1 mg in 1 ml, 20–40 ml/day is a common dose. The woman who goes into labour taking 20 mg methadone daily will experience abstinence symptoms, unless the drug is continued during labour and in the puerperium. The infant may also be adversely affected (see page 116).

(3) *Supportive therapy.* Regular supportive interviews with the patient on maintenance therapy are used to guide the woman away from her drug-oriented life-style. Once mutual trust has been established, it may be possible to convert her treatment from methadone maintenance to a slow withdrawal regimen as an outpatient. The period on a stable dose is followed by a gradual reduction over 2–3 months.

Management in the third trimester
A patient who remains on injectable narcotic drugs throughout her pregnancy jeopardizes the life of her unborn child. Even at a late stage she must be persuaded to renounce the needle and take drugs by mouth. Dose reduction is not encouraged, as this may affect the fetus adversely.

THE FUTURE OF MOTHER AND BABY

The ex-heroin addict or the mother on methadone maintenance can usually be trusted to care for her own baby. In the unit at Charing Cross Hospital, mothers and their babies have been followed up regularly over a number of years. The children make good progress and appear to thrive in the relaxed atmosphere provided for them. A crisis in the mother's life or a relapse into illicit drug use can occur. It is often only a temporary problem. In general, we have been greatly encouraged by the ability of some mothers to rear their young successfully. Tylden (1973) reports a contrary experience.

OTHER NARCOTIC DRUGS OF MISUSE

Following break-ins at warehouses and drug stores, several other narcotic drugs have become available to the narcotic and polydrug abuser, such as (a) pethidine (meperidine), (b) dextropropoxyphene (propoxyphene) and (c) dipipanone (pipadine).

Since 1975, dipipanone has been particularly popular among addicts in the UK, where the drug is marketed with the antiemetic cyclizine as Diconal. Many young women obtained these tablets from their family doctors who were unaware of the potential misuse of this preparation. Typically, the youngster would present late, just before closing time, complaining of backache, to wheedle a prescription out of the tired doctor. The dipipanone tablets, obtained by deception, were then crushed and injected intravenously. In the pregnant girl, the problems created by the misuse of Diconal and the other opioids are similar to those encountered in heroin addiction (see page 111).

OPIOID ANTAGONISTS

(1) *Pentazocine* (*Fortral*). This drug is not often used by narcotic addicts as it may precipitate both withdrawal symptoms and hallucinatory experiences in susceptible individuals. Pentazocine dependence is occasionally seen.

(2) *Buprenorphine* (*Temgesic*). A partial agonist and antagonist. Experience with this drug is still limited.

Sedatives including alcohol

The abuse of many non-opioid sedatives, including alcohol, may lead to states of intoxication and dependence. Abrupt withdrawal of the drug is followed by an abstinence syndrome. Physical dependence in the mother exposes the fetus and neonate to the hazards of an acute withdrawal state. The expectant mother often conceals her drug use. An epileptic fit may be the first evidence.

Most sedatives depress rapid eye movement (REM) sleep. This may return to normal as tolerance develops. On withdrawal, a rebound effect occurs, leading to a marked increase in REM sleep. This is associated with vivid dreams and nightmares. The patient cannot tolerate this disturbed sleep, asks for more drugs and thus establishes a vicious circle.

Sedatives are generally metabolized in the liver, where they induce microsomal enzyme-oxidizing systems. In this way, cross-tolerance may develop, a factor of importance when medication and alcohol are taken regularly.

BARBITURATES

The illicit use of barbiturates by young women is usually one aspect of polydrug abuse. The narcotic-dependent girl may substitute large doses of barbiturates for heroin if her drug of first choice is not available on the black market. Occasionally, a barbiturate is the preferred drug. The former dangerous practice of intravenous barbiturate use is now seldom seen.

Clinical features

The patient may be seen in a quiet, contented state with drooping eyelids and a glassy stare. Concentration and attention are ill-sustained. Her judgement is poor and, as she becomes more drowsy, her speech slurs and she becomes ataxic. Large doses may lead to coma and death. Illicit barbiturate use at the time of confinement will expose the mother to an abstinence syndrome indistinguishable from the confusional state which characterizes alcohol withdrawal (delirium tremens).

Management of mother
(1) *Admission to hospital* is mandatory, since barbiturate withdrawal may lead to status epilepticus. (2) *drug treatment* initially is pentobarbitone 200–400 mg 4–6 hourly to suppress withdrawal symptoms. This dose may be reduced by 100 mg daily. The patient will be weaned off the drug in 2–3 weeks. (3) *Supportive therapy* – after discharge from hospital, the expectant mother will need regular supervision to support her in the resolve to stay abstinent.

Effect on the fetus
Regular use and abuse of barbiturates carries an increased risk of fetal malformation. The abnormalities described include neural tube defects, hare-lip and congenital dislocation of the hip.

Effect on the neonate
Unlike the infant born to a narcotic-dependent mother, this baby usually has a high Apgar score at birth and is of normal weight. During intra-uterine life, barbiturates stimulate fetal liver microsomal enzyme systems. As a consequence, bilirubin conjugation is accelerated and physiological jaundice is rare in these infants. For the first 3–7 days of life, they appear to progress normally. This may prove to be dangerously misleading, as the baby could be sent home before the withdrawal symptoms have had time to develop (Desmond *et al.*, 1972). It is suggested that functional immaturity of the neonatal hepatic and renal systems may hinder drug excretion and delay the onset of withdrawal symptoms. *Acute symptoms* include hyperactivity, hyperacusis, shrill cry, tremors, sleeplessness, hypertonus and hyperphagia. *Subsequent symptoms*, in a less acute form, may persist for some weeks. These babies have a low threshold to stimuli and sleep only for short periods. They are more hungry than ordinary infants.

Management. The baby should be nursed in quiet surroundings, with frequent feeding and mild sedative drugs.

BENZODIAZEPINES
It is not always appreciated that the use of these drugs may promote tolerance, abuse and physical dependence. Oswald and Priest (1965) have shown that benzodiazepines, like barbiturates, depress REM sleep. On sudden withdrawal of the drug, a compensatory increase in paradoxical sleep occurs. This is associated with vivid dreams and nightmares. The abstinence syndrome in the mother is milder but similar to that of sudden barbiturate withdrawal.

Effect on the fetus
Diazepam may increase the risk of hare-lip and cleft palate, but this is uncertain.

Effect on the neonate
In the newborn, two syndromes have been described: (1) *an acute withdrawal syndrome*, indistinguishable from narcotic withdrawal states – the onset may be delayed by up to 3 days and residual effects may last several months (Hill and Stern, 1979); (2) *hypotonia*, hypothermia, respiratory depression and anorexia (Forfar, 1981).

MEPROBAMATE

Physical dependence on meprobamate may develop if the daily dose exceeds 1 g. The drug has come under suspicion as a possible teratogen (Forfar, 1981). In most respects meprobamate behaves like other sedatives. Perhaps there are no reports of withdrawal symptoms in the neonate because the drug has lost some of its popularity.

METHAQUALONE

In the UK this drug is no longer marketed in a combination with the antihistamine diphenhydramine (Mandrax). The latter was a common sedative drug of abuse.

ALCOHOL

Alcohol dependence, once believed to be the prerogative of the male, is showing an alarming increase in women. This syndrome, classically affecting women of middle age, is now seen in younger patients. The obstetrician will meet this problem with increasing frequency.

Boys and girls start drinking in adolescence. Women have a poor head for alcohol and tend to become dependent on a lower dose and after a shorter period of heavy drinking than men.

The patient accustomed to high blood alcohol concentrations may show abstinence symptoms as that level falls, even though she is still drinking. Sudden withdrawal may lead to a confusional state (delirium) (see page 130).

Effect on the fetus
Alcohol passes the placenta freely with serious consequences for the fetus. Persistent heavy drinking increases the risk of fetal malformation. Hare-lip, limb, cardiac and visceral abnormalities have been described. The clustering of major malformations with microcephaly, typical facial stigmata, low birth weight and slow post-natal growth have been described by Jones *et al.* (1973) as 'the fetal alcohol syndrome'.

Effect on the neonate
Alcohol withdrawal symptoms may occur in the neonate born to a mother abusing alcohol until delivery. The infant may be irritable, tremulous and have feeding difficulties.

Stimulants

AMPHETAMINES

The potential for abuse of this group of drugs is now widely recognized. Amphetamines are no longer prescribed to help the overweight woman to reach her ideal weight nor to treat her depression; hence, therapeutic dependence is rare.

The addict usually obtains the drug by illegal means. Tolerance develops quickly. Very large doses may be used orally or by intravenous injection.

Clinical features
The pregnant woman abusing amphetamines will be cheerful, energetic and managing on little sleep. Her appetite is depressed and as a result she is likely to be in a state of poor nutrition. She may carry a baby small for her dates. A consistently raised blood pressure may give rise to diagnostic difficulties if the misuse of

amphetamines is not suspected. Falling blood levels of the drug are associated with a depressed mood, lethargy and increased appetite. In this 'down phase' the patient may be verbally aggressive and difficult to handle. The increase in REM sleep, observed after amphetamine withdrawal, supports the view that the patient's symptoms are due to an abstinence syndrome. The problems encountered during the withdrawal phase are seldom serious.

Effect on the fetus
Amphetamines are probably teratogenic (Forfar, 1981). The abnormalities which have been described involve the urogenital and cardiovascular systems. The risk of hare-lip and limb deformities is increased.

Management
It is not appropriate to prescribe amphetamines for withdrawal symptoms. Referral for psychiatric assessment is a wise precaution, as amphetamine abuse can give rise to serious psychiatric disturbances.

COCAINE

Cocaine may be sniffed or taken orally for its stimulant effect. The narcotic-dependent woman may add cocaine to her usual intravenous narcotic 'fix'. The problems encountered are similar to those of amphetamine abuse.

Hallucinogens

LYSERGIC ACID DIETHYLAMIDE (LSD)

Most of the comments about LSD are also true of other hallucinogens. LSD is derived from ergot. These substances tend to be taken by polydrug users for the pleasure they derive from the potential psychedelic effect. LSD is taken in very small doses; 200 µg will produce a reaction. It is rapidly metabolized by the liver, leaving little evidence in its wake. A great variety of sensations and experiences are described. The users are unable to anticipate their subjective experience and discuss both good and bad 'trips'.

LSD does not lead to physical dependence. Its effects are autonomic, sensory and emotional. The autonomic response is mainly sympathomimetic. The sensory responses are perceived as alterations in the quality and intensity of normal sights, sounds and smells, or may be diminished to the point where the subject feels detached and unreal. The emotional experience can vary from ecstasy to terror and is, to some extent, dependent on the user's mental state. LSD users may describe 'flashbacks', in which a previous, often unpleasant, LSD experience recurs, even though they have had not further exposure to the drug. LSD can precipitate a schizophrenic illness in the constitutionally predisposed. The genetic dangers are very real. *In vitro*, LSD has been shown to cause breakages in chromosomes which pose a theoretical risk of congenital abnormality.

CANNABIS

This differs from other drugs under discussion as the resin of cannabis, produced in the flowering tops of the plant, is a mixture of substances. The most important active constituent is tetrahydrocannabinol. Marijuana is prepared from the dried plant and contains other plant material mixed with resin. Hashish is stronger, the resin being more concentrated. Cannabis, in its many different forms, may be smoked occasionally, regularly or be used as part of the polydrug addict's armamentarium.

The pharmacological properties do not give rise to concern in the occasional users. Heavy regular use, however, may lead to an unrealistic attitude to life. This may express itself as profound lethargy. Ante-natal appointments, like most other commitments, are liable to be ignored.

Reports of cerebral atrophy in heavy cannabis users have not been substantiated, nor is there conclusive evidence of chromosome damage (Matsuyama and Jarvik, 1977). Work on animal models suggests a teratogenic potential, but there are no studies in man which confirm an untoward effect on the fetus.

Tobacco

Infants born to mothers who smoke regularly have cord-blood carboxyhaemoglobin concentrations of 2–10% (Hill and Stern, 1979). The risk of prematurity, stillbirth and neonatal death are considerably increased and are directly related to the number of cigarettes smoked.

There is a clear relationship between smoking and low birth weight. At delivery, a low Apgar score is usually noted. More sinister still are the findings from the Davie, Butler and Goldstein (1972) study that the low birth weight is followed by a persistent lag in growth. This physical deficit is associated with lower intellectual attainments.

Depressive illness

The obstetrician, in the course of his career, will see many patients who complain of feeling depressed. Unhappiness and despair are appropriate reactions to frustration and loss. The misery is understood by both patient and doctor. Family and friends rally round to support the patient. Usually she adapts to the new situation, and her distress resolves. It is only when her personality resources are very limited that this normal reaction to adversity comes to medical attention. It is very important to distinguish the stage of simple unhappiness from a depressive illness. The patient suffering from a depressive illness shows a general reduction in her capacity to function normally. Early diagnosis is important, as untreated the patient suffers much unnecessary distress and cannot fulfil her normal role in the family. Although not a common problem during pregnancy, depressive illness carries some risk of suicide. In practice, the clinical presentation of the depressed patient is variable.

Psychiatrists over the past 50 years have been debating the classification of depression. Their deliberations have been most ably reviewed by Kendell (1976). In obstetrics, the classification by Pollitt (1978) into psychological and physiological depression offers practical guidance. Being based on biological principles, it points naturally to the appropriate treatment.

Psychological depression

This is characterized by an abnormally prolonged reaction to unfavourable life-events.

ÆTIOLOGY

Predisposition
An immature personality.

Precipitating factors
These include:

1. *Frustrations.* At work or caring for an elderly relative.
2. *Losses.* Include bereavement, loss of paramour, redundancy, loss of status through unemployment or leaving a familiar setting for a new environment.
3. *Persistent adverse social conditions.* Include inadequate housing or no home at all, debts and low income.
4. *Psychosocial factors.* The socially disadvantaged state of women, their helplessness and their dependence may contribute to the higher rate of depression in the female. Marriage would appear to protect the mental health of men, but seems detrimental to their wives.
5. *Marital difficulties.* Factors, such as those listed above, either operating singly or in combination, may lead to psychological depression.

CLINICAL FEATURES

The patient complains of misery and depression. A gloomy mood dominates the picture. Characteristically, the patient communicates her distress to those around her and may resort to impulsive behaviour. Suicidal threats or attempts may be made to elicit help.

MANAGEMENT

(a) Regular support from a social worker may be all that is required; (b) modification of the environment, where possible eliminating those factors which led to her depression, may be helpful; (c) a mild night sedative, prescribed for a few nights only, should restore sleep. Refreshed, the patient will be more able to adapt to her circumstances.

CASE HISTORY

Mrs P., 20 years old, was an only child and rather spoilt. Her father tended to be conspicuous by his frequent absences on business travel. Often he would return bearing exotic presents for his daughter, who learned to associate father's reappearance with interesting gifts. Mother had difficulty in displaying any real affection towards her daughter who nevertheless continued to hold her in esteem, until adolescence was to open her eyes. At that point, mother slipped from her imaginary pedestal, never to be reinstated. Father, on the other hand, continued to be idolized, mainly from afar. At school she proved to be popular neither with her contemporaries nor the staff. Academically, she might have done quite well, but failed to reach her potential. After leaving school she lived in a superficial social whirl. Physically attractive and well groomed she readily found partners at the many parties she attended. Relationships formed in this manner always proved to be short-lived. She succeeded easily in avoiding the sexual experience she dreaded.

She met her future husband, a man 12 years her senior, while on holiday. They married, and she seemed to find happiness in the challenge and excitement of matrimony. Her mature and benevolent husband allowed her to ignore their sexual difficulties. Much to their surprise, Mrs P. conceived almost at once. The baby had not been planned. From the very first she found it difficult to come to terms with her pregnancy. While battling against her lack of maternal feelings, she was struck a cruel blow: her father died quite unexpectedly.

Mrs P. found herself unable to accept her loss. She became depressed and cried a great deal. No longer did she take pride in her appearance or their home and spent most of the day in bed. Unable to cope with life, she asked for her pregnancy to be terminated. This request was strenuously resisted by her husband, an attitude Mrs P. simply could not comprehend. After all, father used to satisfy every wish. She persisted with her demand for an abortion on psychological grounds. An experienced obstetrician recognized her depressive illness and arranged a psychiatric assessment. Psychotherapy was recommended. It was fortunate that Mrs P. was able to relate to her therapist, in whom she saw a father-figure. After several interviews with him she recovered her composure and was soon able to resume her normal activities. In due course, the baby arrived. The pleasure and excitement surrounding the successful birth of her daughter did not last. When called upon to take charge of the baby she tearfully protested that she was too exhausted. In order to prevent a recurrence of her depression, her husband wisely solved the immediate problem by engaging a nurse to care for the baby.

COMMENT

An emotionally deprived childhood may impede the development of a mature personality. The case history describes such a patient with personal and sexual difficulties. Unaccustomed to adversity, she could not adapt to life without her father. Unable to grieve appropriately, she developed a psychological depression.

Physiological depression

This is the severer form of depression. The illness is associated with a disturbance of normal homeostatic processes, which leads to the physiological abnormalities characterizing the disorder (see page 123). In the young woman, loss of energy and drive may be the presenting symptoms. Her thinking often revolves around the belief that she has been a failure as a wife and mother, but in the younger person these thoughts rarely reach delusional strength. It is curious that in this severe depressive illness the mood disturbance itself may not be profound, and the patient may be more distressed by the anxiety, phobias or somatic symptoms.

The woman who presents without an overt mood disturbance and is able to hide her distress under a smiling facade may be misdiagnosed. To avoid this pitfall the physician must elicit the existence of the physiological disturbances by direct questions (see page 123).

AETIOLOGY

Predisposition
1. *Genetic factors.* It is generally accepted that heredity is an important factor. A possible X-linked pattern of inheritance has been postulated, but remains speculative.

ifluence of gender. Women are more prone to develop depressive illness, at :ast in the setting of the Western world.

The over-conscientious personality. The patient with a strict upbringing, who has learned always to consider others, tends to inhibit her own emotions. She is thus more likely than others to develop a depression.

Precipitating factors

1. *Biochemical aspects.* The catecholamine hypothesis has gained ground and offers a biological explanation. At first, a relative deficit of one or more neurotransmitters at specific central synapses was thought to be the complete answer. Further work suggests that catecholamines, indole amines and adrenergic–cholinergic systems may all be involved.
2. *Psychological stress.* This may also trigger a physiological depression. Characteristically, the illness will progress under its own momentum, even when the stress has been eliminated.
3. *Hormonal influence.* The incidence of depression in women is increased at times of hormonal change. The premenstrual and puerperal times are typical examples. Some patients are sensitive to the depressant effect of the 'pill'. The menopause is also a possible contender, but more controversially so (see Chapter 8). Depression following major surgery points to the possibility of a 'hormonal stress' factor. Myxoedema and Cushing's syndrome are further examples. However, no clear relationship to hormonal change at the cellular level has been demonstrated.
4. *Viral infections.* Influenza, glandular fever and hepatitis are common precipitants.
5. *Drugs.* Reserpine, which depletes brain amines, is fortunately seldom used nowadays for the treatment of hypertension or pre-eclampsia. Systemic steroids are offered frequently. Chlorpromazine and its depot preparations are less well known for their depressive effects. Rarer still, and even less well documented, are some antibiotics.
6. *Weight loss.* Depression may be precipitated by an over-zealous weight-reducing regimen.
7. *Time zone trauma.* Jet-lag may predispose to physiological depression.
8. *No known precipitant.* This represents the largest group of patients.

CLINICAL PRESENTATION

Experience suggests that this type of depression is quite common during pregnancy. A typical letter of referral may commence: 'Mrs X broke down and cried during her ante-natal interview . . . . I am surprised, since she has always appeared composed and competent before . . . .' Occasionally, the patient presents with unexplained physical symptoms mimicking organic disease. More commonly she complains of being unable to cope with her responsibilities. Often, the patient herself has searched in vain for a possible cause. This further increases her unhappiness. 'I have everything going in my favour. I wanted the baby so much, and now I cannot cope. I try to pull myself together, but I just cannot get the work done. If the door bell or the phone rings, I panic, I just don't want to see friends. When my husband comes home in the evening I feel a little better, but even he means less to me than he should.' The patient is perplexed by her symptoms, particularly if she does not feel particularly low in mood.

CLINICAL FEATURES

Mood change
This is intense and prolonged, colouring the patient's whole existence. She may be quite unable to display emotion, as shown by loss of facial expression.

Altered activity
Her normal energy may be replaced by lethargy and lack of sexual drive. This results in neglect of social interaction and withdrawal from the mainstream of life. Profound retardation or, on occasion, overactivity and agitation may occur.

Depressive thought content
The patient views her life – past, present and future – through very dark spectacles. She can only recall her failures. It is not surprising that these sombre thoughts may attain a delusional quality. Preoccupation with these unpleasant ideas leads to loss of interest and lack of concentration.

Delusions
These tend to be of guilt or unworthiness.

Somatic complaints
These are common and may be the presenting symptoms.

Physiological changes
(a) *Specific rhythm disturbances.* The patient feels at her worst in the mornings and improves a little as the day advances. (b) *Sleep disturbance.* This is characterized by early morning waking after a fitful night. The patient wakes tired and distressed. (c) *Autonomic disturbance.* Hypotension, bradycardia and hypothermia are common. Diminished peristalsis results in constipation. Loss of appetite may lead to lack of appropriate weight gain. A dry mouth may be particularly troublesome. (d) *Disturbance of metabolism.* This may involve electrolytes, cholesterol and the basal metabolic rate. (e) *Hormonal change.* May partially explain the loss of libido.

MANAGEMENT

The patient's full co-operation is essential for successful treatment.

Simple explanation
A discussion of the physiological nature of the disturbance, the precipitating factors, excellent prognosis and available treatment will help the patient to establish a good therapeutic relationship with her doctor. Without a sound rapport, a patient who blames herself for her illness is unable to accept medical advice.

Drug therapy
The need for drug therapy must be explained thoroughly and weighed against any theoretical risk to the fetus. It is important to stress (a) that the drug must be taken regularly to achieve adequate blood levels, and (b) that 2–3 weeks may elapse before beneficial effects become evident. Otherwise the patient may abandon her treatment prematurely, especially when troubled by undesirable side effects.

A tricyclic antidepressant drug like amitriptyline (see page 135) may be used. A common therapeutic dose lies between 150 and 200 mg/day. The drug is given in d doses. The largest dose, perhaps 75 mg, is given at night, as it has a marked ve action. Side effects are less troublesome if treatment is started on a lower building up to a therapeutic level. A patient whose dominant symptoms include lethargy and lack of drive may respond better to a monoamine oxidase inhibitor (MAOI). Phenelzine 15–30 mg 2–3 times daily or isocarboxazid 10–20 mg 3 times daily may prove effective. MAOIs should not be taken after 1600 hours (4 p.m.), to avoid wakefulness at night.

If treatment is successful, the patient will be much improved in 3–4 weeks. The initiation of antidepressant therapy provides few problems. The skill of managing the patient's illness lies in knowing when to reduce the dose and stop treatment. It is accepted generally that tricyclics as well as MAOIs should be continued for 2–3 months after the patient is symptom-free. Withdrawal of the drug should be gradual. The drug treatment of depression is dealt with more fully on page 135.

Electroconvulsive therapy (ECT).

If drug therapy does not control symptoms in 2–3 weeks, or should the patient admit to active suicidal intent, shock therapy is indicated. ECT poses only a negligible risk to the fetus. The anaesthetist will take special care to oxygenate the patient fully prior to and after the fit. The convulsion is modified by the intravenous administration of suxamethonium bromide, a depolarizing short-acting muscle relaxant. Good muscular relaxation is particularly important between the 8th to 16th weeks of gestation. The view of Trethowan (1979) is that ECT in pregnancy is safer than medication.

Assessment of suicide risks

Suicide in pregnancy is rare, but each patient must be assessed carefully for any potential risk.

CASE HISTORY

Mrs C, aged 31, was a trained nurse. She had reached the 26th week of her pregnancy when she attended for a routine examination. She complained of early morning headaches since an attack of influenza some 3 weeks previously, which had not responded to analgesics. At an attempt by the obstetrician to elicit further details, Mrs C. dissolved into tears. Her obstetrician was concerned, as she had been known to him as a healthy, calm and conscientious colleague. She was referred the same day for psychiatric assessment.

Mrs C. was distressed, as she could not understand why headaches incapacitated her so severely. For the last 4 days she had slept fitfully, and woken exhausted at 0400 hours (4 a.m.) and had dreaded the next day. Every task became a chore. She felt slowed down and irritable, had lost her appetite and was concerned that her weight had not increased over the previous 2 months. Normally an active and creative person, she found herself sitting in a chair doing nothing. Although feeling better towards the evenings and managing to cook a meal, she blamed herself for neglecting her responsibilities. The history revealed that her father suffered from recurrent depressive episodes.

COMMENT

The history illustrates several features of physiological depression. Presenting symptoms of headache and lethargy were associated with a disturbance of normal homeostatic mechanisms. Sleep, appetite and weight were affected and the diurnal emphasis of symptoms was noted. A positive family history, the recent virus infection and her conscientious personality may be regarded as precipitating or contributing factors.

Drug treatment with MAOIs proved effective. Medication was gradually withdrawn 1 month after symptomatic relief, before the onset of labour.

Recurrent forms of depressive illness

These may occur at predictable times of the year or be quite irregularly spaced, with freedom from attack for several years (unipolar affective disorder). Alternatively, depressive episodes alternating with manic or hypomanic attacks may happen at different times (bipolar affective disorder).

Mania and hypomania

Mania is usually brought to the attention of the doctor by a distraught relative or friend. The patient herself does not seek medical advice. She is delighted with her state of elation. Hypomania is the term used for the less dramatic forms of mania.

CLINICAL FEATURES

Mood and behaviour
Early in the illness increased self-confidence, boundless energy and a buoyant mood dominate the picture, provided the sufferer's every whim is granted. If she is crossed, her infectious gaiety may change very suddenly to irritability, anger and verbal abuse. Haughtiness may similarly change to open hostility. Money is spent freely, but not wisely. One patient returned from a shopping trip with 21 different hats. Casual sexual affairs add to the general confusion.

Thought and speech
In mania there is characteristic pressure of thought and speech. Ideas rapidly overtake one another. The listener is able to recognize only a tenuous connection between the many ideas expressed in rapid succession. 'Clang association' may be noted: 'Good, goody its godly'. Grandiose ideas progress to delusions which often bear religious overtones.

Psychomotor activity
Constructive overactivity is soon replaced by purposeless commotion, as projects proliferate. The patient starts one task after another, but is quickly distracted – nothing is completed. Her room is a spectacle of total disarray.

Untreated, the patient finds progressively less time to eat or sleep; finally, exhaustion supervenes. As the illness progresses, it may prove difficult to differentiate the psychotic features of mania from schizophrenia. Much reliance must be placed on the chronological unfolding of events, as reported by members of her immediate circle.

MANAGEMENT

In the pregnant state early diagnosis and treatment is particularly important. Untreated, the illness would compromise the health of both mother and fetus.

Admission to hospital
This is required for most patients, even against their wishes.

Drug treatment
Treatment with lithium carbonate is effective in about 75% of patients, but full benefits are not seen for the first 7–10 days. The drug was first used in 1949 prior to the discovery of chlorpromazine. Johnson, Gershon and Hekimian (1968) conducted a controlled study of 28 manic patients. They compared chlorpromazine in doses of 200–1800 mg daily with lithium carbonate in amounts sufficient to maintain the serum lithium concentration at 1.0 mmol/l or greater. Complete control of symptoms was obtained in 78% of cases treated with lithium as against 36% of those treated with chlorpromazine. Patients prefer treatment with lithium, as it leaves them more alert and free from anticholinergic side effects. For the effect of lithium on the fetus and special problems of lithium therapy, see page 140.

Twenty to thirty per cent of patients do not respond to lithium, or are too disturbed to await the onset of its beneficial effects. In these patients chlorpromazine may be substituted or used in conjunction. Pimozide, with a maximum dose of 32 mg daily, has also been used successfully in the treatment of mania (Cookson, Silverstone and Wells, 1979). This drug causes less drowsiness than does chlorpromazine, but it is slower to show its beneficial effects. Further details of neuroleptic drugs are given in *Table 5.1*.

Insomnia

As the end of pregnancy approaches, many women sleep badly. It is important to enquire into this aspect of their well-being, as there may be no spontaneous complaint. A sleep deficit can very easily build-up. A tired mother would find the demands of labour and subsequent infant care unduly stressful. The cause of her insomnia needs careful evaluation. It is necessary to establish her actual sleep pattern; has she difficulty in getting to sleep because she is anxious? Does she wake frequently because the fetus is too lively, or because of physical discomfort? Early morning waking may be the first symptom of a depressive illness (see page 123).

MANAGEMENT

General measures
A well-ventilated, adequately heated room, a bed-board under the mattress, extra pillows and a hot drink from a vacuum flask may all be helpful.

Tape recorded relaxation exercises
These may help the tense or anxious patient to fall asleep without the use of drugs.

Drug therapy (see page 141).

Schizophrenia

Schizophrenia is characterized by defects in thinking, mood, perception and feeling. Interpersonal relationships are disturbed. Schizophrenia remains the most serious psychiatric illness, with a lifetime expectancy of 0.9% in the general

TABLE 5.1. Major tranquillizers

	Phenothiazines			Thioxanthenes	Butyrophenones
	Aliphatic compound	Piperazine compound	Piperidine compound		
For oral administration	1. Chlorpromazine (Largactil) in divided doses 100–800 mg/day 2. Promazine hydrochloride (Sparine) 75–500 mg/day	Trifluoperazine (Stelazine) in divided doses 5–50 mg/day	Thioridazine hydrochloride (Melleril)* 30–100 mg/day increasing to 150–600 mg/day in divided doses	Not suitable	1. Haloperidol (Serenace) in divided doses 1.5–40 mg/day 2. Pimozide* (Orap) 2–10 mg/day
For i.m. and i.v. use	Chlorpromazine 100–150 mg i.m.	Trifluoperazine 1–3 mg i.m.	—	—	Haloperidol 10–30 mg i.v.
Depot preparation	—	Fluphenazine (Modecate) 25–75 mg i.m. every 2–4 weeks	Pipothiazine (Piportil) 50–200 mg i.m. every 4 weeks	Flupenthixol (Depixol) 20–100 mg i.m. every 2–4 weeks	—
Extrapyramidal side effects	++	+++	+	+	++++
Drowsiness	+++	+	+	0	++
Endocrine dysfunction	++	+	++	+	+
Oedema and weight gain	+++	++	++	0	0
Toxicity Cardiac	++	+	++	0	+
Liver	+++	+	+	0	+
Blood	++	+	++	0	+
Anticholinergic side effects	++	+	+	0	+
Photosensitivity	++	0	+	0	0–+
Pigmentary retinopathy	0	0	+	0	0
Altered seizure control	++	+	rare +	0–+	0–+

* Drug not used in pregnancy

population. The introduction of neuroleptic drugs (see page 133) in the 1950s has led to successful treatment. Patients are now discharged after a short stay in hospital and treatment is continued within the community. This policy has led to an increase in the number of pregnant women on maintenance therapy (for details see page 133). These mothers commonly remain well during their pregnancy (Baker, 1967). Mothers with a past history of schizophrenia or suffering only from minor disability appear to be protected from relapse by their pregnancy. Post-partum recrudescence will be met more frequently.

Special problems of a patient with a history of schizophrenia

The patient who has recently recovered from a schizophrenic illness remains vulnerable. She may be remote and aloof. Her natural shyness and undemanding behaviour allow her to fade into the background. The attitude of the ante-natal clinical staff is crucial to the patient's well-being. From her very first clinic attendance the staff should be alerted to the patient's needs. A special effort on their part may be required to gain her confidence. The mother who prefers solitary pursuits will need extra encouragement to join the organized activities which are available, such as parenthood classes and relaxation groups. The patient's tendency to remain aloof, as already noted, is likely to be reflected in her marriage. Her husband becomes accustomed to a distant relationship with his wife. Thus she may be deprived of his interest and involvement in her preparation for childbirth. He may remain uninterested and unconcerned, unless actively encouraged to be more supportive.

Diagnostic difficulties

Psychiatrists differ in their diagnostic criteria for schizophrenia. Variation is most marked at an international level. The reliability of their diagnosis has fluctuated from 50–60% in a US–UK study, using prepared cinematic records (Sandifer *et al.*, 1968), to 92% correspondence when a standardized, structured interview was used by psychiatrists with a common training (Wing *et al.*, 1967).

CLINICAL FEATURES

The first episode of the illness may occur from the mid-teens onwards. The onset may be acute and florid, or slow and insidious. The following history will demonstrate some important clinical features of schizophrenia.

CASE HISTORY

Mrs S. aged 29 years, was a housewife, 26 weeks into her first pregnancy. She had a past history of schizophrenia and had been discharged from a psychiatric hospital on maintenance therapy.

Present complaint
In the course of a few days she had become withdrawn. She seemed perplexed and unable to cope with her routine responsibilities, complaining 'I am in a muddle'. Mrs S. had also stopped decorating the baby's nursery, a task that had given her much pleasure the previous week. Two restless nights with little sleep were

followed by refusal to eat. She would drink only black coffee, advising her husband to do likewise, believing that the milkman had left poisoned milk. Noting these symptoms the husband came to the conclusion that all was not well.

Personal and social history
This was unremarkable except for a persistent pattern of social withdrawal.

Past health
This had been good. The schizophrenic illness had been her only set-back. Since her previous breakdown she had been on maintenance flupenthixol intramuscularly, 40 mg every 3 weeks. The drug had been stopped, perhaps rather unwisely, when the pregnancy was diagnosed.

Mental state examination
1. *General appearance and behaviour.* The patient looked dishevelled – she had not washed or combed her hair.
2. *Orientation.* She knew the time, date and place where she was interviewed.
3. *Mood.* She was miserable, with no evidence of flattening of mood or inappropriateness.
4. *Speech.* Her speech was hesitant, but relatively normal.
5. *Thought disorder.* Mrs S. was unable to focus on the important points of the conversation, demonstrating a formal thought disorder. She showed two other abnormalities of thinking: (a) thought-blocking – sudden cessation of her speech occurred in mid-sentence; (b) thought-withdrawal – 'My thoughts are just taken out of my head. That's why I can't think.'
6. *Delusions.* Mrs S. demonstrated her abnormal belief that the milkman had poisoned the milk, refusing food and drinking only black coffee.
7. *Hallucinations.* No evidence of abnormal perception could be demonstrated.

Management
1. *Hospital admission.* The patient readily agreed to be admitted to hospital.
2. *Case notes.* The case records of her past illness were traced and revealed useful information. Mrs S. had responded quickly to treatment with chlorpromazine and had been discharged on maintenance therapy. No evidence of personality deterioration was noted at that time.
3. *Drug therapy.* Mrs S. again responded to drug therapy. She had lost all her florid symptoms by the end of the first week. Intramuscular flupenthixol 40 mg was restarted and continued at 3-weekly intervals as maintenance therapy (see page 133).
4. *Occupational therapy and social activities.* Both these approaches helped Mrs S. to mix with other patients and to restore her rather limited self-confidence.
5. *Counselling.* (a) The patient – the importance of maintenance therapy was discussed and stressed. She was introduced to her health visitor and social worker, both of whom offered to visit her regularly after discharge. (b) The husband – initially he needed reassurance and advice. Prior to his wife's discharge from hospital we were able to discuss with him how he could give support, stressing the need for consistent but 'low key' involvement. (c) The couple – they were encouraged to accept that they need time to adjust to the new demands of parenthood and were advised to practise a suitable method of contraception.

Discussion
1. *Diagnosis*. The frequently difficult differential diagnosis of schizophrenia, as mentioned on page 128, is not relevant here. Mrs S. showed florid symptoms in the absence of disorientation and significant systemic disease.
2. *Prognosis*. The acute onset and dramatic symptoms carry a relatively good prognosis for the attack. Relapse may occur. The patient is particularly vulnerable post-partum. Recurrent attacks of schizophrenia tend to damage the personality. This deterioration may be aggravated with each succeeding recurrence. If marked, it may interfere with her ability to be an effective wife and mother. Her maternal feelings may be strong and she might daydream of a large family, but repeated pregnancies could be detrimental to the whole family unit and constitute an unacceptable risk.

Organic mental reactions

This group includes a number of different clinical syndromes, caused by damage to or temporary impairment of brain cells. The obstetrician is most likely to see a patient suffering from an acute confusional state (delirium).

Acute confusional state

This state is characterized by an altered and fluctuating level of awareness. Thinking, perception and memory are disturbed. The onset of the delirium is acute.

AETIOLOGY

The causes of acute confusional states are many and varied. The abrupt withdrawal of alcohol or of sedatives, the toxic effects of drugs, metabolic or endocrine disturbances, post-anaesthetic or postoperative complications, and serious infections, may all be underlying factors.

CLINICAL FEATURES

Clouding of consciousness leads to disorientation. The patient is unable to grasp and retain the impressions which normally allow her to judge the passage of time and her whereabouts. She may misidentify herself, her relatives and staff.

Delirium interferes with the patient's capacity for logical thought and speech. This facet of the illness makes it difficult for her to co-operate. Positive disturbances of perception occur in this setting. Illusions and hallucinations are common. The latter may be auditory, visual or tactile. The patient is often terror-stricken by the experience. Her sense of extreme fear may lead to precipitate inappropriate actions. She may run from the ward or jump through a window.

MANAGEMENT

Physical examination and investigation
The patient who presents in a delirium requires a complete physical examination and investigation to discover the cause. Treatment of the underlying pathological

process is started as soon as possible. Correction of any electrolyte imbalance is important. Avitaminosis will respond to an intravenous multivitamin preparation. Infection must be treated promptly.

Medication
Delirium can usually be controlled adequately with phenothiazine (see *Table 5.1*). If the patient is unable to take oral medication, chlorpromazine 50–100 mg may be given by deep intramuscular injection every 6–8 h. Should this dose cause hypotension, haloperidol 5–10 mg intravenously or intramuscularly may be substituted. Chlordiazepoxide 80–240 mg daily or chlormethiazole 2–6 g daily should be used only in the delirium of alcohol- or drug-induced withdrawal states. Such a seriously disturbed patient may need treatment by continuous infusion of chlormethiazole (see page 142).

Nursing
The patient should be nursed in well-lit surroundings, as sensory deprivation may enhance existing confusion and disorientation. Excessive noise is avoided by accommodating the patient in a quiet corner of the ward. A delirious patient ought not to be left alone. Ideally, the same special staff should be assigned to nurse the patient, who may be restless and terrified. She may lash about or fall out of bed. The obstetric nurse should be reminded of these very real dangers. Accidents can be forestalled by placing a mattress next to the patient's bed and by protecting any sharp corners with blankets.

Mental handicap

This is characterized by a deficiency of intellectual function from childhood. It ranges in its severe form from those who cannot care for themselves and are unable to lead independent lives, to others who are educationally subnormal and merge into the community at large. The obstetrician is likely to meet the less severely handicapped patient.

The stable girl of low intelligence

The patient may enjoy a relatively normal existence. Often she lives with her parents and either helps in the house or earns her own living. Her job will be limited to simple routine tasks. She is slow to learn a new routine, but once it is mastered she will carry it out quite reliably. Perhaps her low intelligence has never been diagnosed. As a child she may have attended an ordinary school. If her demeanour was acceptable she may have been able to pass her school years quietly and inconspicuously at the bottom of the lowest stream. Her reading and writing skills may be limited to a few short, simple words.

This woman's ante-natal care is not likely to pose special problems, provided due allowance is made for her learning difficulties. Indeed she may only come to particular notice through her inability to sign consent forms or to fill in the ever-increasing load of research questionnaires.

MANAGEMENT

Assessment
Her general behaviour and social competence are more important than her level of intelligence in determining how much support the patient requires.

Training
The patient's own mother may be willing to assist, or a period in a residential 'mother and baby unit', where she will be shown the routine of caring for an infant, may be helpful. Her own attempts of mothering will be supervised until she has mastered the necessary skills. This training may be sufficient for the patient to accept responsibility for her baby. Regular supervision would be essential, as this mother would not be able to cope with a crisis effectively, nor with any situation requiring a change in routine.

Birth control
Some method of birth control, which does not depend on patient co-operation, is desirable to prevent repeated, inappropriate pregnancies. An intrauterine device or sterilization might be considered. It is essential that the patient is able to understand the implications of the selected procedure and can give informed consent.

The unstable girl of low intelligence

The patient presents the obstetrician with a more serious problem. The girl may have been leading a nomadic, promiscuous existence and have failed to seek medical advice until labour is established. Poverty and ignorance may contribute to a poor nutritional state. Severe anaemia is not uncommon. Emotionally she is quite unprepared for the delivery or for the care of the infant. Before any plan for the future of mother and baby can be formulated, she may have absconded, abandoning her newborn infant. Adoption may then be the only practical answer to an intractable problem.

Psychotropic drugs in pregnancy

The thalidomide tragedy has firmly disposed of the belief that the placenta acts as an impregnable barrier which protects the fetus from harm. More recently, a further problem has become manifest. It has been shown that some drugs, harmless during fetal development, may exert their deleterious effect at a later stage. They may interfere with the functioning of fully-formed fetal organs late in pregnancy and even affect the neonate after birth (Forfar, 1981).

The human embryo is most sensitive to the teratogenic effects of drugs from the 2nd to 8th week of gestation, a time of differentiating structures and of organ formation. Therefore, drugs taken during this phase may cause fetal damage while the pregnancy is quite unsuspected.

In theory, this hazard could be diminished or even eliminated entirely if the importuning patient were resisted more firmly. This line of action may prove difficult with patients who expect a prescription for drugs to relieve every minor emotional discomfort. The mother-to-be should certainly be counselled against self-medication. General practitioners and specialists need to exercise special care when psychoactive drugs have to be prescribed to women of child-bearing age. However, the potential risk must be seen in perspective. The indications for drug therapy may be unequivocal. A patient suffering from schizophrenia requires medication whether she is pregnant or not. On the other hand, very often the indications for drug therapy are less clear. A compromise must then be reached to safeguard the mother's mental health without endangering the welfare of her developing baby. In the future, preconception clinics may become the primary source of guidance on these issues.

Major tranquillizers

The anti-psychotic drugs (major tranquillizers and neuroleptics) exert their action by interfering with dopaminergic pathways in the mesolimbic and mesocortical systems. The drugs are used to control the florid symptoms of schizophrenia, such as delusions, hallucinations and disturbed behaviour.

PHENOTHIAZINES (see also *Table 5.1*)

1. Aliphatic compounds: chlorpromazine (Largactil); promazine (Sparine).
2. Piperazine compounds: trifluperazine (Stelazine); fluphenazine (Modecate).
3. Piperidine compounds: thioridazine (Melleril); pipothiazine (Piportil).

THIOXANTHENES

Flupenthixol (Depixol; Fluanxol).

BUTYROPHENONES

Haloperidol (Serenace; Haldol).

DIPHENYLBUTYLPIPERIDINES

Pimozide (Orap).

Dosage
The dosage of these drugs is adjusted to suit individual requirements. Initially, large doses of phenothiazines are required to control florid symptoms. Many schizophrenic women stay surprisingly well during pregnancy. A gradual reduction of the maintenance dose may be attempted. However, the drug should not be discontinued, as the risk of relapse is high (see page 128). Most patients dislike taking phenothiazines, as they object to the many side effects, drowsiness in particular. Not surprisingly, patient compliance is poor. This has led to the development of long-acting intramuscular preparations, which is a welcome advance.

1. CHLORPROMAZINE
    (a) *Principal indications.* Schizophrenia; mania; acute confusional states.
    (b) *Dose.* 400–800 mg/day are required to control florid symptoms. Once this has been achieved, maintenance therapy on a much lower dose (100–200 mg/day) may be adequate.

2. PROMAZINE

(a) *Principal indications.* Control of agitation in: schizophrenia, mental handicap and hypomania (rarely).

(b) *Dose.* 75–500 mg/day.

3. TRIFLUPERAZINE

(a) *Principal indications.* This drug has an alerting action and may therefore be useful in a schizophrenic patient without florid symptoms.

(b) *Dose.* 5–50 mg/day.

4. FLUPHENAZINE. This depot preparation is given intramuscularly. A dose of 25–75 mg may be required every 2–4 weeks. Extrapyramidal side effects are common and may require the concomitant administration of antiparkinsonian drugs: (a) procyclidine (Kemadrin) 15–30 mg/day; (b) orphenadrine (Disipal) 50–150 mg/day.

5. FLUPENTHIXOL. The only thioxanthene in general use. Like fluphenazine, this depot preparation is given by intramuscular injection. The dose is tailored to the patient's needs. 20–100 mg may be given every 2–4 weeks to maintain remission. Extrapyramidal side effects are less troublesome than with fluphenazine.

6. HALOPERIDOL (HALDOL or SERENACE). A butyrophenone is a dopamine antagonist. It can be given orally or by injections.

(a) *Principal indications.* Schizophrenia; mania; acute confusional state.

(b) *Dose.* 1.5–40 mg/day orally.

(c) *Side effects.* Similar to phenothiazines. Extrapyramidal effects are more marked.

(d) *Effect on the fetus.* No abnormalities have been reported.

(e) *Effect on the neonate.* No adverse reports.

7. PIMOZIDE (ORAP)

(a) *Principal indications.* Schizophrenia; mania.

(b) *Dose.* 2–10 mg/day.

(c) *Side effects.* As for phenothiazines (see below).

Side effects of all major tranquillizers

Dopamine blockade of the nigro-striatal pathway leads to extrapyramidal side effects. Action on the tubero-infundibular axis results in an elevated plasma prolactin level.

1. *Extrapyramidal:* akathisia; dystonia; oculogyric crises –; tardive dyskinesia.
2. *Endocrine:* increase in serum prolactin; menstrual irregularities.
3. *Autonomic*
    (a) Anticholinergic: blurred vision; dry mouth; stuffy nose; retention of urine.
    (b) Sympathomimetic: hypotension.
4. *Central nervous system:* drowsiness.
5. *Drug interactions:* the effect of drugs which depress the central nervous system is potentiated, e.g. morphine, alcohol, anaesthetics, barbiturates.
6. *Dermatological:* photosensitization, causing skin eruptions.
7. *Haematological:* agranulocytosis (1 in 10 000).
8. *Hepatic:* cholestatic jaundice.

Antidepressants

All antidepressants increase the concentration of monoamine transmitter substances at the neuronal level in the central nervous system. They preserve brain amines from either destruction or reabsorption. The greater availability of amines raises the level of adenosine monophosphate (AMP) at the post-synaptic membrane. AMP facilitates neurotransmission. Antidepressants are believed to act selectively in conserving specific biogenic amines. There are no absolute contraindications to the use of antidepressants in pregnancy. Four main groups of drugs are in general use (*Table 5.2*):

1. Tricyclics.
2. Tetracyclics.
3. Monoamine oxidase inhibitors (MAOIs).
4. Others – nomifensine, L-tryptophan, etc.

1. TRICYCLICS. These drugs are structurally related to phenothiazines. They are thought to exert their action by preventing the reabsorption of transmitter substances from the neuronal cleft. Imipramine was the first drug of this group; since then, many others have been introduced. Clinically, they fall into three groups: (a) drugs with a marked sedative effect; (b) drugs with a more alerting action; (c) intermediate compounds.

   (a) Tricyclics with a marked sedative effect include: amitriptyline (Tryptizol) 75–200 mg/day; trimipramine (Surmontil) 50–150 mg/day; doxepin (Sinequan) 30–150 mg/day.

   (b) Tricyclics with an alerting action include: imipramine (Tofranil) 75–150 mg/day; nortriptyline (Aventyl) 75–150 mg/day.

   (c) Tricyclics of intermediate action include: dothiepin (Prothiaden) 75–150 mg/day; clomipramine (Anafranil) 30–150 mg/day; lofepramine (Gamanil). This drug has been introduced more recently. Lofepramine appears to be as effective as amitriptyline and has fewer autonomic side effects (Pugh *et al.*, 1982). Gokelma (1983) reported no significant effects on the heart. These findings suggest that lofepramine may prove to be clinically useful in the treatment of moderate to severe depression.

Principal indication
Physiological depression.

Dosage
Although average doses have been supplied in the text, marked variation in tolerance is encountered. It is a common failing to take insufficient care in the adjustment of the dose to individual need, which results in therapeutic failure. The dose may be too high or too low for maximum beneficial effect. Blood level estimations are helpful if difficulties arise. Most active drugs have some side effects; with tricyclics they can be minimized by starting treatment on a low dose. Sedative tricyclics are best prescribed in a single nightly dose. When they are used in this way, drowsiness is a positive benefit, as it will induce sleep. The onset of the antidepressant effect can be expected only after 1–4 weeks of regular, adequate treatment. All too often these drugs tend to be abandoned before the expected improvement could have occurred.

TABLE 5.2. Antidepressants

Drug	Dose	Anticholinergic side effects	Cardiovascular

TRICYCLIC		Dry mouth
		Constipation
		Blurred vision
		Glaucoma
		(Mild confusion)
		(Poor memory)
		(Possible drug
		interactions)
			Postural hypotension
			Alteration in cardiac
			conduction
			ECG:
			  Longer Q–T interval.
			  flattened T-wave;
			  quinidine-like effect,
			  AV conduction is
			  prolonged → heart block
			Arrhythmias

Imipramine (Tofranil)	25–50 mg t.d.s. Start 10 mg t.d.s.	+ +	+ +
Amitriptyline (Tryptizol)	Start 25 mg t.d.s. → 150 mg t.d.s. or 75–100 mg o.n.	+ + +	+ + +
Doxepin (Sinequan)	10–50 mg t.d.s.	+ +	0
Dothiepin (Prothiaden)	25–50 mg t.d.s. or 100 mg o.n.	+ +	+ +
Trimipramine (Surmontil)	50–100 mg o.n.	+ + +	+ +
Nortriptyline (Aventyl; Allegron)	25 mg t.d.s.	+ +	+ +
Clomipramine (Anafranil)	10–50 mg t.d.s. or 50 mg o.n.	+ + +	+ +
TETRACYCLIC Mianserin (Bolvidon; Norval)	10–20 mg t.d.s. or 40 mg o.n.	0	0
NEW COMPOUND Nomifensine (Merital)	Start 25 mg b.d.; raise to 50 mg t.d.s.	0	0
MAOIs			Orthostatic hypotension with no adaptation in time Dose-related anti-anginal effect. Oedema

Non-hydrazines:
  Tranylcypramine
  (Parnate)
	10–30 mg a.m. +
	10–30 mg mid-day
		+ +	+ +

+ 1 mg trifluoperazine = Parstelin	1–2 tablets a.m. + 1 tablet mid-day	+ +	+ +
Hydrazine derivatives: Phenelzine (Nardil)	15–30 mg, 2–3 times daily	+ +	+ +
Isocarboxazid (Marplan)	10–20 mg t.d.s.	+	+

Central nervous system	Metabolic/endocrine	Gastro-intestinal (due to anticholinergic effects)	Genito-urinary	Teratogenicity
Drowsiness Lightheadedness Confusional reaction of atropine type Fine tremor	Weight increase Craving for carbohydrates due to lowering of blood glucose	Constipation Hiatus hernia exacerbated Acid in stomach decreased	Increased bladder and sphincter tone	
0	–	++	++	+
+++	++	++	++	Isolated reports Reports in animals
++	?	+	0	Not known
+	+	++	++	Not known
+++	++	++	++	Not known
0	+	++	++	Not known
++	Raised prolactin	++	++	Not known
Drowsiness ++	Not known	0	0	Not known
+	0	0	0	Not known
Initial restlessness or hyperactivity Insomnia	Liver toxicity Hydrazine derivatives clinically like viral hepatitis	Interaction with foodstuffs – cheese, yeast extracts, sympathomimetic amines	+	May activate schizophrenic illness
+	++	+++	+	++
++	++	+++	+	++
++	+++	++	++	+
+	+++	++	0	0

Side effects
1. Cardiovascular system: conduction abnormalities in a damaged myocardium; postural hypotension.
2. Central nervous system: convulsions; epileptogenic threshold lowered.
3. Anticholinergic effects: constipation; blurred vision; urinary retention; dry mouth.
4. Hepatic: hepatitis occurs very rarely.

Effect on the fetus
No convincing evidence of teratogenicity has been found (Orgegozo and Loiseau, 1977).

Effect on the neonate
There are isolated reports of breathing difficulties, irritability and tachycardia in the infant, especially with imipramine (Forfar, 1981).

2. TETRACYCLICS. The main advantages over the tricyclics is a reduction in anticholinergic side effects, especially with mianserin. These drugs cause some drowsiness and are usually given in a single dose at night. Two drugs are in common use. Mianserin may cause leucopenia, and the white cell count should be monitored after 4–6 weeks. The drug is apparently low in cardiotoxicity. Maprotiline is similar to the tricyclics.

(a) Mianserin (Norval; Bolvidon) 30–150 mg/day.
(b) Maprotiline (Ludiomil) 25–150 mg/day.

Principal indication
Similar to tricyclic drugs.

Effect on the fetus
Hill and Stern (1979) report an increased risk of fetal malformations.

Effect on the neonate
No adverse effects have been reported.

3. MONOAMINE OXIDASE INHIBITORS (MAOIS). As the name suggests, these drugs inhibit the enzyme monoamine oxidase, which plays a part in metabolizing brain amines. A similar action in the bowel allows tyramine, contained in some foods, to be absorbed in an unchanged state. Blackwell *et al.* (1967) found that 4% of the general population lack the isoenzyme for tyramine degradation. Tyramine has a sympathomimetic action; therefore, a rise in blood pressure may occur, provoking a hypertensive crisis when MAOIs are taken. Hence, tyramine-rich food substances must be avoided by women taking MAOIs. The dietary restrictions comprise cheese, Oxo, Marmite and similar meat or vegetable extracts. Game and pickled herrings also contain high levels of tyramine. Chianti wine must also be denied. The physician needs to remain alert to drug interactions with sympathomimetic compounds and opioids. Pregnancy is not a contraindication to the use of MAOIs.
  However, treatment with these drugs should be completed before delivery, to *avoid* interaction with anaesthetic agents. Unexpected surgical complications or a premature delivery could pose problems, but the forewarned anaesthetist would take appropriate action.

There are two main groups of MAOIs:

(a) Hydrazines: phenelzine (Nardil) 30–90 mg/day; isocarboxazid (Marplan) 10–20, 3 times daily.
(b) Non-hydrazines: tranylcypramine (Parnate) 20–30 mg/day; Tranylcypramine + trifluoperazine (Parstelin) 2–3 tablets/day.

Principal indications
(a) *A depressive illness* in which lethargy and loss of drive are dominant features.
(b) *If a depression has not responded* to the more stimulating tricyclic drugs in adequate doses after 4–6 weeks.

Dosage
Average doses have been given. These are always administered in divided doses. MAOIs are alerting drugs; therefore, they should be taken before 1600 hours (4 p.m.).

Side effects
1. Autonomic: similar to tricyclics.
2. Central nervous system: restlessness, hyperactivity, insomnia.
3. Liver: hepatitis (rare).
4. Haemopoietic: blood dyscrasia (very rare).
5. (a) Interaction with food substances: cheese, Marmite, Bovril and other yeast extracts, Chianti wine. (b) Drug interactions: antihypertensives, tricyclics, sympathomimetics, pethidine and some anaesthetic agents.

Effect on the fetus
MAOIs are not teratogenic in man. Phenelzine has been shown to be teratogenic in the rat.

Effect on the neonate
No problems have been reported.

4. OTHER ANTIDEPRESSANTS
(a) Nomifensine (Merital). This drug is thought to differ from other antidepressants in its mode of action – blocking the re-uptake of 5-hydroxytryptamine (5-HT), dopamine and other biogenic amines. Unlike the tricyclics and maprotiline, it has no epileptogenic effect. It tends to have an alerting effect and should not be taken at bedtime.
(b) Viloxazine (Vivalan). Viloxazine (Vivalan 100–400 mg daily) produces nausea in about 20% of patients, but does not cause drowsiness (except in overdose).
(c) Trazodone (Molipaxin). Trazodone (Molipaxin 100–600 mg daily) has an early onset of anxiolytic action. Drowsiness is the main side effect, with occasional dizziness.
(d) L-Tryptophan (Optimax WV; Pacitron). This is a dietary amino acid and a natural precursor of 5-HT. A rise in free plasma tryptophan raises the concentration of 5-HT in the extracellular fluid around the neuronal synapses. L-tryptophan alone, or in combination with either tricyclic or MAOIs has been used in the treatment of depression.

Lithium carbonate (Priadel, Phasal)

The mode of action of this drug remains controversial. It is believed to diminish the amount of noradrenaline available at central adrenergic receptors, by promoting its intraneuronal inactivation. In addition, it affects the water–electrolyte balance, especially the distribution of sodium. It is a moot point whether lithium prophylaxis should be continued during pregnancy. Exposure of the fetus to lithium in the early weeks of gestation carries a definite teratogenic risk.

Principal indications
(1) Mania.
(2) Prophylaxis: (a) bipolar depressive illness; (b) recurrent depression.

Dosage
The effective dose is one that maintains serum lithium levels between 0.6 and 1.0 mmol/l. Higher levels lead to toxicity. During pregnancy, the plasma clearance of lithium is accelerated. To maintain therapeutic blood levels of lithium, the dosage may require an upward adjustment. Post-partum, the maternal lithium level will rise rapidly, unless the dosage is reduced. Careful laboratory control is essential.

Side effects
1. Central nervous system: tremor, muscle fatigue and weakness, ataxia, drowsiness.
2. Endocrine: non-toxic goitre, hypothyroidism, weight gain.
3. Gastrointestinal: nausea, vomiting, abdominal discomfort, diarrhoea.
4. Urinary system: polyuria leading to polydipsia.

Signs of toxicity
The central nervous system is affected principally. Hypertonia and hyperreflexia are warning signs. They are followed by impaired consciousness and seizures.

Effect on the fetus
Lithium has been shown to be teratogenic in animal studies. In man the evidence is less convincing. However, Mignot, Devic and Dumont (1978) found an increase in cardiovascular abnormalities, which were 7.8% instead of the expected 0.4%. Orgegozo and Loiseu (1977) also report a higher incidence of congenital heart disease.

Effect on the neonate
Hypotonia, hypothermia, cyanosis and respiratory distress have been reported. The fetal thyroid is sensitive to lithium; hypothyroidism may develop in the baby.

Anxiolytics and hypnotics

Anti-anxiety preparations are the most frequently prescribed drugs in both the UK and the USA, yet in the management of anxiety states and insomnia, drug therapy remains a controversial subject. Arguments for restricting the use of drugs as the front-line management of anxiety and insomnia are persuasive. Anxiolytic drugs have a place in the treatment of the mother whose anxiety is interfering with her ability to cope with life. Insomnia in pregnancy requires careful evaluation. The obstetrician may decide to prescribe a hypnotic for a limited therapeutic trial. If therapy is not effective, a change of medication may succeed. This approach is preferable to allowing the patient to escalate the prescribed dose. Hypnotics may be prescribed by the obstetrician or the family doctor, but not by both concurrently.

BENZODIAZEPINES

Benzodiazepines are probably the drugs of first choice in the treatment of anxiety states and insomnia. The subjective feelings of anxiety are generated within the limbic system of the cerebral hemispheres. Overactivity in this structure is held in check by gamma-aminobutyric acid (GABA). Benzodiazepines act by enhancing the effectiveness of GABA receptors. Treatment with this group of drugs poses few problems. However, continuous use may lead to dependence. Withdrawal symptoms in the mother are unusual, if the drug is only used for short periods. Overdose with benzodiazepines is rarely fatal. In pregnancy particularly, these drugs are preferable and safer than small doses of major tranquillizers. Benzodiazepines of varying durations of activity are available. They may thus be used as anxiolytics or hypnotics.

Average doses have been given in the text. The dose required must be tailored to the needs of each patient. The aim of treatment is to relieve symptoms without causing undue drowsiness.

Drugs suitable for the treatment of anxiety
1. Diazepam (Valium) 2–5 mg, 2–3 times daily.
2. Chlordiazepoxide (Librium) 5–10 mg, 3 times daily.
3. Oxazepam (Serenid-D) 10–15 mg. Has a shorter duration of action.

Drugs suitable for the treatment of insomnia
1. Temazepam (Normison; Euhypnos) 10–20 mg.
2. Nitrazepam (Mogadon) 5–10 mg.
3. Flurazepam (Dalmane) 15–30 mg.
4. Lormetazepam (Noctamid) 0.5–1 mg.
5. Flunitrazepam (Rohypnol) 0.5–1 mg.

Effect on the fetus (see page 116)

Effect on the neonate (see page 116)

BARBITURATES

The use of these drugs in pregnancy is not advisable.

Dangers
1. The *risk of dependence* is high.
2. *Even low doses* may lead to a withdrawal syndrome.
3. The *risk of fetal malformations* is increased.
4. *Overdose* is often fatal.

Effect on the fetus (see page 116)

Effect on the neonate (see page 116)

OTHER DRUGS USED IN THE TREATMENT OF ANXIETY

1. Meprobamate (Equanil). The use of meprobamate carries a considerable risk, and it is best avoided. The problems encountered are the same as for barbiturates.
2. Propranolol (Inderal). Propranolol diminishes sympathetic overactivity by blocking central and peripheral beta-adrenergic receptors. Use in pregnancy is controversial; if used, the drug should be phased out well before the onset of labour.

Principal indications
Anxiety states with a marked somatic component.

Dosage
10–30 mg 3 times daily, starting with a low dose.

Contraindications
1. Metabolic acidosis.
2. Cardiovascular: cardiac failure; conduction defects.
3. Asthma.

Side effects
1. Respiratory: bronchospasm.
2. Cardiovascular: bradycardia; hypotension; cold extremities.
3. Endocrine: altered response to stress.

Effect on the fetus
No specific teratogenic effect is known. However, there have been reports of growth retardation and decreased placental size (Hill and Stern, 1979).

Effect on the neonate
Hypoglycaemia, bradycardia and respiratory distress may occur.

3. Chlormethiazole (Heminevrin). Chlormethiazole should be used with care as it has a high potential for dependence.

Principal indications
1. Alcohol withdrawal states.
2. Abstinence syndromes following abrupt drug withdrawal.

Dosage
500–1000 mg may be required 4–6 hourly. If oral medication is impracticable, an intravenous infusion of 0.8% chlormethiazole can be substituted. The danger of dependence is real; the drug should be phased out in 5–9 days.

Side effects
1. Mucous membranes: nasal irritation associated with sneezing. Conjunctival irritation.
2. Gastrointestinal: nausea.

Effect on the fetus
No specific problems have been reported.

Effect on the neonate
In pre-eclamptic mothers treated with a combination of chlormethiazole and diazoxide, neonatal problems have been described e.g. hypotonia, decreased ventilatory effort and apnoea. Neonatal difficulties have not been reported when chlormethiazole has been used alone. Many other sedatives are available. None has any particular advantage in the treatment of the pregnant woman.

Suicide

Suicide in pregnancy

United States and UK sources are largely in agreement that suicide in pregnancy is unusual. Rosenberg and Silver (1965) examined coroners' records in California for the years 1961–63 and found that of 207 suicides in women aged 16–50 years, only 3 were pregnant. The number of the identified pregnant suicides was just below the expected number if pregnancy and suicide were independent. Sim (1968) reported only 1 pregnant suicide in Birmingham over a 12-year period. Weir (1965) identified, from coroners' records in the London boroughs and the City of London from 1948 to 1962, 1012 suicides in the age group 15–44 years. Fifty-one were pregnant. He noted that, below the age of 25, the risk of suicide during pregnancy was slightly increased, whereas above that age pregnancy seemed to confer some protection. Above the age of 25 years, inability to conceive was sometimes related to suicide. However, the assertion from these studies that pregnancy protects against suicide is challenged by the work of Goodwin and Harris (1979). Their research was based not only on coroners' records, but included interviews with physicians and the study of hospital records.

Attempted suicide in pregnancy

Workers in Australia, Sweden and the UK have shown that attempted suicide in pregnancy is more common. However, it is still relatively infrequent. The action is not necessarily related to the pregnant state.

PREVENTION OF SUICIDE

It is dangerous to assume that the patient who threatens suicide or talks about it will not be at risk. A simple question 'Do you feel able to carry on?' or 'Do you think life worth living?' will establish the patient's true feelings and plans. The actively suicidal mother should be admitted to a psychiatric unit for further management.

Conclusions

Relative freedom from psychological disturbance in pregnancy is an oversimplified concept and applies only to psychotic illness. Most women face up to the common anxieties of pregnancy with equanimity. Pre-conception clinics, parenthood classes and a supportive obstetric environment help others to master their anxieties.

Minor neurotic disturbances are common. Thus depression, anxiety, phobias or obsessional behaviour may all occur in pregnant women. Appropriate symptoms in response to stress have been differentiated from symptoms which interfere with the mother's ability to continue her daily activities, and may constitute a neurotic illness. Active treatment is discussed. Obsessional symptoms may not be easy to evaluate and, like major psychotic illness and drug addiction, warrant specialist referral. Drug dependence, a perennial problem, has been covered in some detail, as the information is not readily available. The so-called 'typical junkie' is rarely seen; the diagnosis is not always obvious and hence often delayed, to the detriment of the mother and her unborn child.

If the common nausea and vomiting of pregnancy does not subside as expected, the clinician may be faced by a diagnostic problem. Anorexia nervosa and especially bulimia nervosa should be considered in the differential diagnosis.

The potential risks of drug therapy, especially in the first 8 weeks of gestation, have been discussed and placed into perspective. Psychotropic drugs have been reviewed in relation to their effect on mother, fetus and neonate. More successful treatment of patients suffering from schizophrenia has increased the number of affected women able to live in the community; hence more patients on maintenance therapy with phenothiazines will wish to have children. Maintenance therapy should be continued throughout pregnancy and the post-partum. The illness is seldom reactivated during pregnancy, but acute relapse in the puerperium is much more common.

References

ASTBURY, J. and WALTERS, A. W. (1979) Amniocentesis in the early trimester of pregnancy and maternal anxiety. *Australian Family Physician,* **8,** 595–599

BAKER, A. A. (1967) *Psychiatric Disorders in Obstetrics.* Oxford and Edinburgh; Blackwell Scientific Publications

BLACKWELL, B., MARLEY, E., PRICE, J. and TAYLOR, D. (1967) Hypertensive interactions between monoamine oxidase inhibitors and foodstuffs. *British Journal of Psychiatry,* **113,** 349–365

BLINICK, G., WALLACH, R. C., JEREZ, E. and ACKERMAN, B. D. (1976) Drug addiction in pregnancy and the neonate. *American Journal of Obstetrics and Gynecology,* **125**(2), 135–142

BRAVERMAN, J. and ROUX, J. F. (1978) Screening for the patient at risk for post-partum depression. *Obstetrics and Gynecology,* **53,** 731–736

COOKSON, J. C., SILVERSTONE, T. and WELLS, B. (1979) A double-blind controlled study of Pimozide vs. Chlorpromazine in mania. *Neuropharmacology,* **18,** 1011–1013

COPPEN, A. J. (1959) Vomiting of early pregnancy. Physiological factors and body build. *Lancet,* **1,** 172–173

COX, J. L., CONNOR, Y. and KENDELL, R. E. (1982) Prospective study of the psychiatric disorders of childbirth. *British Journal of Psychiatry,* **140,** 111–117

CRISP, A. H. (1974) Primary anorexia nervosa or adolescent weight phobia. *Practitioner,* **212,** 525–535

DALTON, K. (1971) Prospective study into puerperal depression. *British Journal of Psychiatry,* **118,** 689–692

DAVIE, R., BUTLER, N. R. and GOLDSTEIN, H. (1972) *From Birth to Seven.* Report of the National Child Development Study. London; Longmans

DESMOND, M. M., SCHWANECKE, R. P., WILSON, G. S., YASUNAGA, S. and BURGDORFF, I. (1972) Maternal barbiturate utilization and neonatal withdrawal symptomatology. *Journal of Pediatrics,* **80,** 190–197

d'ORBAN, P. T. (1976) Child stealing: a typology of female offenders. *British Journal of Criminology,* **16,** 275–281

FAVA, G. A., KELLNER, R., MICHELACCI, L., TROMBININ, G., PATHAK, D, ORLANDI, C. and BOVICELLI, L. (1982) Psychological reactions to amniocentesis: a controlled study. *American Journal of Obstetrics and Gynecology*, **145**(5), 509–513

FORFAR, J. O. (1981) Community paediatrics. 1. Drugs and the fetus. *Update*, May, 1469–1483

FRASER, A. C. (1976) Drug addiction in pregnancy. *Lancet*, **2**, 896–899

FROMMER, E. A. and O'SHEA, G. (1973) Antenatal identification of women liable to have problems in managing their infants. *British Journal of Psychiatry*, **123**, 149–156

GOKELMA, Y. (1983) Heart-effects of Lofepramine in depressed patients with and without heart diseases. Paper presented at VII World Congress of Psychiatry, Vienna

GOODWIN, J. and HARRIS, D. (1979) Suicide in pregnancy: the Hedda Gabler syndrome. *Suicide and Life Threatening Behaviour*, **9**(2), 105–115

HAMILTON, M. (1984) Symptoms and treatment of anxiety. *Mims Magazine*, March, 44–51

HARVEY, W. A. and SHERFEY, M. J. (1954) Vomiting in pregnancy. *Psychosomatic Medicine*, **16**, 1–9

HILL, R. M. and STERN, L. (1979) Drugs in pregnancy; effects on the foetus and new-born. *Drugs*, **17**, 182–197

JOHNSON, G., GERSHON, S. and HEKIMIAN, L. J. (1968) Controlled evaluation of lithium and chlorpromazine in the treatment of manic states. *Comprehensive Psychiatry*, **9**, 563–573

JONES, A. C. (1978) Life change and psychological distress as predictors of pregnancy outcome. *Psychosomatic Medicine*, **40**, 402–412

JONES, K. L., SMITH, D. W., ULLELAND, C. N. and STREISSGATH, A. P. (1973) Pattern of malformation in offspring of chronic alcoholic mothers. *Lancet*, **1**, 126–127

KENDELL, R. E. (1976) The classification of depression: a review of contemporary confusion. *British Journal of Psychiatry*, **129**, 15–28

KENDELL, R. E., RENNIE, D., CLARKE, J. A. and DEAN, C. (1981) The social and obstetric correlates of psychiatric admissions in the puerperium. *Psychological Medicine*, **II**, 341–350

KENDELL, R. E., WAINWRIGHT, S., HAILEY, A. and SHANNON, B. (1976) The influence of childbirth on psychiatric morbidity. *Psychological Medicine*, **6**, 297–302

KRON, R. E., KAPLAN, S. L., FINNEGAN, L. P., LITT, M. and PHOENIX, M. D. (1975) The assessment of behavioural change in infants undergoing narcotic withdrawal; comparative data from clinical and objective methods. *Addictive Disorders*, **2**, 257–275

KUMAR R. and ROBSON, K. (1978). Neurotic disturbance during pregnancy and the puerperium: preliminary report of a prospective survey of 119 primiparae. In *Mental Illness in Pregnancy and the Puerperium* (Sander, M., Ed.). London; Oxford University Press

LITTLE, B. C., HAYWORTH, J., BENSON, P., BRIDGE, L. R., DEWHURST, SIR J. and PRIEST, R. G. (1982) Psychophysiological ante-natal predictors of post-natal depressed mood. *Journal of Psychosomatic Research*, **26**(4), 419–428

MACGILLIVRAY, I. (1983) *Pre-eclampsia: The Hypertensive Disease of Pregnancy*. Philadelphia; W. B. Saunders

MARKS, I. M. (1969) *Fears and Phobias*. New York; Academic Press

MATSUYAMA. S., and JARVIK, L. (1977) Effects of marihuana on the genetic and immune systems. National Institute for Drug Abuse, Research Monograph Series, Vol. 14, pp. 179–193

MEARES, R., GRIMWADE, J. and WOOD, C. (1976) A possible relationship between anxiety in pregnancy and puerperal depression. *Journal of Psychosomatic Research*, **20**, 605–610

MIGNOT, G., DEVIC, M. and DUMONT, M. (1978) Lithium et grossesse. *Journal of Gynaecology, Obstetrics and Biology*, Reprint 7, 1303–1317

NILSSON, A. and ALMGREN, P. (1970) Problems of antenatal depression. *Acta Psychiatrica Scandinavica*, Supplement 220

NORDMEYER, K. (1946) Zur Ätiologie der hyperemesis gravidarum. *Deutsche Medizinische Wochenschrift*, **71**, 213

ORGEGOZO, J. M. and LOISEAU, P. (1977) Effets teratogènes et oncogènes des médicaments du système nerveux central. *Neurologie*, **27**, 2225–2233

OSWALD, I. and PRIEST, R. G. (1965) Five weeks to escape the sleeping pill. *British Medical Journal*, **2**, 1093–1095

PAFFENBARGER, R. S. JUN. (1964) Epidemiological aspects of parapartum mental illness. *British Journal of Preventive and Social Medicine*, **18**, 189–195

PAYKEL, E. S., EMMS, E. M., FLETCHER, J. and RASSABY, E. S. (1980) Life events and social support in puerperal depression. *British Journal of Psychiatry*, **136**, 339–346

POLLITT, J. (1978) The depressed patient. *Practitioner*, **220**, 205–212

PUGH, R., BELL, J. COOPER, A. J., DUNSTAN, S., GREEDHARRY, D., POMEROY, J., RAPTOPOULOS, P., ROWSELL, C., STEINERT, J. and PRIEST, R. G. (1982) Does lofepramine have fewer side effects than amitriptyline? Results of a comparative trial. *Journal of Affective Disorders*, **4**, 355–363

PUGH, T. F., JERATH, B. K., SCHMIDT, W. M. and REED, R. B. (1963) Rates of mental disease related to childbearing. *New England Journal of Medicine*, **268**, 1224–1228

ROSENBERG, A. J. and SILVER, E. (1965) Suicide, psychiatrists and therapeutic abortion. *California Medicine*, **102**, 407–411

RUSSELL, G. (1979) Bulimia nervosa: an ominous variant of anorexia nervosa. *Psychological Medicine*, **9**, 429–448

SANDIFER, M. G., HORDERN, A., TIMBURY, G. C. and GREEN, L. M. (1968) Psychiatric diagnosis: a comparative study in North Carolina, London and Glasgow, *British Journal of Psychiatry*, **114**, 1–9

SANDLER, M. (1978) In *Mental Illness in Pregnancy and the Puerperium* (Sandler, M., Ed.), pp. 9–24. Oxford; Oxford University Press

SIM, M. (1968) Psychiatric disorders of pregnancy. *Journal of Psychosomatic Research*, **12**, 95–100

SNAITH, R. P. (1983) Pregnancy related psychiatric disorder. *British Journal of Hospital Medicine*, **29**(5), 450–456

STANDLEY, K., SOULE, B. and COPANS, S. A. (1979) Dimensions of prenatal anxiety and their influence on pregnancy outcome. *American Journal of Obstetrics and Gynecology*, **135**, 22–26

STONE, M., SALERNO, L. J., GREEN, M. and ZELSON, C. (1971) Narcotic addiction in pregnancy. *American Journal of Obstetrics and Gynecology*, **109**(5), 716–723

TOD, E. D. M. (1964) Puerperal depression: a prospective epidemiological study. *Lancet*, **2**, 1264–1266

TRETHOWAN, W. H. (1979) *Psychiatry*, 4th ed. London; Baillière

TYLDEN, E. (1968) Hyperemesis and physiological vomiting. *Journal of Psychosomatic Research*, **12**, 85–93

TYLDEN, E. (1973) The effects of maternal drug abuse on the foetus and infant. In *Adverse Drug Reaction Bulletin*, No. 38, pp. 120–123 (Davies, D. M., Ed.). Newcastle upon Tyne; Regional Postgraduate Institute for Medicine

WEIR, J. G. (1965) Study of 65 pregnant suicides in London. In *Medicina Psychosomatica in Obstetrica et Gynaecologia*, pp. 397–399. Proc. 2nd International Congress Psychosomatic Medicine in Obstetrics and Gynaecology, Vienna, July 1965

WELNER, A. (1982) Childbirth-related psychiatric illness. *Comprehensive Psychiatry*, **23**(2), 143–154

WING, J. K., BIRLEY, J. L. T., COOPER, J. E., GRAHAM, P. and ISSAACS, A. D. (1967) Reliability of a procedure for measuring and classifying 'present psychiatric state'. *British Journal of Psychiatry*, **113**, 499–515

WOLKIND, S. and ZAJICEK, E. (1981) *Pregnancy – a Psychological and Social Study*. London and New York; Academic Press

Chapter 6

The puerperium

Brice Pitt

Introduction

It has long been recognized that the period after the travail of giving birth is hazardous to the physical and mental health of the newly delivered mother. Before the era of modern obstetrics there was a serious risk to life from post-partum haemorrhage and eclampsia just after delivery, and a little later puerperal sepsis used to be a terrible scourge. The 'churching' of women after childbirth is in part a recognition that they have been fortunate to come safely through the perils of giving birth.

Hippocrates described a woman who became mentally deranged shortly after bearing twins. She died a few days later, and may well have been suffering from delirium as a manifestation of puerperal fever. Celsus, Galen and Soranus also recorded cases of post-partum psychosis (Boyd, 1942). With the development of psychiatry and mental hospitals in Europe in the eighteenth and nineteenth centuries, the frequent association between childbirth and insanity was noted with particular interest. Hamilton (1962) lists over 300 references to the topic in the scientific literature of the time. The psychoses of the post-natal period were generally regarded as specific clinical entities peculiar to that time. Those arising within the traditional six weeks of the puerperium were designated 'puerperal psychoses', while those developing later in the post-partum year, while the mother was still producing breast milk, 'lactational'.

In the twentieth century, the concept of the specific puerperal (or lactational) psychosis has lost ground, and finds only a few defenders (among them Hamilton, 1962, and Hays and Douglass, 1984). It is now generally upheld that major mental illness occurring after childbirth is just the same as that arising unrelated to childbearing in women of comparable age. However, modern epidemiological studies, e.g. that of Pugh et al. (1963), have plainly shown that there is a significant risk of serious mental illness not only in the puerperium but for nine months after delivery, although the risk is greater the nearer to the time of giving birth. The legal concept of infanticide, which in the past in England allowed a mother who killed her baby within a year and a day of its birth to be found guilty of a lesser (non-capital) crime than murder, was a humane recognition of diminished responsibility due to mental derangement during this time.

147

The mental illness most prominent among those admitted to mental hospitals and psychiatric wards in the post-partum period is severe depression or melancholia. With the advances of obstetrics in recent decades the risk of maternal mortality has so dwindled that the occasional suicide of a desperately depressed mother must now be reckoned among its important causes. Indeed, as the threats to physical health have now been so greatly reduced, those which jeopardize mental and emotional stability have been highlighted and should have a prominent place among the concerns of the contemporary obstetrician.

The lay public have been aware for a long time that many women 'fail to thrive' after having a baby, and that (while few are sick enough to 'go away' for psychiatric treatment) tears, exhaustion and a distinct lack of *joie de vivre* are commonplace. It is not infrequently remarked that a particular woman 'hasn't been the same' since she had her last baby. Psychiatrists have long realized that the origin of many of their female patients' depressions, anxiety states, phobic disorders or orgasmic dysfunctions appears to have been in the puerperium. In recent years these impressions have been confirmed by epidemiological studies, like that of Kendell (1978) using the Camberwell register of psychiatric contacts by women delivering in that London borough to indicate morbidity before and after childbearing. It is now known that some 50% of women suffer very mild emotional upsets in the early puerperium ('the blues'), about 10% more protracted and distressing states of depression (lasting weeks, months or even years), and perhaps one in four or five per thousand develop serious derangement amounting to psychosis. Anxiety states and possibly psychosomatic conditions such as asthma, epilepsy, migraine, colitis, eczema and psoriasis may also develop or worsen in the puerperium. These matters are not just of concern to doctors; the emotional disorders of the puerperium, along with many other aspects of obstetrics, are rapidly becoming feminist issues.

This chapter considers the nature of those different disorders, the relationship between them, their frequency, clinical manifestations, treatment and prognosis, and offers some hypotheses on their causation.

Incidence

Puerperal psychosis

Statistics for puerperal psychosis are usually based upon returns for admissions to psychiatric wards and may thus underestimate the frequency of these disorders. In any case the figures reported vary a good deal, from the more usual 1 per 1000 births (Osterman, 1963; Sim, 1963) to the exceptional 6.8 per 1000 in a Scandinavian study (Janssen, 1964). The previously mentioned New England survey by Pugh *et al.* (1963) showed that puerperal admissions significantly exceeded those at other times in the childbearing years, whereas pregnancy itself was a time of relative immunity to psychiatric admissions. The risk, greatest (after a two-day 'latency period') in the days and weeks after giving birth, dwindled subsequently, until at 9 months post-partum it was no greater than at other times. The excess of admissions was very largely accounted for by those with a diagnosis of affective or emotional disorder, serious depression or its opposite, mania. Dean and Kendell (1981) noted that admissions for functional psychoses in the first 3 months post-partum increased 16-fold. Karnosh and Hope (1937) drew particular attention to the 'latency period' of 2 days after delivery. Paffenbarger (1964) reported that 46% of 126 patients becoming mentally ill within 9 months of giving birth became ill in the first week, and 76% in the first month.

It must be remembered that prompt psychiatric intervention, especially in lying-in wards, and resourceful deployment of the community psychiatric team aborts many cases of puerperal psychosis and enables others to be managed successfully at home, so that the likely incidence of puerperal psychosis is of the order of 1 in 200 births (0.5%). Before the introduction of antibiotics, puerperal delirium was commonly reported. For example, Skottowe (1942) found this diagnosis in almost half of a series of women admitted with puerperal psychosis. Whether this was a true manifestation of, say, puerperal sepsis or whether it was then assumed that confusional features, not uncommon in the early stages of puerperal psychosis even today, must have been due to such an infective or toxic factor is hard now to say. Be that as it may, less than 20 years later Seager (1960) found no delirious patients in his series, and this is now a very rare diagnosis indeed, except in underdeveloped countries where obstetric facilities may be in short supply.

In the 1950s, schizophrenia or schizo-affective psychosis appeared to be the commonest major puerperal mental illness (e.g. Madden et al. 1958; Martin, 1958), but this may have been a passing diagnostic fashion, because previously (e.g. Boyd, 1942) and subsequently (e.g. Prothere, 1969) affective disorders have led the field. The clinical picture is typically mixed at the outset of a puerperal psychosis, which allows some controversy about the diagnosis, but the subsequent course is usually that of an affective illness, either mania (Brockington et al., 1978) or depression. In the Edinburgh study of Dean and Kendell (1981), 49 (69%) of 71 women admitted to psychiatric wards within 3 months of giving birth were depressed, 9 (13%) manic, 4 had schizo-affective disorder and only 1 was schizophrenic.

It is worth noting here that admissions for post-abortion psychosis are only one-fifth as common as for puerperal psychosis (Brewer, 1978).

Maternity 'blues'

At the opposite extreme to the severity of puerperal psychosis is the trivial and transitory disorder of mood which occurs typically on the third or fourth day post-partum and lasts perhaps only a few hours, and certainly no longer than a couple of days. This phenomenon, generally named 'the blues', 'third or fourth day', 'mother's maternity' or 'baby blues', is of negligible clinical importance but has attracted interest as a possible model of the more serious disorders in those, say, who are genetically or constitutionally predisposed. Considering how mild and fleeting the symptoms are, it is a little surprising that estimates of the frequency of the condition should be fairly consistent. In recent studies (Kane et al., 1968; Yalom et al., 1968; Davidson, 1972; Pitt, 1973; Nott et al. 1976; Harris, 1980; Stein, 1980), they range from 50% to 76%.

Puerperal depression

Between the poles of psychosis and 'the blues' lie an important group of troubled women who are far from deranged but considerably afflicted by anxiety (taking the form of excessive worry or distressing bodily symptoms) and even more by depression. Whereas psychosis usually arises within a month of delivery, these symptoms often develop later. Before 1960, reports on such disorders were scant because the bias was towards hospital admissions. In the early 1960s, however, two general practice surveys (Ryle, 1961; Tod, 1964) agreed that 3% of their patients suffered quite serious depression in the puerperium. Using a prospective epidemiological approach, Pitt (1968) found a much higher number; 10.8% suffering at least moderate depression of 1 month's duration before their attendance at the post-natal clinic in a random sample of women having their babies in a London teaching hospital. Neugebauer (1983) has argued, however, that this figure of just over 10% is an underestimate, and that the correct proportion should be nearer 20%. In another such hospital, using a similar technique, Kumar and Robson (1978) found a remarkably similar number (11%), while the comparable prospective general practice study by Dalton (1971) found over 7% of the women surveyed to be suffering from puerperal depression. Incidentally, a further 6.2% of Pitt's patients had developed new symptoms of anxiety or psychosomatic disorder.

Using questionnaires and rating scales with a cut-off point above a certain morbid score (rather than the clinical identification of cases), Jacobson, Kaij and Nilsson (1965) and Nilsson and Almgren (1970) in Scandinavia and Blair et al. (1970) in England found from 18% to 25% of their subjects to have developed troublesome symptoms of emotional disorder in the puerperium. Paykel et al. (1980) found mild to moderate depression in 20% of their series. Using Goldberg's Standard Psychiatric Interview, Cox, Connor and Kendell (1982) identified severe post-natal depression in 13% of their 105 women. Watson et al. (1984), in a prospective study of 128 women, identified affective disorder in the sixth postnatal week in 12%.

These various levels of morbidity are rather neatly brought together by the study of Rees and Lutkins (1971) who used the Beck Depression Inventory to screen pregnant women (and their husbands) before and after their babies were born. The controls were approximately age-matched nulliparous women working in a local factory. The childbearing women were significantly more liable to depression than their nulliparous controls, both in pregnancy and the puerperium. Fathers were less depressed than their wives, but more than the factory women. At a score of 25 on the Beck Inventory, indicating quite severe depression, there were approximately 3% of mothers in the puerperium, consistent with the findings of Ryle (1961) and Tod (1964). Ten per cent scored between 17 and 25, indicating moderately severe depression and consistent with the findings of Pitt (1968), Kumar and Robson (1978), Cox, Connor and Kendell (1982) and Watson et al. (1984). Mild depression suggested by scores between 10 and 17 occurred in 30% of women puerperally, which is rather in keeping with the findings of the Scandinavians (Jacobson, Kaij and Nilsson, 1965; Nilsson and Almgren, 1970; and also Blair et al., 1970; Paykel et al., 1980). Thus, from this study it looks as if there may be a continuum of depression ranging from relatively mild to fairly severe, affecting in all about one-third of puerperal women, although whether 'the blues' and psychotic melancholia are part of this continuum is not altogether clear.

Another study worth quoting in some detail is that of Kendell (1978), as it almost decides the question of whether there is a true increase in psychiatric morbidity in the puerperium, or whether more notice may be taken of emotional disturbance at this time because there is more observation, interest and concern than is the lot of the women who have not just had a baby. The Camberwell register indicates all psychiatric contacts, new and old, made by residents of that London Borough, and by examining the register it was possible to ascertain how often Camberwell women saw a psychiatrist in the 2 years before and the 2 years after they had a baby. It was found that there was a prominent, and highly significant, increase in psychiatric contacts in the 3 months after childbirth. For example, during this period there were more episodes of psychosis (predominantly depressive) than in the whole of the previous 2 years. Depressive illnesses as a whole, not only the psychotic, showed a peak in these 3 months post-partum. There was a generally higher rate of psychiatric contacts in the 2 years after childbirth than in the preceding 2 years.

Oddly, although pregnant women seem significantly unlikely to see a psychiatrist either as inpatients or for outpatient assessment, there is ample evidence that anxiety and depression of neurotic degree (although not psychosis) are just as common in pregnancy as in the puerperium. Thus, in the Rees and Lutkins (1971) study, quoted above, the pregnant women were significantly anxious and less depressed than they were in the puerperium. The study by Pitt (1968) found more subjects anxious and depressed before than after delivery, and Jarrahi-Zadeh *et al* (1969) and Davidson (1972) found depression more frequently in pregnancy than in the puerperium. Nilsson and Almgren (1970) recorded 'mental adaptational difficulties' in 17% of their subjects during pregnancy and 18% in the puerperium, and Kumar and Robson (1978) found 10% of their subjects to have developed depression in early pregnancy compared with 11% in the post-natal period. Elliott *et al.* (1983) measured psychological change during pregnancy and the post-partum year and found the greatest difference between late pregnancy and the puerperium; this change was in the direction of improvement. Different attitudes to, expectations of and supports for the anxious, depressed pregnant women may determine why she is less likely to present as a psychiatric 'case' and have implications for the better management of the distressed puerperal patient (see below).

Clinical forms and features

Puerperal psychosis

With the systematic clinical studies of the mentally ill at the end of the nineteenth century, especially those of the German school and the great codifier Kraepelin (1913), the concept of puerperal psychosis as a distinct clinical entity was ever more hard to sustain. Thus, Bleuler (1911) remarked that schizophrenia could arise in the puerperium where it had no special features, and Kraepelin himself noted that mania might be precipitated by childbirth, but only where it was already latent. An important American study (Strecker and Ebaugh, 1926) had no difficulty in ascribing 50 successive cases of mental illness in the puerperium to the conventional categories of manic-depressive psychosis, schizophrenia or toxic-exhaustive (delirious) states. Their conclusion that there was no such entity as post-partum psychosis has been generally upheld subsequently, the view being that childbirth simply precipitates a particular psychosis to which there is an hereditary or constitutional predisposition. This subject has been comprehensively reviewed by Brockington, Winokur and Dean (1982).

Dissenters point to confusion, in the absence of any obvious toxic or infective factor, as a typical early feature of the supposedly functional puerperal psychosis. Marcé (1858) first noted this in this historic treatise on mental illness in childbearing women, and the accuracy of his observation has been confirmed by many others, e.g. Janssen (1964). A shifting in the early stages from the picture of one mental illness to that of another, e.g. schizophrenic symptoms at the onset of what turns out to be depression, is also said to be characteristic, e.g. by Nyssen (1955). Hamilton, whose 1962 monograph has already been quoted, and Brockington *et al.* (1978), collaborated in a blind diagnostic study in which the former was sent transcripts of the mental states of 135 patients, including 50 with post-partum psychosis, after all obvious clues to the post-partum state had been removed. Hamilton correctly identified 27 of them at the expense of 26 false guesses, and his success was apparently highly significant.

However, Stengel, Zeitlin and Rayner (1958) observed that all the features 'characteristic' of post-partum psychosis (among which can be included the two-day 'latency period' and the acute onset after a night or two of sleeplessness) are also characteristic of postoperative psychosis. It seems probable, indeed, that they are typical of any acute psychosis developing after a major stress or life-event. The only truly (and inevitable) typical feature of post-partum mental illness is that the disturbed thoughts and feelings are focused on the baby.

Despite the frequent difficulty in making a clear diagnosis at the onset of psychosis developing after childbirth, eventually the condition can nearly always be classified as depressive, manic, schizophrenic, paranoid or delirious. These five forms of puerperal psychosis are briefly described below.

SEVERE DEPRESSION

Severe depression or melancholia (a word no longer in vogue but still useful in designating an unquestionably morbid and serious mood disturbance) has the typical features of 'endogenous depression': profound despondency worse in the mornings, guilt, suicidal tendencies and early waking. Sometimes, talk and action are slowed and retarded, but in other cases agitation is extreme.

For example, the writer was asked to give an opinion on the management of a young unmarried primiparous women whose anxiety, already apparent before she gave birth to a normal healthy little boy, intensified subsequently to the consternation of others in the lying-in ward and her cohabitee. The ward sister attributed her condition at first to 'the blues', but later realized that there was more to it than that and called the ward doctor. He was a locum who had started work that day and did not know the patient. He spoke to her briefly at the foot of the bed and prescribed a hypnotic to be given that night. The young mother appeared more composed, but suddenly made a dash for the lavatory and locked herself in. It was then found that the baby was missing. She failed to open the door to the nurses and her boyfriend, and when eventually it was forced open, the window was open and she was gone. A search was made in the hospital grounds, and eventually she was found with multiple injuries four floors below the ward. The baby in her arms was dead. Ironically, when questioned about the tragedy a year later she was quite bland; in the fall she had sustained serious damage to her frontal lobes.

Nowadays, when mother and baby are very rarely both lost as a result of childbirth, severe depression looms large as the main contemporary cause of such a double disaster. Infanticide seems less an act of overt aggression than a kind of euthanasia: the mother feels so negative about herself and her world that she is impelled to remove her baby from it as a deed of compassion.

Loss of appetite and immense fatigue are other features of puerperal melancholia. There is a feeling of utter misery and hopelessness which circumstances by no means warrant. As this is the most readily treatable mental illness in the puerperium, its early diagnosis is extremely important. It is uncommon, yet a busy obstetric unit with 3000 deliveries a year might well have six or more cases in the same period. Midwives and obstetricians need then to be alert to such significant signs as insomnia, despair and extreme distress.

Hemphill (1952) noted a tendency to severe premenstrual tension subsequent to recovery from severe post-natal depression.

MANIA

Mania, although opposite to depression, is never far from it. In psychodynamic terms it may be seen as a massive, strenuous denial of being depressed. In fact, it is the other side of the same coin – 'bipolar' depression. All manic mothers will become depressed, although only a minority of those who are depressed show any mania. In the puerperium the manic mother is over-confident, especially about child care. Suddenly she 'knows all there is to know' and more. She has abundant energy and little need for food or rest. She is extremely talkative, but will not listen. Her boisterous *bonhomie* is only infectious in the short term; a little of her company goes a long way. She is overbearing, irritable, or even aggressive if thwarted, and may briefly dissolve into tears or profound dejection. She is erotic, flirtatious and inclined heedlessly to spend a lot of money if she gets the chance. She is bursting with ideas and plans, but as she tries to implement several at once and is readily distracted, her day is too short and nothing of value is achieved. She lacks judgement and self-criticism, and for all her confidence her baby is liable to neglect from her 'lick and promise' approach. Allowed its natural course, mania usually runs for weeks and then ends in depression.

SCHIZOPHRENIA

Schizophrenia developing acutely in the puerperium causes a major disruption of the personality, with jumbled thoughts, cryptic and incoherent utterances, delusions, hallucinations, emotional blunting or lability and bizarre, unpredictable behaviour as prominent features. The delusions, often ill-informed, may be grandiose, and the notion that the baby is another Christ or Messiah is fairly common still. The hallucinations are mainly auditory – one or two, or a tumult of voices talking to and about the subject. Visual hallucinations, if they occur, take the form of strange visions. The schizophrenic mother often feels herself to be possessed, and influenced from afar. Others can read her thoughts, and she theirs. She may appear remote, withdrawn and dreamy, or erratic and excitable. (Ophelia's mad scene in *Hamlet* is fairly typical, including the mixture of affective features – lofty disinhibition and fits of depression – which are commonly seen in puerperal schizophrenia.) The schizophrenic's baby is in jeopardy from her mother's unreliable oddness, although the danger of neglect is greater than that of injury.

PARANOIA

Paranoia is usually classified under schizophrenia, but takes a very characteristic form in the puerperium. The paranoid mother believes that she and her baby are in danger. She thinks that every conversation that she witnesses but cannot hear is about her. When people laugh, they are laughing about her. Such remarks as she overhears, or are addressed directly to her, she interprets as hostile and threatening. She may be frankly hallucinated, hearing voices which no one else can hear. She and the baby are targets of a huge plot, involving all those on the ward, staff and fellow patients, and probably extending far beyond. They are trying to poison her, and take away her baby. Occasionally she feels that her baby is no longer hers, but has been replaced overnight by a changeling. Nevertheless, her care of the baby is usually good, her maternal capacity being impaired little, if at all. Her attitude to the midwives and doctors is brusque, affronted, sullen or plainly hostile, and they may respond in kind. Again, there is always the chance that the mother diagnosed as paranoid who refuses drugs may get them in her food, so not infrequently the paranoia becomes less delusional!

Immigrant women, especially those who do not know the language or the culture, are significantly at risk from paranoia. This is not surprising, especially in the strange environment of a hospital, where it is very easy to get hold of the wrong end of the stick. They usually fare best if discharged early to their own homes.

PUERPERAL DELIRIUM

Finally, puerperal delirium is now very rare except in the Third World. It is the mental manifestation of serious physical disorder – infection, eclampsia, blood loss, manutrition – causing cerebral impairment. Confusion, drowsiness, incoherence, restless spells, agitation and predominantly visual illusions and hallucinations are the classical features. All fluctuate a good deal according to the patient's general condition, e.g. symptoms are often worse towards evening, when pyrexia tends to increase. Delirium lasts only as long as the underlying illness, and ends in recovery or death. A famous such patient in literature was Tolstoy's Anna Karenina.

Maternity 'blues'

Hamilton (1962) asked domiciliary midwives what they considered to be the features of this mild, commonplace emotional disturbance in the early puerperium. They gave the following, in order of frequency: fatigue, crying, anxiety (usually over the baby), confusion, headaches, insomnia, hypochondria, and hostility to the husband! Pitt (1973) used these observations for a rating-scale in his study of 'the blues' at The London Hospital, and found that tearfulness, depression and anxiety are the principal features, and that 'confusion', i.e. relative impairment of concentration, memory and learning, was a probable significant accompaniment. Hamilton's other features, however, were as common in the controls who did not suffer 'the blues'. Of the 100 women Pitt interviewed between the seventh and tenth days post-partum, 50 were diagnosed as having 'the blues'. Of these, 33 (66%) developed the condition within 4 days of parturition, 13 (26%) on the third day. Most subjects described tears and despondency lasting from barely an hour to most of the day on from 1 to 3 days, but 6 subjects went on to develop puerperal depression; this was not significantly more, however, than the controls. Most women could find a reason for their distress – they were worried about their babies, or homesick – but objectively they seemed to have no more to worry them than the controls. There was, however, a significant difference between control and study groups in respect of finding breast-feeding difficult: an equal majority in each group were breast-feeding, but mothers suffering from 'the blues' tended to find it harder.

While Nott *et al.* (1976) found that women worst affected tended to have been no less depressed at the end of pregnancy, Yalom *et al.* (1968) observed three times as much tearfulness in the first 10 days after delivery as in a similar period in the eighth month of pregnancy, and for reasons which would not normally have produced tears at the other times.

The cognitive impairment is of interest as possibly indicating an organic factor, but seems to be very largely subjective. True, Robin (1962) found that psychological testing in the early puerperium suggested impairment of conceptual thought, but Jarrahi-Zadeh *et al.* (1969) noted a better performance of the Porteous Maze and Trial Making Tests at this time than at the end of the pregnancy, although complaints of mental 'fogginess' were commoner.

Puerperal depression

The main disorder intermediate between 'the blues' and severe melancholia is a state of weary, irritable despondency, varying from day to day and tending to worsen towards afternoon and evening. The depression is rarely of suicidal intensity, but is unfamiliar, mysterious and utterly spoils the experience of new motherhood. Guilt is secondary to irritability, and is never delusional. There is much anxiety, especially over the baby. Carne (1966) described how a vomiting baby may be a presenting sign of a mother's depression, and worries about all aspects of feeding, stools, crying, breathing and failure to thrive presented again and again to the general practitioner, health visitor or at the well baby (welfare) clinic may have equal significance. Irritability and exasperation are mainly directed towards the spouse and other children, but the baby is not exempt. Anxiety is often accompanied by anger, and an infant which keeps crying and cannot say what is wrong may be seen as a persecutor. Impulses to hit the baby very hard are common, and although rarely acted upon, puerperal depression is an occasional cause of non-accidental injury.

Despite utter weariness at the day's end there is difficulty in getting off to sleep. The husband who seeks to put things right by making love is likely to be rebuffed: depression diminishes libido. Appetite is usually low, but sometimes depressive over-eating – finding transitory comfort in food – increases weight, girth and self-disgust.

Normal confidence and competence are lost. The new mother is dismayed to find, on her return from hospital, that she cannot cope. Obviously, the addition of a baby to the home requires a new routine, but she cannot find one which enables her to get anything done, and feels that she is floundering against time. She may give up everything except the basic care of the baby, and let herself and the home go – often to her baffled husband's consternation. Some women describe puerperal depression as 'like being premenstrual all the time'.

Despite the extensive common knowledge of puerperal depression freely available in women's programmes on the radio, and in pages in newspapers and magazines, many women fail to recognize the disorder in themselves. As most have not suffered depression previously, they think something is physically wrong with them – anaemia, perhaps, or disordered glands – to explain their extraordinary fatigue. Those who do recognize their depression may be ashamed to admit it for fear of being thought ungrateful, unmotherly or making a fuss about nothing. If the delivery was safe and the baby well, what have they to be depressed about? Should they not be delighting in the joys of motherhood? Or, everyone knows that women get a bit depressed after having a baby, its called 'the blues', so why should they think that they require special attention? Partly for these reasons, only 5 of 33 mothers with puerperal depression, in the study by Pitt (1968), appeared to have had any treatment for it in the post-partum year.

It should be emphasized that these symptoms are by no means unique to the puerperium. They are characteristic of so-called neurotic or reactive depression, which presents more frequently to the general practitioner than the psychiatrist. A difference, however, is that whereas non-puerperal neurotic depression keeps recurring, usually under stress, many puerperal depressives have no previous history (Dalton, 1971; Kumar and Robson, 1978) and are less likely to relapse except after another birth.

Other disorders

Pitt (1968) found that just under 11% of the random sample of women who had their babies in The London Hospital during the period of his survey developed depression in the puerperium. A further 6% were classified as doubtfully depressed, and therefore excluded from the study group. They included:

1. Anxiety states unaccompanied by depression.
2. Anxiety and depression purely reactive to the baby's ill health.
3. Prolonged fatigue in the absence of other evidence of depression or anaemia.
4. The development or recurrence of possibly psychosomatic disorders such as migraine, rhinitis, epilepsy and psoriasis.
5. Diminution of libido as a single symptom.

Writing anecdotally, from experience, it seems that puerperal anxiety accompanying puerperal depression sometimes develops into phobic disorders. Some young mothers become housebound, for fear of going out. Others cannot stay indoors alone, and either call or keep their husbands at home as much as they can or have to go round to their mothers' or sisters' or a friend's home, leaving the housework until their husbands are at home. Others are able to go out only with the baby. The phobia may not then be apparent until the child is of school age, when the mother is afraid to let him go and be left on her own.

Loss of sexual interest, or orgasmic dysfunction (frigidity), is an all too common sequel of childbearing. Again and again one hears that a wife has gone off sex, or beome less keen, since she had the last, or even the first, baby. There are various possible reasons, but often none seems adequate as an explanation for what can become a major marital problem:

1. Continuing or only partly resolved depression.
2. Perineal soreness, say after an episiotomy; or laxity of the pelvic muscles, following pregnancy and delivery, which may make intercourse less enjoyable.
3. The fear of conceiving again, which can be very strong despite the availability of effective contraception.
4. Resentment of the husband, perhaps for his lack of support during pregnancy and the puerperium; or a feeling that having procreated, he has served his turn!

Causation

Thomas and Gordon (1959) put forward three theories to explain the occurrence of puerperal mental illness:

1. Childbirth is a cause of significant stress originating in physical factors such as hormonal disturbance or haemorrhage, or in psychological factors which can cause external stress, such as that produced by an unwanted pregnancy, or internal stress, such as that produced by difficulty in adjusting to the maternal role.
2. Childbirth is just one of any number of possible precipitants against a background of a constitution, inherited or acquired, which predisposes to psychosis indistinguishable from that unrelated to childbirth.
3. There is a personality or physical defect ('Achilles heel') relating specifically to sexual and reproductive life.

The merits of these three hypotheses will be discussed briefly, at the end of this section, but the reader may bear them in mind as the relative importance of constitutional, physical, psychological and social factors is now considered.

Constitutional factors

FAMILY AND PREVIOUS HISTORY OF MENTAL ILLNESS

Puerperal psychotics closely resemble women who develop psychosis unrelated to childbirth in respect of a family and previous history of mental illness. Fifty-three per cent of the series by Sim (1963) had such a family history. Thuwe (1974) showed that the children of women admitted to mental hospitals with a first attack of mental illness developing within the puerperium were significantly liable to mental illness too, and that nature was a more likely factor than nurture. Protheroe (1969) observed that the risk of affective illness among the relatives of patients with puerperal affective illness was very like that in those related to non-puerperal affective patients. Martin (1958) concluded from her survey of 75 patients admitted with post-partum mental illness that the only sure causative factor was heredity.

Similarly, a previous psychiatric history is found no less often for puerperal than for non-puerperal psychotics and far more often than in puerperal women free from mental illness. Seager (1960) indeed found a rather higher incidence of previous mental illness in puerperal than non-puerperal psychotic women, while Janssen (1964) found that the puerperal patients had more previous puerperal mental illness and the same order of previous psychiatric hospital care, although the non-puerperal mentally ill had had more outpatient psychiatric contact. In an uncontrolled study, Sim (1963) found previous puerperal psychosis in 27.6% of his puerperal subjects, and of mental illness in 44% altogether.

This, then, is the picture for psychosis. That for the milder disorders may be different. Neither Pitt (1973) nor any other workers have found a significant family or previous history in sufferers from 'the blues', and a family history is not characteristic of puerperal 'neurotic' depression. The evidence that such depressives are liable to have a previous history, however, is conflicting.

Neither Pitt (1968), Dalton (1971) nor Kumar and Robson (1978) found such a previous history, but Tod (1964) found a previous history in 55% of his (probably more severe) puerperal depressives, and in only 7% of their normal puerperal controls. Paykel et al. (1980) found a previous psychiatric history in 63% of their mild to moderately depressed puerperal subjects, and in only 13% of those who were not depressed: the difference is highly significant. Braverman and Roux (1978) used a previous history of post-partum depression successfully as a predictor of that disorder. Watson et al. (1984) found a highly significant association between depressive illness in the puerperium and a previous psychiatric history.

PREVIOUS PERSONALITY

Many undesirable traits have been attributed to those women subject to puerperal mental illness – inadequacy, immaturity, vulnerability, low self-esteem, shyness, aggression and denial – although these are hard to measure and the evidence is largely anecdotal and impressionistic. However, those experienced in the field agree most on the prominence of obsessional traits, especially in puerperal depressives.

For example, Sim (1963) described the typical previous personality of a puerperal patient: 'She is almost certainly married, with a moral code which precludes pre-marital intercourse. She marries reasonably young. Her school and employment records are effective and on the whole above average. Her personality is generally pleasant. The baby is generally planned, and she is a good mother. Her family too are of this stamp, and this will be reflected in their incidence of mental breakdown, which is usually of a depressive nature. She may show a degree of vulnerability to the commoner precipitating factors of breakdown such as bereavement, infection, operation and childbirth.'

Douglas (1963) describes a rather similar personality for puerperal depressives treated in the Cassel Hospital – 'good', compliant and over-controlled. Because they have learnt to do as they are told and suppress their rebellious and angry feelings, they are good patients at the ante-natal clinic but severely challenged by the demands of so primitive a being as a little baby. Pitt (1968) seemed to go some way towards verifying this when he found that puerperal depressives had significantly higher scores for neuroticism and introversion on the (shortened) Maudsley Personality Inventory than their normal puerperal controls, but probably the fact that they were depressed when completing the questionnaire was a distorting factor. Using the Eysenck Personality Inventory, Kumar and Robson (1978) found no association between neuroticism then and subsequent puerperal depression, but Watson et al. (1984) definitely did.

Nilsson and Almgren (1970) concluded that their subjects with 'post partum adaptational difficulties' were liable to deny their reproductive function, because they contacted the ante-natal clinic later and reported dysmenorrhoea and morning sickness less often than others. They also tended to see relatively little similarity between themselves and their mothers, more with their fathers, prefer masculine characteristics, to have had difficulties in sexual adjustment and not to regard motherhood as a primary aim.

Hayworth et al. (1980) found an association between extrapunitively hostile women (so assessed in pregnancy) and post-partum depression.

AGE

There is a little evidence (Janssen, 1964; Paffenbarger, 1964) that women admitted to psychiatric hospitals for puerperal mental illness tend to be somewhat older than normal puerperal controls, but Seager (1960) and Protheroe (1969) found no such difference.

As for the milder disorders, Kumar and Robson (1978) found a significant excess of puerperal depressives aged over thirty, but Paykel *et al.* (1980) found their depressed mothers to be younger than those not depressed, while Tod (1964) and Pitt (1968) found no difference.

Parity

Although post-partum mental illnesses most often follow a first baby (Fondeur *et al.*, 1957; Paffenbarger, 1964; Protheroe, 1969), anyone who ever has a baby has at least one and there is probably avoidance of subsequent childbirth by some of those who were ill after the first (Janssen, 1964). Dean and Kendell (1981), however, argued that there is a truly increased morbidity after a first birth.

Yalom *et al.* (1968) and Nott *et al.* (1976) found 'the blues' most often in primiparous women, but Pitt (1973), Handley *et al.* (1980) and Stein (1980) did not. Half of those suffering puerperal depressions, in the study of Tod (1964), did so after the birth of a third baby.

Overall, there is a lack of consistent evidence to link post-partum mental illness with any particular parity. Many women who are well after giving birth the first time develop major or minor mental disorder after a subsequent delivery.

Somatic factors

Childbirth is so great a physiological event, and the incidence of mental illness (after the two-day 'latency period') in the two weeks afterwards is relatively so high, that it is natural to conclude that some somatic aspect of the former is very likely to precipitate the latter.

HORMONAL CHANGES

As women are notoriously liable to mood changes in the course of the menstrual cycle (Dalton, 1960; see also Chapter 4) to say nothing of the menopause, and as the hormonal changes at parturition are greater than either of these (and far more sudden), they are often regarded as responsible both for puerperal psychosis and 'the blues'. Imbalance between oestrogen and progesterone following the third stage of labour (Malleson, 1953) is especially favoured. Reviewing this topic, Gelder (1978) considers that 'the blues' being so common and following delivery so closely are the most likely puerperal disorder to be hormonally induced, probably by progesterone withdrawal at the end of pregnancy. He was, however, unable to demonstrate that women more severely affected by 'the blues' suffered a bigger drop in progesterone post-natally than those with fewer and milder symptoms. However, women with 'the blues' could be more sensitive to hormonal change: for example, the study showed that those who suffered most from 'the blues' were more likely to report premenstrual tension (Nott *et al.*, 1976).

Although Gelder feels that puerperal psychosis is less likely to be hormonally determined, he notes the resemblance to postoperative psychosis, and suggests that changes in adrenal steroids resulting in differing levels of free cortisol could affect predisposed subjects in both situations.

The moderate disorders, such as puerperal depressions, which usually begin later than 'the blues' and psychosis, seem least likely to be hormonally caused, although

Dalton (1971) found that women developing depression tended to be euphoric at the end of pregnancy and claims that this means that they are especially sensitive to progesterone; they get 'high' when the level is high and then suffer prolonged withdrawal symptoms which manifest themselves as depression after delivery.

Linn and Polatin (1950) blamed the precipitate fall in the level of gonadatrophin. Bower and Altschule (1956) postulated rebound over-production of steroids after the loss of the placenta. Railton (1961) thought a lowering of the level of circulating corticoids was possibly relevant. Ballachey et al. (1958) and Grimmell and Larsen (1965) suspected relative hypothyroidism in the puerperium.

However, while all these theories are somewhat plausible, there is no firm evidence for any, and no endocrine treatment of post-partum mental illness, e.g. with progesterone, steroids or thyroxine, has gained acceptance.

An endocrine factor is largely responsible for psychosis associated with the hypopituitarism of Sheehan's syndrome (Schneeberg and Israel, 1960) but this is very rare.

AMINE THEORY

The work of Coppen, Eccleston and Peet (1973) on tryptophan was confirmed in childbearing subjects by Stein et al. (1976), who likewise found low levels of free tryptophan in the plasma of those most depressed (with 'the blues'). Handley et al. (1977) found a seasonal variation, free tryptophan being some 50% lower in the latter part of their study, from January to April. (If this is relevant, it could be one reason why women break down after one birth, yet not after another; a study giving particular attention to the date of delivery has yet to be made.)

They also found that those who failed to show a rapid rise in total tryptophan on the first 2 days after delivery were significantly liable both to 'the blues' and to complaints of depression in the next few months (Handley et al., 1980).

OBSTETRIC COMPLICATIONS

Except in the now rare delirious states, obstetric complications are surprisingly irrelevant to puerperal mental disorder (Tetlow, 1955; Protheroe, 1969). Pitt (1968), Dalton (1971) and Kumar and Robson (1978) found no higher incidence of complications among their puerperal depressives, while Paykel et al. (1980) even reported rather less. Dean and Kendell (1981), however, found that women admitted to psychiatric wards within 3 months of giving birth were significantly more likely to have had a caesarean section.

Psychological factors

The psychological impact of childbearing is so great that psychological theories vie with hormonal theories as the main cause of puerperal psychiatric disorders.

Apart from the anxiety and effort of labour, suddenly there is a major change from two-persons-in-one before delivery to two quite separate individuals afterwards, demanding considerable psychological adjustment.

BONDING

The work of Klaus and Kennell (1976) has shown the probable importance of bonding (the mother's intense attachment to her baby) in weathering this change and getting the relationship between mother and baby off to a good start. It is believed to be important that the mother be awake and alert to welcome her baby into the outside world, and that time be given at the time of birth for skin-to-skin contact between them. It is claimed that extra contact in the early puerperium has measurable effects on maternal behaviour (e.g. more attention and responsiveness to the baby, more eye-to-eye contact) months or even a year later. Caesarian section, heavy anaesthesia, an infant needing intensive care and the practice of taking the baby away after its birth and not returning it to the mother until some hours later are all thought to be obstacles to bonding. 'Leboyer' deliveries (Leboyer, 1974), which involve stroking the newborn baby while it lies on the mother's abdomen or at her breast immediately after delivery (along with hushed, twilit births, warm baths and not cutting the cord straight away), have the advantage that they should encourage bonding.

However, there is no evidence yet that bonding is a protection against puerperal mental disorder. Robson and Kumar (1980) found that while depression reduced maternal attachment, the presence or absence of early bonding was irrelevant to the subsequent development of puerperal depression. Bonding must make the heavy commitment of motherhood more of a pleasure than a chore, and in its absence the baby may be regarded as strange, ugly, messy, demanding and disconcertingly dependent, but it is not known to what extent this reduced quality of the maternal experience contributes to depression or psychosis.

INTERNAL AND EXTERNAL FACTORS

Victorhoff (1952) and Tetlow (1955) describe adoption psychoses, and Victorhoff (1952), Thomas and Gordon (1959) and Wainwright (1966) found 'puerperal psychosis' in fathers. It is difficult to invoke a primary somatic factor in any of these! But what is the nature of the psychological stress of childbirth? Is it external – a mishap like an illegitimate pregnancy or a perinatal death – or is there an internal factor which makes a normal experience an ordeal?

Internal psychological factors
The consensus of psychodynamic theories about internal factors, e.g. Bergler (1959), Lomas (1959) and Douglas (1963), is that vulnerable women are unable to accept the full responsibilities of their biological role, experience a reactivation of early conflicts (especially over their mothers) in pregnancy, find the demands of childbearing more than they can meet and are decidedly ambivalent about their offspring, although their hostility is usually covert. The views of Deutsch (1947) on the importance of female masochism are unlikely to find favour with many women these days, but help explain why some feel that by having a caesarean section or epidural anaesthesia they have cheated! Such theories are not implausible, but difficult to objectify and to prove.

External psychological factors
External stresses, on the other hand, are easier to measure:

1. *Illegitimate pregnancy.* In the studies of Tetlow (1955) and Janssen (1964) illegitimate pregnancy was followed significantly more often by psychosis, but this was not the case in those of Seager (1960), Paffenbarger (1964) and Protheroe (1969). Nilsson and Almgren (1970) did not find that their 'post

partum adaptational difficulties' were associated with being single at the time of conception or delivery.

2. *Unplanned pregnancy*. It is not easy to be sure whether and to what extent a pregnancy is unplanned, although possibly about 40% still are. Kumar and Robson (1978) found that puerperal depressives originally had doubts about going through with the pregnancy significantly more often than those who were not depressed, but this was not the finding of Pitt (1968). Breen (1975) found, in fact, that more of those women who were deemed 'ill-adjusted' to the birth of a first child had planned their pregnancies than those who were moderately or well adjusted. Thus, as is so often the case in this intriguing and perplexing field, the evidence is inconsistent and contradictory.

3. *Peri-natal death*. Internal factors, such as risk-taking and ambivalence, make a contribution to unplanned and illegitimate pregnancies, but peri-natal death of the baby is more obviously a totally unintended mishap and the evidence that it increases the risk of psychiatric disorder is, not surprisingly, pretty firm. Thus, Paffenbarger (1964) and Janssen (1964) both found significantly more such losses among puerperal psychotics than their normal obstetric controls, while in the study by Tod (1964) puerperal depressives more often had a history of stillbirth or bearing a congenitally abnormal baby. Clarke and Williams (1979) found that whereas only 4% of women with live babies showed moderate depression (as indicated by a Beck scale score of 17 or more) up to 6 months post-partum, 20% of those who had lost their babies were so depressed in the early puerperium. Later, however, the number dropped to 13%, and 6 months after the delivery there was no difference between the depression of younger mothers (under 24) with live babies and that of those who had lost theirs.

4. *Premature babies*. Caplan (1960) and Kaplan and Mason (1960) have well described the special difficulties of the mothers of premature babies. Paffenbarger (1964) found that mentally ill mothers had a significantly shorter pregnancy and lighter babies than those who were normal.

5. *Marital stress*. The state of a marriage is hard to measure, but marital stress is of probable relevance. Uncontrolled studies by Lomas (1960) and Daniels and Lessow (1964) described a situation where the wife breaks down because of a lack of maternal feeling, while the passive, habitually dominated, husband cannot give the strong support needed. A couple intensely dependent upon each other, each seeing the other as a tower of strength, are undone by the intrusion of the baby whose strenuous demands expose the patient's inadequacies. Controlled studies of puerperal depression give some support to these observations. Kumar and Robson (1978) found more marital tension in their patients than the controls, and Paykel *et al.* (1980) found that depressed mothers had significantly less support from and communication with their husbands. Watson *et al.* (1984) reported more marital dissatisfaction among subjects with post-natal affective disorder.

6. *Loss of parent*. Frommer and O'Shea (1973) found that twice as many women who had lost either parent because of death, desertion or separation by illness became puerperally depressed as those who had not been so deprived. Nilsson and Almgren (1970) described insufficient contact with the mother during childhood in those with 'post partum adaptational difficulties'. Kumar and Robson (1984) note childhood separation from the father in post-natal depressives.

7. *The baby*. It is as difficult to confirm or refute the notion that the baby itself is a

significant stress, causing depression, as it is to substantiate or discard hormonal theories. 'The blues' may be seen as a model for both. The first 2 days after delivery bring rest, relief and a sense of achievement, but on the third day and thereafter the baby is very much there to be looked after. A baby in the womb is a physical burden, but demands no maternal skill at all. Once out, however, it must be fed, changed, washed, comforted and guarded – not just for a few days but for years. Especially after the first baby, the impact of motherhood may account for some tears and misgivings in the early puerperium. Some babies seem fundamentally insecure. While it is generally supposed that anxious mothers make their babies anxious and fretful, thus increasing parental anxiety and setting up a vicious circle (e.g. the theory of 'three month colic' in *The Naked Ape* (Morris, 1963), it may well be that primarily unhappy, unsettled, sleepless, inconsistent 'cry-babies' can induce maternal anxiety which may not be allayed until the infant has developed enough to talk.

Social factors

Culture and social class have little bearing on a puerperal mental illness (Fondeur *et al.* 1957; Janssen, 1964), except where they affect obstetric standards. Paykel *et al.* (1980), however, found more depressive mothers to be inadequately housed. Their finding that these mothers also lack the support of their husbands or a confidante was anticipated by Gordon, Kapostins and Gordon (1965) and Gordon and Gordon (1960), who noted that a recent move, the absence of the husband at the time of the birth and lack of support from him and others were important determinants of the 'maternity psychiatric syndrome' in predisposed women.

Pitt (1971) unexpectedly showed that domiciliary births were more often followed by depression than hospital deliveries. The conclusion was that women seeking a home confinement at that time were a highly self-selected group, including not only very maternal, competent and confident women opposed to the 'medicalization of motherhood', but others who were simply terrified of hospital.

Cox (1978, 1979) studied women of the Buganda tribe in Uganda and, despite major difficulties in applying Western concepts of psychiatric illness to this group, was able to demonstrate levels of morbidity in pregnancy and the puerperium of approximately 17% and 8%, respectively – remarkably similar to the largely middle-class London women in the study by Kumar and Robson (1978). The anthropologists Stern and Kruckman (1983) postulate that a failure to 'structure' or make special the post-partum period and a lack of social recognition of the role transition for the new mother contribute to post-partum depression in the USA.

Conclusions

Returning to the three hypotheses of Thomas and Gordon (1959), mentioned at the beginning of this section, it appears that there is some evidence for all three:

1. Childbirth itself does seem to be a significant stress since it provokes a significantly high morbidity – not only for psychoses but for lesser mood disorders as well.
2. The close similarity of puerperal to non-puerperal *psychoses* in respect of a family and previous history of mental illness suggest that in these disorders childbirth is just one precipitant among several possible others.

3. Particularly in respect of the milder disorders, there appears to be in some women a peculiar vulnerability to childbirth, for so many puerperal depressives have never suffered depression before, or only after previous childbirth. The 'Achilles heel' idea, however, is probably too narrow. There is unlikely to be a single factor, but a number which together cause a special sensitivity to parturition and its aftermath.

Elsewhere, the writer had attempted a profile of the women at risk from puerperal depression (Pitt, 1981): 'It looks, then, as if a woman who lost her mother before the age of 11 (Frommer and O'Shea, 1973) with a previous history of depression (especially puerperal), with very mixed feelings about pregnancy, whose husband is unloving and unsupportive, who is poorly housed, lacks confidantes and suffers four or more unpleasant life-events shortly before or during her pregnancy (Paykel et al., 1980) and who becomes particularly anxious as the time of her delivery draws near (Tod, 1964; Meares, Grimwade and Wood, 1978), is a strong candidate for puerperal depression. Her plasma cortisol may be raised in the 38th week of pregnancy and her total tryptophan fails to rise just after delivery (Handley et al. 1980).'

Whether forewarned is forearmed will be considered in the next section.

Prevention

While it is not certain that post-partum mental illness can be prevented, there should be an alert awareness of risk and the significance of early symptoms so that the diagnosis may be made early and treatment started as soon as possible.

When the pregnant woman is first seen at the ante-natal clinic, a comprehensive history should be taken, including family history, personality, the social and marital situation, previous illnesses and reactions to childbearing, present state of mind and attitude to the current pregnancy, and any special problems.

Women thought to be at risk need extra support through pregnancy and the puerperium, not least to enable them to express their doubts, misgivings and negative feelings without fear of criticism. Gordon, Kapostins and Gordon (1965) showed that systematic education of pregnant mothers reduced post-partum morbidity. Best results were obtained where husbands attanded with their wives. They were informed about the responsibilities of motherhood, advised to get help from dependable friends, to make the acquaintance of couples recently experienced in parenthood, to restrict unimportant tasks, not to move house soon after giving birth, to bother less with keeping up appearances, to get plenty of rest, to avoid extra responsibilities and reduce those they already had while maintaining outside interests, and to arrange paid help and baby-sitters at an early stage. Except in the rare instance where previous childbirth has regularly been followed by severe mental illness, termination of a wanted pregnancy is rarely advised; as Sim (1963) pointed out, puerperal psychosis is not wholly predictable and early treatment is usually very effective. Therefore, even if there is a strong family and previous history of mental illness it should be possible for a wanted pregnancy to proceed provided that observation of the mother's mental state is particularly close. If the pregnancy is unwanted, on the other hand, the risk of psychiatric disorder post-partum can be added to the case for termination.

Treatment

Psychosis

The first step in management must be diagnosis. Puerperal psychoses are unlikely to be missed eventually, but can develop very swiftly, and the significance of severe sleeplessness, anxiety, perplexity and gloom in the early days after delivery, especially in those with a previous or family history of psychiatric illness, should not be overlooked. The danger of missing the early signs of psychosis is especially that the patient may commit suicide if her disorder is not noticed.

Deeply depressed or disturbed mothers and those who are plainly failing because of their mental state to look after their babies adequately need admission to a psychiatric ward, preferably taking their babies with them to reduce depression and guilt over their failure to cope and to encourage bonding and successful mothering. Mother and baby units (Bardon *et al.*, 1968; Margison and Brockington, 1982) still exist, but many general psychiatric wards are now prepared to admit one or two mothers with their babies. The other patients usually accept the infants gladly. The staff encourage the mothers to do at least something for their babies daily, under sufficient supervision, increasing the amount of mothering in line with improvement in the mental state.

Where already established, breast-feeding could and should be continued. It is an excellent way of getting mother and baby together, and of the psychotropic drugs commonly employed it is only if lithium carbonate is necessary (in treatment of the mother's mania or bipolar depressive illness) or benzodiazepines are used that there is a significant quantity of the drug in the milk. The antidepressants and major tranquillizers are secreted in very tiny amounts indeed.

Antidepressants (usually tricyclic – dothiepin, trimipramine, amitriptyline or clomipramine in doses of 75–150 mg/day) are very effective in the treatment of severe depression (or melancholia), but take at least 2 weeks to work. For the most pressing problems, e.g. anguish with strong suicidal tendencies or retardation and food refusal, electroplexy gives swift relief. The risk of pulmonary embolus associated with this treatment (Impastato and Gabriel, 1957) has been eliminated by the modern practice of giving muscle relaxants after anaesthesia before electroconvulsive therapy. Tranquillizers may be given to relieve agitation, say haloperidol 0.5 mg 3 times per day, or thioridazine 50–100 mg three times per day, but preferably not benzodiazepines if the mother is breast-feeding her baby.

The more sedative major tranquillizers – haloperidol up to 9 mg per day, thioridazine or chlorpromazine up to 600 mg per day, in divided doses – are given to manic patients, whose overactivity is thus lessened, although normal mood may not be restored for several weeks. Lithium carbonate is an alternative or complementary treatment – say 750–1000 mg per day, aiming at a serum lithium of about 0.6 mmol/l – but not in breast-feeders.

Tranquillizers are also given for schizophrenia – chlorpromazine (as above), or trifluoperazine, up to 30 mg per day. The latter is especially useful in the treatment of paranoid psychoses.

The treatment of delirium is that of the underlying disorder, e.g. rest and antibiotics for puerperal sepsis, with enough sedation (in the form of major tranquillizers) to ensure such rest, and a good night's sleep.

The background to these physical and pharmacological treatments is psychotherapy, to explain, encourage, reassure, increase insight into feelings the mother would rather disown but cannot (e.g. hostility to her baby) and enable her to talk about them frankly and get them into perspective: having such feelings, after all, is one thing – acting upon them is another. Therapeutic community wards, where patients and staff meet in groups very frequently, provide an excellent psychotherapeutic setting for puerperal mental illness, but there is also certainly a place for individual person-to-person therapy. Hayman (1962) has noted what rapid progress can be made in psychotherapy at this time: presumably because so much is changing, results can be achieved in months which might otherwise take years.

The relief of obvious environmental stress is clearly important, where possible, and the social worker is also involved with the spouse and family, who are caught up in the crisis of puerperal psychosis. Existing supports (e.g. a helpful mother or neighbour) need to be strengthened, others sought (e.g. getting the husband some time off work when this wife comes home), the needs of any other children met, and the patient relieved, if possible, of most responsibilities save for the baby and herself.

Unhelpful, uncomprehending, hostile, disparaging or rejecting attitudes need to be tackled, and it is sometimes desirable to start marital therapy. Frequent visiting, especially by the husband, is encouraged from the day of the patient's admission, and usually after a week or two she will spend her weekends at home. When she is finally discharged the general practitioner and health visitor should already be fully in the picture. Support and surveillance should also be provided by a community psychiatric nurse, who works with the health visitor, and the psychiatrist at an outpatient clinic or a day hospital. A home help can be valuable in doing the heavy housework and giving encouragement and sympathy.

Most mothers who become psychotic in the early puerperium can, however, be managed in the lying-in wards and later, with the resources mentioned in the previous paragraph, at home, without admission to a psychiatrist ward. If the psychiatrist is brought in early he may well be able to reassure both patient and staff. Drug treatments as described above can then be started, and usually the patient's discharge home need not be delayed. Indeed, if she is paranoid, sooner is usually better than later!

Maternity 'blues'

'The blues' really need no specialized treatment at the time, but it should be noted that mothers who are prepared for them at ante-natal classes are less likely to be disconcerted when they are affected and more able to accept reassurance that they are a familiar occurrence. A sympathetic word of encouragement and explanation by the midwife or doctor at the time is thus that much more effective.

Puerperal depression

It is important not to confuse 'the blues' with neurotic puerperal depression. Too often a woman who has felt wretchedly low for weeks is told that all she has is 'the blues', which is unhelpful and wrong. Far too often the condition remains undiagnosed (Pitt, 1968), and the depressed mother suffers in silence or expresses her feelings in bodily symptoms or disturbed family relationships.

Yet the simple question, 'have you felt depressed since you had your baby?' on the occasion of the post-natal examination (frequently six weeks post-partum) often allows a grateful outpouring of troubled feelings. There are also many tears, which are in part a sign of previously bottled-up depression, but which also show what a relief it is to be able to talk frankly, especially to the doctor or midwife, who is now seen as recognizing that women can get depressed after childbirth, rather than expecting them always to be joyful and appreciative. Time is needed for sympathetic listening to this abreaction followed by an explanation that although far from negligible this depression is pretty common, no reflection on maternal worth, and will pass. Arrangements need to be made for continuing support by the general practitioner, health visitor, social worker or sometimes a psychiatrist until the depression is over. At the follow-up sessions there is still the need for the patient to talk out bad feelings of despair, bitterness, guilt, inadequacy, envy or hostility, without being rebuked or too hastily silenced by reassurance. The husband may also need to be seen.

Probably an important reason why *pregnant* women appear to cope pretty well with their depression (which is just as common as in the puerperium) is because they are so well supported – not only by their families, the doctors and the midwives, but also by each other at the ante-natal clinics. Recognizing how often such support is lacking after delivery, some women have set up mutual support groups. Wellburn (1980), who herself suffered puerperal depression, describes post-natal support groups run by the National Childbirth Trust, and there is now in England an Association for Post Natal Illness for those who have been or are depressed.

Medication has a place in the treatment of the more severe, protracted or troublesome forms of puerperal depression. Dothiepin 75–100 mg daily is a generally useful antidepressant, but phenelzine (though a monoamine oxidase inhibitor, and thus requiring dietary and medical restrictions) is often of value, at a dose of 15 mg 3 times a day.

Anxiety may be eased by a benzodiazepine (e.g. lorazepam 1 mg 3 times a day) if the mother is not breast-feeding, or haloperidol 0.5 mg 3 times a day otherwise.

Prognosis

The prospect of recovery from puerperal psychosis is good. Janssen (1964) found that patients admitted to psychiatric hospitals with puerperal mental illness had a shorter stay than their non-puerperal controls. Protheroe (1969) found a better prognosis for affective than for schizophrenic puerperal psychosis, 86% of those admitted with the former making complete recoveries. The duration of a puerperal affective psychosis is rarely more than 2–3 months, whereas in schizophrenia residual symptoms (rarely sufficient, however, to prevent discharge home) may persist for years.

The risk of relapse after subsequent birth is usually given as 14–20% (Fondeur *et al.*, 1957; Martin, 1958; Protheroe, 1969). However, this is the risk of readmission, and the actual *incidence* of subsequent puerperal psychosis, which is then treated very early so that admission is avoided, may well be higher. Janssen (1964) noted a tendency for his patients to avoid getting pregnant again, and for depressives in particular to relapse puerperally rather than at other times. Protheroe (1969), however, failed to confirm this. Martin (1958) did not find that waiting 2 years for the next baby reduced puerperal relapse, but it seems commonsense that a women who has suffered puerperal psychosis should wait until she is properly recovered and her child is no longer an infant before she seeks another pregnancy. If she does become pregnant again, she should be carefully and frequently assessed until the new baby is at least 3 months old, and proper treatment should be given promptly at the first sign of relapse.

Far more of Janssen's puerperal patients were under psychiatric care outside the puerperium than their controls (who did not suffer from puerperal mental illness) in a follow-up period of at least 7 years, while 50% of Protheroe's patients had a subsequent non-puerperal episode.

Paradoxically, the prognosis for recovery from less severe puerperal depression may not be so good. There have been very few follow-up studies, but Pitt (1968) was able to trace 85% of his patients after a year, and found that while 57% of these had fully recovered, taking from a few weeks to several months to do so, 43% had not, describing such symptoms as loss of sexual responsiveness and other interests, irritability, ready depression and fatigue. This meant that at least 1 in 25 of the random sample of pregnant women followed into the puerperium seemed the worse for her experience a year later. No special features distinguished those who recovered fully from those who did not. However, hardly any of either group had received any treatment.

In another study, 16 women with very troublesome puerperal symptoms were followed up 4½ years later by semi-structured interviews, while their children were assessed in play sessions (Uddenberg and Englesson, 1978). Half the women reported repeated or prolonged spells of impaired mental health, poor relationships with spouse and baby and rejection of the maternal role. They were also described more negatively by their children.

Wolkind, Coleman and Ghodsian (1980) report a particularly poor prognosis for depression arising relatively late in the post-natal year (after 4 months) over the course of the next 4 years. These studies indicate how little justification there is for complacency about these 'neurotic' states arising in the puerperium. Diagnosis, treatment and support are all much in need of improvement, and further research into who is at risk, why and what may help them is vital.

Conclusions

The puerperium is a time of relatively high psychiatric risk. Milder emotional upsets (neuroses) are no commoner than in pregnancy, but may last much longer. Serious mental illness (psychosis) occurs more often post-partum than at any other period before the climacteric (and five times more frequently than after abortion). Only these serious disorders are significantly associated with a previous or family psychiatric history. Depression is by far the commonest puerperal psychosis, followed by mania.

It is unclear whether the hormonal upheaval of parturition or problems of relating to the new baby are the significant stress, but the evidence tends to favour the baby rather than the birth. Early loss of a parent, recent distressing life-events and lack of support contribute to depression.

Maternity 'blues' is as trivial as it is common, but more prolonged depression is a troublesome complication of the puerperium in at least 1 in 10 mothers and needs recognition, counselling, support and, sometimes, medication.

Psychosis (melancholia, mania, schizophrenia, paranoia or delirium) follows 1 in 200 births, but less than half necessitate admission to a psychiatric ward. Admission of the baby with the mother is desirable. Breast-feeding can be continued, despite the use of most psychotropic drugs.

The prognosis of mental illness developing in the puerperium is rather better than at other times. After depression, there is a greater risk of relapse following subsequent childbirth.

References

BALLACHEY, E. L., CAMPBELL, D. G., CLAFFEY, E., ESCAMILLA, R., FOSTER, A., HAMILTON, J. E., HARTER, J. M., LITTERAL, A. B., LYONS, H. M., OVERSTREET, E. W., POLIAK, P. P., SCHAUPP, K. L. JR., SMITH, G. and VORIS, A. T. (1958) Response of post partum psychiatric symptoms to triodothyronine. *Journal of Clinical and Experimental Psychopathology*, **19**, 170

BARDON, D., GLASER, Y. I. M., PROTHERO, D. and WESTON, D. H. (1968) Mother and baby unit; psychiatric survey of 115 cases. *British Medical Journal*, **25**, 755–758

BERGLER, E. (1959) Psychoprophylaxis of post partum depression. *Postgraduate Medicine*, **25**, 164–168

BLAIR, R. A., GILMORE, J. S., PLAYFAIR, H. R., TIDSALL, M. W. and O'SHEA, C. (1970) Puerperal depression: a study of predictive factors. *Journal of the Royal College of General Practitioners*, **19**, 22–25

BLEULER, E. (1911) *Dementia Praecox or the Group of Schizophrenias* (translated by J. Zinkin). New York; International Universities Press

BOWER, W. H. and ALTSCHULE, M. D. (1956) Use of progesterone in the treatment of a post partum psychosis. *New England Journal of Medicine*, **254**, 157–160

BOYD, D. A. (1942) Mental disorders associated with childbearing. *American Journal of Obstetrics and Gynecology*, **43**, 148–163, 335–349

BRAVERMAN, J. and ROUX, J. F. (1978) Screening for the patient at risk for post partum depression. *Obstetrics and Gynaecology*, **52**, 731–736

BREEN, D. (1975) *The Birth of a First Child: Towards an Understanding of Femininity*. London: Tavistock Press

BREWER, C. (1978) Post abortion psychosis. In *Mental Illness in Pregnancy and the Puerperium* (Sandler, M., Ed.). Oxford; Oxford University Press

BROCKINGTON, I. F., SCHOFIELD, E. M., DONNELLY, P. and HYDE, D. (1978) A clinical study of post partum psychosis. In *Mental Illness in Pregnancy and the Puerperium* (Sandler, M., Ed.). Oxford; Oxford University Press

BROCKINGTON, I. F., WINOKUR, G. and DEAN, C. (1982) Puerperal psychosis. In *Motherhood and Mental Illness* (Brockington, I. F. and Kumar, R., Eds). London/New York; Academic Press/Grune and Stratton

CAPLAN, G. (1960) Patterns of parental response to the crisis of premature birth. *Psychiatry*, **23**, 365–374

CARNE, S. (1966) The influence of the mother's health on her child. *Proceedings of the Royal Society of Medicine*, **59**, 1013–1014

CLARKE, M. and WILLIAMS, A. J. (1979) Depression in women after peri-natal death. *Lancet*, i, 916–917

COPPEN, A., ECCLESTON, E. G. and PEET, M. (1973) Total free tryptophan concentration in the plasma of depressive patients. *Lancet*, ii, 1415–1416

COX, J. (1978) Some socio-cultural determinants of psychiatric morbidity associated with childbearing. In *Mental Illness in Pregnancy and the Puerperium* (Sandler, M., Ed.). Oxford; Oxford University Press

COX, J. (1979) Psychiatric morbidity and pregnancy: a controlled study of 263 semi-rural Ugandan women. *British Journal of Psychiatry*, **134**, 401–405

COX, D., CONNOR, Y. and KENDELL, R. E. (1982) Prospective study of the psychiatric disorders of childbirth. *British Journal of Psychiatry*, **140**, 111–117

DALTON, K. (1960) *The Premenstrual Syndrome*. London; Heinemann

DALTON, K. (1971) Prospective study into puerperal depression. *British Journal of Psychiatry*, **118**, 689–692

DANIELS, R. S. and LESSOW, H. (1964) Severe post partum reactions: an interpersonal view. *Psychosomatics*, **5**, 21–26

DAVIDSON, J. R. T. (1972) Post partum mood change in Jamaican women: a description and discussion on its significance. *British Journal of Psychiatry*, **121**, 659–663

DEAN, C. and KENDELL, R. E. (1981) The symptomatology of puerperal illness. *British Journal of Psychiatry*, **139**, 128–133

DEUTSCH, H. (1947) *The Psychology of Women*, Vol. 11, *Motherhood*. London; Research Books

DOUGLAS, G. (1963) Puerperal depression and excessive compliance with the mother. *British Journal of Medical Psychology*, **36**, 271–278

ELLIOTT, S. A., RUGG, A. J., WATSON, J. P. and BROUGH, D. I. (1983) Mood changes during pregnancy and after the birth of a child. *British Journal of Clinical Psychiatry*, **22**, 295–308

FONDEUR, M., FIXSEN, C., TRIEBEL, W. A. and WHITE, M. A. (1957) Post partum mental illness. *Archives of Neurology and Psychiatry*, **77**, 503–512

FROMMER, E. and O'SHEA, R. (1973) Ante natal identification of women liable to have problems in managing their infants. *British Journal of Psychiatry*, **123**, 149–156

GELDER, M. (1978) Hormones and post partum depression. In *Mental Illness in Pregnancy and the Puerperium* (Sandler, M., Ed.). Oxford; Oxford University Press

GORDON, R. E. and GORDON, K. (1960) Social factors in the prevention of post partum emotional problems. *Obstetrics and Gynecology*, **15**, 433–438

GORDON, R. E., KAPOSTINS, E. E. and GORDON, K. (1965) Factors in post partum emotional adjustment. *Obstetrics and Gynecology*, **25**(2), 158–166

GRIMMELL, K. and LARSEN, V. (1965) Postpartum depressive symptoms and thyroid activity. *Journal of the American Medical Women's Association*, **20**, 542–546

HAMILTON, J. A. (1962) *Postpartum Psychiatric Problems*. St. Louis; Mosby

HANDLEY, S. L., DUNN, T. L., BAKER, J. M., COCKSHOTT, C. and COULD, S. E. (1977) Mood changes in the puerperium and plasma tryptophan and cortisol concentrations. *British Medical Journal*, **2**, 18–22

HANDLEY, S. L., DUNN, T. L., WALDRON, G. and BAKER, J. M. (1980) Tryptophan, cortisol, and puerperal mood. *British Journal of Psychiatry*, **136**, 498–508

HARRIS, B. (1980) Maternity blues. *British Journal of Psychiatry*, **136**, 520–521

HAYMAN, A. (1962) Some aspects of regression in non-psychotic puerperal mental breakdown. *British Journal of Medical Psychology*, **35**, 135–145

HAYS, S. P. and DOUGLASS, A. (1984) A comparison of puerperal psychosis and the schizophreniform variant of manic depression. *Acta Psychiatrica Scandinavica*, **69**, 177–181

HAYWORTH, J., LITTLE, B. C., BONHAM CARTER, S., RAPTOPOULOS, P., PRIEST, R. G. and SANDLER, M. (1980) A predictive study of post partum depression – some predisposing characteristics. *British Journal of Clinical Psychology*, **53**, 161–167

HEMPHILL, R. E. (1952) The incidence and nature of puerperal mental illness. *British Medical Journal*, **2**, 1232–1235

IMPASTATO, D. J. and GABRIEL, A. R. (1957) Electroshock therapy during the puerperium. *Journal of the American Medical Association*, **163**, 1017–1022

JACOBSON, L., KAIJ, L. and NILSSON, A. (1965) Post partum mental disorders in an unselected sample: frequency of symptoms and predisposing factors. *British Medical Journal*, **1**, 1640–1643

JANSSEN, B. (1964) Psychic insufficiencies associated with childbearing. *Acta Psychologica Scandinavica*, Suppl. 172

JARRAHI-ZADEH, A., KANE, F. J., VAN DE CASTLE, R. L., LACHENBRUCH, P. A and EWING, J. A. (1969) Emotional and cognitive changes in pregnancy and the early puerperium. *British Journal of Psychiatry*, **115**, 797–805

KANE, F. J., HARMAN, W. J., KEELER, M. H. and EWING, J. A. (1968) Emotional and cognitive disturbance in the early puerperium. *British Journal of Psychiatry*, **114**, 99–102

KAPLAN, D. M. and MASON, E. A. (1960) Maternal reactions to premature birth viewed as an acute emotional disturbance. *American Journal of Orthopsychiatry*, **30**, 539–547

KARNOSH, L. J. and HOPE, J. M. (1937) Puerperal psychoses and their sequelae. *American Journal of Psychiatry*, **94**, 537–550

KENDELL, R. E. (1978) Childbirth as an aetiological agent. In *Mental Illness in Pregnancy and the Puerperium* (Sandler, M., Ed.). Oxford; Oxford University Press

KLAUS, M. H. and KENNELL, J. A. (1976) *Maternal-Infant Bonding*. St. Louis; Mosby

KRAEPELIN, E. (1913) *Lectures on Clinical Psychiatry. Puerperal Insanity* (translated by T. Johnstone). London; Baillière, Tindall and Cox

KUMAR, R. and ROBSON, K. (1978) Previous induced abortion and ante natal depression in primiparae. *Psychological Medicine*, **8**, 711–715

KUMAR, R. and ROBSON, K. (1984) A prospective study of emotional disorders in childbearing women. *British Journal of Psychiatry*, **144**, 35–47

LEBOYER, F. (1974) *Birth Without Violence*. London; Wildwood House

LINN, L. and POLATIN, P. (1950) Psychiatric problems of the puerperium from the standpoint of prophylaxis. *Psychiatric Quarterly*, **24**, 375–384

LOMAS, P. (1959) The husband–wife relationship in cases of puerperal breakdown. *British Journal of Medical Psychology*, **32**, 117–123

LOMAS, P. (1960) Dread of envy as an aetiological factor in puerperal breakdown. *British Journal of Medical Psychology*, **33**, 61–66

MADDEN, J. J., LUHAN, J. A., TUTUER, W. and BIMMERLE, J. F. (1958) Characteristis of post partum mental illness. *American Journal of Psychiatry*, **115**, 18–24

MALLESON, J. (1953) An endocrine factor in certain affective disorders. *Lancet*, **ii**, 158–164

MARCÉ, L. V. (1858) *Traité de la folie des femmes enceintes, des nouvelles accouchées et les nourices*. Paris; Baillière

MARGISON, F. and BROCKINGTON, R. F. (1982) Psychiatric mother and baby units. In *Motherhood and Mental Illness* (Brockington, I. F. and Kumar, R., Eds.). London/New York; Academic Press/Grune and Stratton

MARTIN, M. (1958) Puerperal mental illness – a follow-up study of 75 cases. *British Medical Journal*, **2**, 773–777

MEARES, R., GRIMWADE, J. and WOOD, D. (1978) A possible relationship between anxiety in pregnancy and puerperal depression. *Journal of Psychosomatic Medicine*, **18**, 605

MORRIS, D. (1963) *The Naked Ape*. London; Jonathan Cape

NEUGEBAUER, R. (1983) Rate of depression in the puerperium. *British Journal of Psychiatry*, **143**, 420–421

NILSSON, A. and ALMGREN, P. E. (1970) Para-natal emotional adjustment: a prospective investigation of 165 women. *Acta Psychiatrica Scandinavica*, Suppl. 220

NOTT, P. N., FRANKLIN, M., ARMITAGE, C. and GELDER, M. G. (1976) Hormonal changes and mood in the puerperium. *British Journal of Psychiatry*, **128**, 379–383

NYSSEN, R. (1955) Introduction à l'étude clinique des psychoses puerpérales. *Bruxelles Médical*, **35**, 1243–1248

OSTERMAN, E. (1963) Post partum psychopathological states. *Acta Psychiatrica Scandinavica*, Suppl. 169, 190–192

PAFFENBARGER, R. (1964) Epidemiological aspects of postpartum mental illness. *British Journal of Preventative and Social Medicine*, **18**, 189–195

PAYKEL, E. S., EMMS, E. M., FLETCHER, J. and RASSABY, E. S. (1980) Life events and social support in puerperal depression. *British Journal of Psychiatry*, **136**, 339–346

PITT, B. (1968) 'Atypical' depression following childbirth. *British Journal of Psychiatry*, **114**, 1325

PITT, B. (1971) Neurotic (or atypical) depression following childbirth. In *Psychosomatic Medicine in Obstetrics and Gynaecology* (Morris, N., Ed.). Basel; Karger

PITT, B. (1973) 'Maternity blues'. *British Journal of Psychiatry*, **122**, 431–435

PITT, B. (1981) Depression and childbirth. In *Handbook of Affective Disorders* (Paykel, E. S., Ed.). London; Churchill Livingstone

PROTHEROE, C. (1969) Puerperal psychoses: a long term study – 1927–1961. *British Journal of Psychiatry*, **115**, 9–30

PUGH, J. F., JERATH, B. K., SCHMIDT, W. M. and REED, R. B. (1963) Rates of mental illness related to childbearing. *New England Journal of Medicine*, **268**, 1224–1228

RAILTON, I. E. (1961) The use of corticoids in post partum depression. *Journal of the American Medical Women's Association*, **16**, 450–452

REES, D. and LUTKINS, S. G. (1971) Parental depression before and after childbirth. *Journal of the Royal College of General Practitioners*, **21**, 26–31

ROBIN, A. (1962) Psychological changes of normal parturition. *Psychiatric Quarterly*, **36**, 129–150

ROBSON, K. M. and KUMAR, R. (1980) Delayed onset of maternal affection after childbirth. *British Journal of Psychiatry*, **136**, 347–353

RYLE, A. (1961) The psychological disturbances associated with 345 pregnancies in 137 women. *Journal of Mental Science*, **107**, 279–286

SCHNEEBERG, N. C. and ISRAEL, S. L. (1960) Incidence of unsuspected Sheehan's syndrome. *Journal of the American Medical Association*, **172**, 20–27

SEAGER, C. P. (1960) A controlled study of post partum mental illness. *Journal of Mental Science*, **106**, 214–230

SIM, M. (1963) Abortion and the psychiatrist. *British Medical Journal*, **2**, 145–148

SKOTTOWE, I. (1942) Mental disorders in pregnancy and the puerperium. *Practitioner*, **148**, 157–163

STEIN, G. S. (1980) The pattern of mental change and body weight change in the first post partum week. *Journal Psychosomatic Research*, **24**, 165–171

STEIN, G. S., MILTON, F., BEBBINGTON, P., WOOD, K. and COPPEN, A. (1976) Relationship between mood disturbances and free and total plasma tryptophan in post partum women. *British Medical Journal*, **2**, 457

STENGEL, E., ZEITLIN, B. and RAYNER, E. H. (1958) Post operative psychoses. *Journal of Mental Science*, **104**, 389–402

STERN, G. and KRUCKMAN, L. (1983) Multi-disciplinary perspectives on post partum depression: an anthropological critique. *Social Science and Medicine*, **17**, 1027–1041

STRECKER, E. A. and EBAUGH, F. G. (1926) Psychoses occurring during the puerperium. *Archives of Neurology and Psychiatry*, **15**, 239–252

TETLOW, C. (1955) Psychoses of childbearing. *Journal of Mental Science*, **101**, 629–639

THOMAS, C. L. and GORDON, J. E. (1959) Psychosis after childbirth: ecological aspects of a single impact stress. *American Journal of Mental Science*, **238**, 363–388

THUWE, I. (1974) Genetic factors in puerperal psychosis. *British Journal of Psychiatry*, **125**, 378–385

TOD, E. D. M. (1964) Puerperal depression: a prospective epidemiological study. *Lancet*, **ii**, 1264–1266

UDDENBERG, N. and ENGLESSON, I. (1978) Prognosis of post partum mental disturbance; a prospective study of primiparous women and their 4½ year old children. *Acta Psychiatrica Scandinavica*, **58**, 201–212

VICTORHOFF, V. M. (1952) Dynamics and management of parapartum neuropathic reactions. *Diseases of the Nervous System*, **13**, 291–312

WAINWRIGHT, W. H. (1966) Fatherhood as a precipitant of mental illness. *American Journal of Psychiatry*, **123**, 40–44

WATSON, J. P., ELLIOTT, S. A., RUGG, A. J. and BROUGH, D. F. (1984) Psychiatric disorder in pregnancy and the first post natal year. *British Journal of Psychiatry*, **144**, 453–462

WELLBURN, A. (1980) *Post Natal Depression*. London; Fontana

WOLKIND, S., COLEMAN, E. and GHODSIAN, M. (1980) Continuities in maternal depression. *International Journal of Family Psychiatry*, **1**, 167–181

YALOM, I. D., LUNDE, D., MOOS, R. H. and HAMBURG, D. A. (1968) Post partum 'blues' syndrome. *Archives of General Psychiatry*, **18**, 16–27

Chapter 7

Termination of pregnancy

Peter C. Olley

Introduction

Distinctive aspects of induced abortion

Induced abortion currently engenders, probably more than any other medical procedure, fierce controversy and debate in society, both within and far beyond the ranks of the medical profession. Compared with other gynaecological operations it possesses certain distinctive features which can make the decision-making especially complex, with social, ethical, religious and legal dimensions to be considered in addition to strictly clinical criteria:

1. There may be legal restrictions on the doctor's clinical judgement, e.g. dictating the latest time of gestation when termination is permissible, or preventing abortion where the only significant indications are social. Under certain circumstances induced abortion may be deemed a criminal act, with the operation liable for prosecution even though performed in appropriate, hygienic clinical surroundings at an early stage of pregnancy by a qualified gynaecologist.
2. Induced abortion is one of a select group of medical procedures where, because of intense motivation of many patients, illegal, undercover, often unqualified commercial abortionists can flourish (the 'back street operators'), or where on occasion the pregnant woman herself may attempt self-induction or threaten suicide if denied medical help.
3. In the usual medical situation the intention is to preserve or prolong life as well as improving its quality. Termination of pregnancy, however, can be held to involve the destruction of human life or at very least abolish the potential for a future independent human existence. Some medical and nursing staff may thus refuse on principle to advise or assist in termination operations. In some countries they can be legally exempted on grounds of conscience without detriment.
4. The practice of induced abortion may be actively opposed on moral and ethical grounds by individuals and by certain social and religious groups (e.g. the Society for the Protection of the Unborn Child, the Roman Catholic Church). Such groups will generally discourage their own members from assisting with or subjecting themselves to termination, and campaign for the procedure to be further limited and perhaps outlawed for society at large. Wide coverage by the

173

news media, mass demonstrations and intensive political lobbying may be employed to influence public opinion and persuade the legislature to maintain or pass restrictive laws.
5. Countering these pressures, other groups may be formed to promote more liberal abortion laws or defend the existing provisions (e.g. the Abortion Law Reform Association). They are likely to use broadly similar propaganda techniques to the anti-abortionists to mobilize public and political opinion in their favour. Thus, many extra-clinical factors and pressures are involved in the decision-making process for induced abortion. By comparison, the indications for most gynaecological procedures, e.g. pelvic floor repair, removal of ovarian cyst, etc., are relatively uncomplicated. It therefore behoves medical practitioners involved in referral, assessment or treatment of women with 'unwanted' pregnancies to have a particularly clear understanding of their own attitudes to induced abortion, a thorough grasp of the principles involved, and an up-to-date knowledge of relevant research findings to inform the decision-making and subsequent management.

An outline of arguments for and against induced abortion

A variety of major and supplementary arguments are put forward by the proponents and opponents of a liberal legal abortion policy. The two sides are frequently composed of loose coalitions of disparate interests with many different motives and shades of opinion represented in each pressure group. Many supporters of one point of view would not assent to all of the arguments advanced in its favour.

THE ANTI-ABORTIONISTS' CASE

Induced abortion is an immoral act, against God's will, involving the destruction of a human being. It implies a gross disregard for the sanctity of human life and its continuation will eventually lead to the corruption of society. Under a liberal abortion policy women may be pressured into having a termination against their will. Induced abortion can be a dangerous procedure for the pregnant women. There are frequent deleterious short- and long-term medical or psychological sequelae of termination of pregnancy. Future childbearing abilities of the aborted woman may be impaired, leading to sterility, miscarriage or low birth weight.

A pregnancy, initially unwanted, may be accepted at a later stage, or after delivery. Most and perhaps all women, even those with gross mental or physical illness, can be supported through pregnancy and beyond if appropriate resources are mobilized.

Adoption is available for those women who are unable or unwilling to look after their child. A liberal abortion policy will discourage the use of contraception and will lead to 'abortion on demand'.

A woman who has had the child will thank the gynaecologist for persuading her to change her mind and be glad she did not have the abortion.

THE PRO-ABORTIONISTS' CASE

The life and health of the pregnant woman and her future quality of life and that of her existing children should be the prime consideration, if necessary overriding the right of the fetus to life.

In the early stages of pregnancy the fetus cannot be considered as a live person – it is incapable of life independent of the mother and at this stage can be regarded as a part of the woman's body.

Continuation of certain pregnancies may have more severe consequences for the woman and her family than an early abortion.

Every child that is born should be wherever possible a healthy, wanted child, received into a home where sufficient material and emotional support can be given to ensure its proper development.

A woman should have the right to determine what happens to her own body, including the continuation or discontinuation of a pregnancy. She should not be forced to give birth against her will, e.g. a pregnancy following a rape. A liberal legal abortion policy will eventually reduce the incidence of criminal abortion and thereby decrease maternal mortality and morbidity.

Children born against the mother's will are liable to psychiatric and behaviour problems, themselves leading miserable lives.

The international scene

ABORTION LEGISLATION

Considerable variation between countries in abortion legislation and practice is apparent. Five main categories of legal status for induced abortion can be distinguished which illustrate the broad gradations of opinion about the procedure; estimated percentages of the world's population in mid-1982 living under these legal systems are recorded in brackets (Tietze, 1983):

1. Prohibited under any circumstance (10%).
2. Allowable only where the mother's life is at risk from the pregnancy (18%).
3. Broader medical indications are permissible, where the mother's physical and/or mental health is being threatened by continuation of the pregnancy (8%).
4. Where social as well as strictly medical conditions can be taken into account in the decision (25%).
5. Abortion on request from the pregnant woman (39%).

During the past 15 years a general trend towards more liberal legislation has occurred so that currently about two-thirds of the world's population live in countries where abortion is legally available for broad social and medical reasons or on request. However, it should be noted that restrictive laws are not necessarily strictly enforced nor is termination of pregnancy necessarily easily available even where there are liberal legal provisions (Ashton *et al.*, 1980). Furthermore, the conditions under which an induced abortion may be obtained may fluctuate in a country over a period of years, with for example a relaxation of legal criteria being followed later by a tightening up of the laws – reformation and counter-reformation. These changes may be due to a particular pressure group having temporarily succeeded in swaying the legislature towards its policy or, as in the case of certain Eastern European countries, due to central governments' concern at a low birth rate.

The state of abortion legislation should be viewed as a dynamic rather than a static situation, ever liable to be influenced by general social change.

Accurate statistics about the incidence of induced abortion throughout the world are difficult to assemble. Some major countries do not publish statistics for legal termination and there is no completely reliable way of estimating the incidence of illegal abortion. Recent estimates, admittedly highly speculative, place the abortion rate at up to 55 million per year with some 70 per thousand women in the childbearing years being involved and corresponding to an abortion ratio of 300 abortions per 1000 live births (Tietze, 1983).

The abortion ratio is a useful statistic which relates abortions during a period to live births occurring in a similar period 6 months later. Thus, overall, it is estimated that for every 4 children born alive there have been between 1 and 2 fetuses aborted. Some countries have periodically reported much higher abortion ratios. For example, in 1964 the abortion ratio in Hungary was nearly 1400 per 1000 live births, so that during a period of abortion on request (1959–73) legal abortions exceeded live births. Subsequently, restrictive legislation operative in 1974 abruptly reduced the number of abortions by about 40%.

In those countries where reliable abortion statistics are gathered, a number of general trends in legal abortion can be discerned over the past decade:

1. There has been a rapid increase in the abortion rates among younger and especially unmarried women. This effect has been variously attributed to a host of factors including earlier maturation, changing patterns of sexual behaviour, the acceptance of abortion as an alternative to forced marriage or illegitimate birth, more liberal abortion laws and altered attitudes to abortion by medical practitioners.
2. The peak age for legal abortion has tended to fall in most countries, although there is still considerable variation in the age distributions from different parts of the world. For instance, in 1980, Finland, Japan and Tunisia recorded about 10% of the abortions occurring in the age group 40 years and over, compared with some 1–2% in Canada and the USA. In the 19 years and under age group the proportion is some 20–30% for Canada, UK, USA and Norway, but about 2% for Tunisia and Japan.
3. There are two main age patterns of legal abortion: (a) countries where the abortion ratio tends to increase steadily from younger to older age groups (e.g. Czechoslovakia, Hungary); (b) areas (Canada, England and Wales, Sweden, USA) where the abortion ratio for young women is moderately high reducing to a low at 20–24 or 25–29 and then increasing steadily to a maximum at 40 years or more.
4. Internationally, parity-specific abortion ratios show three distinct distributions: (a) a steady increase from those with none or only 1 prior birth to those with 5 or more (e.g. Singapore); (b) an increase from low rates for childless women to a maximum at 2 or 3 prior births (e.g. Czechoslovakia, Hungary); (c) high abortion ratios among nulliparous women falling to a minimum at 1 prior birth, increasing to a maximum at 4 prior births and declining again at higher parities (e.g. England and Wales, Finland, Sweden, USA).

In Europe and North America there has been a general decline in abortion ratios at higher parities, i.e. abortion for the grand-multiparous woman has become less important. This phenomenon probably reflects the long-established small family norm in these areas, with many women who go on to have larger families being opposed to abortion. High abortion ratios among childless women are due to the large proportion of unmarried women in this group, whereas parity-specific statistics for married women show low ratios for nulliparous wives, with the majority of married women obtaining abortions having previously given birth to 2 or more children, and a maximum at 1 prior birth (England and Wales, Hungary) (Tietze, 1983).

Thus, international abortion practice, despite several uniform trends in recent years, still retains several broad but distinct patterns, e.g. in North America and Western Europe, the European Communist bloc and Third World countries. These reflect, among other factors, differences in the societies, age structures, norms for family size, and abortion laws.

The British Abortion Act 1967

Principal features of the Act

This moderately liberal Act conveniently illustrates many important aspects of abortion legislation and their implications for decision-making. It came into force in England, Wales and Scotland in April 1968, but does not apply to Northern Ireland where the prevailing attitudes were in favour of more restrictive provisions.

The Act makes abortion legal 'if two registered medical practitioners are of the opinion, formed in good faith:

(a) that the continuance of the pregnancy would involve risk to the life of the pregnant woman or of injury to the physical or mental health of the pregnant woman or any *existing* children of her family, greater than if the pregnancy were terminated,

or

(b) that there is a substantial risk that if the child were born it would suffer from such physical or mental abnormalities as to be seriously handicapped.'

One of the above practitioners will usually, although not necessarily, be the gynaecologist carrying out the termination.

The so-called 'social clause' in the Act further qualified these essentially medical indications for abortion by stating: 'In determining whether the continuance of pregnancy would involve such risk of injury as is mentioned in paragraph (a) . . . account may be taken of the pregnant woman's actual or reasonably foreseeable environment.'

Some opponents of the Act felt this clause introduced undue flexibility, allowing unacceptably wide interpretations of terms such as 'reasonably foreseeable environment' to be made, so that abortion on purely social grounds became possible, thereby paving the way to 'abortion on demand'. Comments from medical protection societies indeed suggest that the social and economic consequences of a continued pregnancy can be considered in evaluating likely adverse effects on the health of the mother and the existing children, and in this connection the mother's marital status and intelligence can also be taken into account.

It should be noted that the environmental influences included in the Act refer to those acting on the mother and the existing children. The foreseeable future social situation for the fetus (e.g. as a child in an economically deprived single parent family) is not mentioned as relevant to an abortion decision. However, the Act is concerned with any medical abnormality in the fetus that might prevent it, if born, from leading an independent existence at an appropriate age. Thus a substantial risk of inherited conditions such as Huntington's chorea, phenylketonuria, or acquired malformations such as might result from maternal rubella, would constitute grounds for legal abortion.

In applying the Act in the majority of cases where there is no substantial risk of fetal abnormality, the medical practitioner must predict the relative risk to life of the mother, or health of the mother and existing children, from continuing the pregnancy, or terminating it. It is not expressly stated that the risks must be substantially greater or that the injury to health must be serious, but simply that the risks from continuing the pregnancy must be judged the greater, before induced abortion is legal. Critics of the Act in fact attempted unsuccessfully to alter these provisions in Parliament so that serious injury to health must be proved.

Emergency abortions are possible under the Act, where one registered medical practitioner is of the opinion in good faith that termination is immediately necessary to save the life or prevent grave permanent injury to the physical or mental health of the pregnant woman. A second opinion is not required in these special circumstances, thereby avoiding undue delay in operating. A standard certificate must be signed and completed by the assessing doctors *prior* to a termination (except in certain emergency situations), listing the main grounds for the abortion, and notification must be made to central health authorities within 7 days of the operation. Rules are also specified restricting the disclosure of this information.

The Abortion Act 1967 also included a conscience clause stating that no person is obliged to participate in any treatment authorized by the Act to which he has conscientious objection, unless the treatment is necessary to save the life of, or prevent grave permanent injury to, the physical or mental health of the pregnant woman. In England and Wales conscientious objection might have to be proved in legal proceedings, whereas in Scotland a statement on oath in Court is considered sufficient. It should however be noted that the clause does not release a medical practitioner from general obligations to his patient. For instance, referral to another doctor should be made where the medical practitioner feels unable, because of conscientious objection, to give an opinion in good faith, or to recommend or carry out the abortion while recognizing that there might be sufficient lawful grounds in that particular case. However, a gynaecologist is not in any way compelled to terminate a pregnancy on a patient duly recommended under the Act by two other practitioners, if in his opinion abortion is contraindicated.

The Act did not change the existing legal time limit of 28 weeks' gestation beyond which, on the grounds of fetal viability, abortion was not permitted. However, many pro-abortionists as well as anti-abortionists have considered this limit to be too extreme, risking the abortion of fetuses capable of independent survival. The former group have been in favour of a 24-week limit. Anti-abortionists in fact pressed unsuccessfully via Private Member's Parliamentary Bills to reduce the limit to 22 or even 20 weeks.

In addition to outlining the grounds for legal abortion and laying down rules for notification, the 1967 Abortion Act was also concerned with regulating the places where an abortion might be performed. These were limited to National Health Service (NHS) hospitals or certain hospitals specially approved for the time being by the Minister of Health or the Secretary of State. Such licences could be reviewed and revoked when necessary if standards of practice were thought to be unsatisfactory.

Impact of the Act

What then has been the effect of introducing such legislation which, although not abortion on request, in practice permits abortion on broad medical grounds, supplemented by social considerations?

Its impact on the existing legal situation was far greater in England and Wales than in Scotland. Under the latter country's different legal system it had been possible prior to 1968 'for a doctor acting in good faith to perform a therapeutic abortion, where after careful study of all the circumstances of the case, and after due consultation with colleagues, he decides that the disadvantages of continuing the pregnancy was greater than those of ending it' (Baird, 1967). In England and Wales, where the legal attitude to abortion derived essentially from the Offences against the Person Act of 1981, and the Infant Life (Preservation) Act of 1929, there was a much more restrictive situation prior to 1968. These Acts, respectively, made punishable any unlawful attempts at abortion, and allowed abortion 'in good faith' to preserve the life of the mother.

Test cases, notably the celebrated Rex v. Bourne case of 1938, subsequently modified the court's interpretation and modestly extended the grounds for legal termination. In the above case a distinguished gynaecologist invited prosecution after aborting a 14-year-old girl pregnant after a rape, and was acquitted by the Court. Justice McNaghten's summing up provided much of the basis for legal abortion in England and Wales until the Abortion Act 1967. Thus, the new legislation represented a radical change for England and Wales, whereas under Scottish Common Law doctors had been terminating pregnancies 'in good faith', protected from prosecution, for 30 years before the 1967 Act. It should be noted that legal abortion in Scotland during this era had mostly involved debilitated grand-multiparous married women from lower socio-economic groups, often to be followed by sterilization, that many Scottish gynaecologists did not avail themselves of their legal rights in this respect and that many doctors were not aware of the fundamental legal differences on abortion between the two areas.

In England and Wales, and in Scotland, in the 5 years following the implementation of the Act, the total number of legal abortions performed rose rapidly to a plateau in 1972–74, declined slightly until 1977 and thereafter has

TABLE 7.1. Legal abortions, totals and rates for England and Wales, and Scotland*, by year and residence (after Tietze, 1983)

	1966	1969	1971	1973	1975	1979	1981
ENGLAND AND WALES							
Total abortions	21 400†	54 800	126 800	167 100	139 700	149 700	162 500
Non-residents	—	5 000	32 200	56 600	33 500	29 100	33 900
Residents	—	49 800	94 600	110 600	106 200	120 600	128 600
Abortion rate/1000 women age 15–44 for residents	—	5.3	10.1	11.7	11.2	12.1	12.6
SCOTLAND							
Total abortions	—	3 700	6 900	8 600	8 400	8 800	10 000
Abortion rate/1000 women age 15–44 for residents	—	3.7	6.8	8.4	8.1	8.2	9.2

* The Scottish figures include residents of Scotland obtaining abortions in England.
† Estimate from Diggory and Simms (1970).

shown a rising trend for all age groups back to the previous plateau level (*Table 7.1*). These recent changes have been ascribed both to increases in the fertility rate, a certain disenchantment with 'safe' contraceptive methods (e.g. oral contraception and intra-uterine devices), the pressure on health authorities to reduce regional variations in the abortion services, the reluctance to continue with an unplanned pregnancy during economic recession, and the reduction of family planning services due to financial stringency (Priest, 1972; Ashton *et al.,* 1983).

TABLE 7.2. Percentage of women currently married at termination, by year (after Tietze, 1983)

	1969	1973	1975	1977	1979	1981
England and Wales	46.2	42.4	40.6	38.8	36.2	33.5
Scotland	52.7	43.9	42.1	39.5	38.1	33.4

TABLE 7.3. Abortion, by year and type of service, for residents of England and Wales (after Tietze, 1983)

	1969	1971	1973	1975	1979	1981
NHS hospitals	33 500	53 500	55 500	50 900	55 600	61 100
Non-NHS premises	16 300	41 100	55 100	55 300	65 100	67 500

The proportion of currently married women at the time of termination has fallen steadily since the Act (*Table 7.2*). Several distinctive differences between abortion practice in the two areas, however, have been preserved. In Scotland, legal abortion takes place predominantly (95%) in NHS hospitals, whereas in England and Wales there is a large private sector with NHS facilities providing only about 40% of the total operations. A considerable proportion of the terminations carried out in England and Wales have been on women not normally resident in the country, although this proportion seems to have declined in recent years (*Table 7.1*) as more European countries bring in liberal abortion legislation. Even so, NHS terminations constitute only about one-half of the total for residents (*Table 7.3*) (Tietze, 1983).

Despite the present uniformity of abortion legislation in the UK, there have been wide regional variations in the legal abortion rates. It has clearly been more difficult to obtain a legal abortion in certain districts than in others, depending to a significant degree on the attitudes of the general practitioners and the gynaecologists in the area. *Table 7.4* illustrates the 1972 figures, showing an almost

TABLE 7.4. Regional variations in abortion rates per 100 live births in Great Britain (1972)

Newcastle	11.0	Oxford	6.6
London and Home Counties	10.6	Wessex	6.1
Wales	9.5	Liverpool	5.4
South West	9.5	Sheffield	5.3
Scotland	9.4	Leeds	4.5
East Anglia	8.1	Birmingham	3.2
Manchester	7.2		

four-fold variation between Newcastle and Birmingham. Ashton *et al.* (1980) have commented on the difficulty in obtaining NHS abortions in Wessex.

Much criticism has been periodically expressed about certain aspects of some private sector abortion facilities. It has been alleged that 'abortion on demand' is practised, that there may be insufficient length of inpatient stay and a lack of after-care in order to deal with the large volume of work. A number of clinics have in fact had their approved status for abortion withdrawn. The geographical anomalies in abortion availability, coupled with concern about the high cost of an abortion in the private sector, led to the foundation of charitable organizations, e.g. the British Pregnancy Advisory Service (BPAS), offering pregnancy testing, advice and counselling on obtaining an abortion, and often their own abortion clinics with modest fees. These clinics tended to be set up in areas where NHS abortions were relatively difficult to obtain. Critics of the 1967 Act have striven without success to separate the advisory services from the charitable abortion clinics.

Submission from organizations such as the British Medical Association and the Report of the Lane Committee on the Working of the Abortion Act (1974) would suggest that despite some reservations the Abortion Act 1967 is regarded by the majority of the medical profession as a useful piece of legislation which does not currently require radical alteration.

The process of decision-making

Issues for examination

A number of issues can be distinguished in the career of the abortion applicant: (a) circumstances that lead up to her becoming pregnant; (b) reasons for the pregnancy to be considered as 'unwanted'; (c) why abortion has been chosen as the solution to the problem; (d) the chain of referral to the gynaecologist; (e) the gynaecologist's decision about abortion and how this is made; (f) the nature of the pregnant woman's response to this decision.

Clearly, an application for termination of pregnancy is usually a late episode in a chain of events in which several different professionals may be involved at one time or another. The pregnant woman herself is entangled in a distinctive web of circumstances and relationships, and a number of other people such as the putative father or the woman's parents may also have an intense, vested interest in the outcome. It is therefore important, in the management of what essentially is a crisis situation, to understand the different roles and predicaments of the various actors in the drama.

Some of the material in this chapter is derived from the author's experience in Aberdeen, Scotland, where a moderately liberal abortion policy (although certainly falling far short of 'abortion on demand') has been in force for more than a quarter of a century. During this period, comprehensive, detailed records on all obstetric and nearly all gynaecological patients have been accumulated and have formed the basis for a series of research studies on fertility behaviour in general, and abortion practice in particular, in a total community of some 200 000 (Baird, 1967; Horobin, 1973). Thus, multidisciplinary studies of abortion can be seen in perspective against other comprehensive information on illegitimate pregnancies, spontaneous abortion, contraception and sterilization, etc., in the city's total population (Aitken-Swann, 1973; McCance, Olley and Edward, 1973; Thompson, 1977). Although abortion practice and attitudes do vary with time and place, many of the basic situations that were encountered in Aberdeen seem to be both universal and perennial and are probably currently replicated in many other Western industrialized societies.

The people involved

THE PREGNANT WOMAN – THE ABORTION APPLICANT

Clearly she is the principal person involved, with the main attention being focused on her history, health and circumstances.

'Unwanted' pregnancy

At the time of assessment for termination, many of the women have firmly decided that their pregnancy is 'unwanted' and wish to have it terminated, but there are exceptions. Some may be undecided or actually in the process of changing their minds, whereas others may have essentially accepted the pregnancy but are being coerced into having an abortion by their sexual partner or their parents. Unwanted by whom? is a highly relevant question. Thus, it is important to determine the patient's *own* attitude to the pregnancy at an early stage in the assessment.

The concept of unwanted pregnancy is itself complex. 'Unwanted' should not be regarded as a term interchangeable with 'illegitimate' or 'unplanned'.

Some unmarried women may be pleased to be pregnant, perhaps to hasten a marriage, to confirm their feminine status or to have the child of an admired consort that they are debarred from marrying. Occasionally, from the outset, pregnancy is embarked upon with the deliberate intent of rearing a child in a single-parent family situation without the male partner. An unplanned pregnancy may also be accepted from the start by the pregnant woman.

Nevertheless, many illegitimate and many unplanned pregnancies are regarded as unwanted by the pregnant woman. Indeed, Bone (1973) found that over one-third of pregnancies to married or stably-cohabiting women were unplanned and about one-half of these were 'sorry it had happened at all'. Regret about pregnancy appears to increase with parity, rising from 5% of those having their first or second child to more than 30% having their third, and over 50% their fourth or later child (Cartwright, 1976). Initial conscious feelings of marked disappointment and anxiety at becoming pregnant are frequently encountered even among married women in stable circumstances expecting their first babies. Frequently, this is only a transient feature and a rejecting view in the first trimester is often replaced by acceptance by the third trimester, illustrating a possible pitfall in assessment for therapeutic abortion. Furthermore, a 'wanted' pregnancy does not always lead to a wanted child or an unwanted pregnancy to a rejected child. Yet another complexity is introduced by psychodynamic writers who aver that a pregnancy apparently accepted at a conscious level may be rejected at a level outside full awareness and result in, for instance, neglect of appropriate antenatal care. An ambivalent attitude to pregnancy has been cited by Chertok, Mondzain and Bonnaud (1963) in cases of hyperemesis gravidarum. Conversely, gross delay in seeking abortion for an 'unwanted' pregnancy may occasionally be interpreted as an underlying desire to continue to term.

Contraceptive practice
Every pregnant abortion applicant (for a few are discovered by the gynaecologist not to be pregnant) has been, in effect, an inefficient contraceptor. However, there is a wide spectrum of individual reasons for this. One group, particularly among the unmarried, will have totally neglected contraceptive measures. For others, notably the married women, there has been a failure of contraception. This may result from the use of an intrinsically inefficient technique, e.g. safe period, spermicidal jelly or the irregular use of an efficient method such as the oral contraceptive pill. A minority of the applicants will claim to have been meticulous users of an efficient method, and even occasionally a woman who has previously undergone a sterilization operation will become pregnant and apply for termination in a bitter and bewildered mood.

Lack of effective contraception is frequently due to ignorance about suitable techniques, fear or distaste for certain methods such as 'the pill' and sometimes difficulty that single women experience in obtaining contraceptives. These deficiencies are largely correctable by the provision of better education and more widely available contraceptive services.

Some religious groups oppose the use of certain effective methods on principle and in some socially disadvantaged subcultures contraception may be tacitly discouraged. Nevertheless, there are many intelligent well-informed women, without specific fear of contraception, who neglect to take precautions, carry them out haphazardly or discontinue them while still at risk. This behaviour may be one example of many in a chaotic, disorganized personality who muddles through life generally, or may be related to adverse side effects experienced with certain techniques such as the pill or intra-uterine devices (IUDs).

However, these factors would seem not to be the whole explanation and deeper psychological motives for inefficient contraception have been suggested for some women. Sandberg and Jacobs (1971) list a variety of such factors in both married and unmarried women. They comment on the denial of personal responsibility for contraception by some women and in some cases the denial that pregnancy was a possibility for them. Sexual intercourse without contraception might also be seen as proof of a deep commitment to the boyfriend or the pleasure may be enhanced by the thrill of risk-taking. In some women there seems to be the underlying need to bolster low self-esteem or confirm their femininity by becoming pregnant. Alternatively, a pregnancy may be used to control a relationship or to express hostility or rebellion towards parents by unmarried women. Pregnancy may also occur during an abnormal mental state of depression or elation, or under the influence of alcohol or drugs, when normal contraceptive measures are neglected.

Thus, there exists a significant group of women at risk of an unwanted pregnancy who are unlikely to be influenced by standard education and information about contraception. They may require special counselling and support to maintain their motivation for regular, consistent contraception, although even these measures may prove unsuccessful.

Alternatives to legal abortion
At the stage of application, the candidate for abortion has voluntarily rejected or downgraded, or has been coerced out of, other possible solutions to the unwanted pregnancy, although these alternatives may be reconsidered at a later time.

Where opportunities for legal abortion are restricted, then illegal procedures by 'back-street operators' or self-induction tend to flourish, with an increased risk of septic or haemorrhagic complications. Woodside (1963), in an interesting study of convicted female abortionists in prison, modifies the common stereotype of the unscrupulous, greedy individual preying on unfortunate women. Several of these abortionists had themselves experienced the problems of an unwanted pregnancy and saw themselves as providing a sort of social service for token payment for working class women in distress.

Accurate estimation of the extent of illegal abortion is difficult. Some 'spontaneous' and many 'septic' abortions are likely to be procured illegally. In Britain, since the 1967 Act, hospital admission for 'septic' abortion has decreased significantly as has the rate of 'spontaneous' abortions for women with illegitimate pregnancies, a probable explanation being a reduction in the number of illegal abortions. There may, however, be a delay of a few years for such changes to develop after the introduction of a liberal abortion programme, as the new legal possibilities percolate slowly through to the people and then start to influence practice.

Resort to illegal abortion or to the final solution – suicide – may be threatened by some applicants if legal abortion is withheld from them. Other possible solutions all entail continuing the pregnancy, with a series of further options for child-rearing. The woman may keep the baby or have it brought up by someone else, either informally or officially fostered or adopted.

Unmarried mothers may rear their babies themselves, with or without support from the putative father or their family. They may marry the putative father or sometimes another man during the pregnancy in order to give the baby legitimacy. Marriage may be deliberately delayed until after childbirth in order to diminish the element of coercion in the situation. On occasion, the baby may be brought up by a relative, often by the woman's own mother, possibly treated as a younger sister and perhaps even officially adopted.

In Britain nowadays, adoption is more and more frequently rejected as an acceptable alternative by pregnant unmarried women, often being regarded as more psychologically traumatic than other options. Consequently, there is a considerable shortage of normal babies available for placement by the adoption agencies. Rearing an unwanted child in adverse circumstances may lead on to child abuse and even neonaticide or infanticide (Resnick, 1970).

The pregnant woman's predicament

The abortion applicant has found herself in a particular set of circumstances which define her pregnancy as undesirable, either to herself or to significant others.

Presenting reasons for termination tend to differ according to marital status and legitimacy of pregnancy. A number of common patterns can be distinguished.

(1) THE UNMARRIED WOMAN. These tend to be young, physically fit, primigravid women, often from the higher socio-economic groups, professing ignorance of, or total neglect of, effective contraception. Lack of available social support and undue distortion of their life situation by having to bear and rear an illegitimate child, potentially leading to serious distress and disorganization, are usually the broad reasons for seeking termination. One or more of the following specific reasons are often advanced in support of induced abortion.

(a) *Marriage is not feasible.* The putative father may be known but considered as unsuitable or too unreliable for marriage. He may have deserted the applicant, denied responsibility for the pregnancy, be untraceable or may even be dead. In fact, he may be prepared to marry but she may have refused. Often the applicant deliberately avoids telling him that she was pregnant. Various unpleasant characteristics of the putative father may have recently been discovered, for example, alcohol abuse, a criminal record or mental instability. Although fond of him, she may feel that a 'shotgun' marriage, possibly involving living in adverse conditions, would be doomed from the start. Under these circumstances she would be uncertain whether he had married her for love. On occasion, marriage between the pair may take place later after childbirth or termination when these pressures have remitted. Pregnancy may have occurred in the context of a casual relationship, with little commitment or affection on either side. The putative father might already be married, a fact which is often unknown to the applicant at the time of conception. On the other hand, the relationship may have been entered into with full prior knowledge of the situation. She may not be prepared to break up another family unit or the married man may refuse to leave his family and may put pressure on her for a termination if she wished to continue the relationship. Occasionally, it is alleged that the sexual partner is unknown and that conception had occurred at a party while the applicant was under the influence of alcohol or drugs, or as a result of rape by an unknown assailant.

(b) *Rejection by the family*. The single woman may fear ostracism or total rejection by her parents or other significant relatives if they should discover her pregnancy. A sister may have previously been in a similar predicament and been denigrated and treated harshly by the family. Girls from certain strict religious backgrounds, or having parents who have specifically threatened dire consequences if they became illegitimately pregnant, may feel particularly ashamed, distressed and depressed at having let them down. They may be unable to contemplate continuing the pregnancy and consider that suicide is the only real alternative to abortion. At the same time they may also be in a state of conflict because of other prohibitions against abortion. However, the prediction of the family's harsh reaction may be quite unrealistic and in the event they may be more accepting than the applicant believes possible.

(c) *Impairing the health of other family members*. She may consider that news of her illegitimate pregnancy might produce a nervous breakdown or physical deterioration in a parent already under stress or suffering ill health, for instance a recently widowed mother with heart disease.

(d) *Adverse effects on careers*. Continuation of the pregnancy at this stage of the applicant's training or job may be seen by her or her family as a major disruption that will ruin further prospects of a chosen career for which considerable sacrifices may already have been made. This will apply particularly to students and those in apprenticeship and professional training. Additionally marriage and responsibility for a child may also be seen as detrimental to the putative father's career, e.g. forcing him to give up a poorly paid but valued apprenticeship for a more immediately lucrative job with fewer eventual prospects. Thus, pressures for termination from the girl's parents, the putative father or his parents may be generated, although the applicant herself may be relatively unmoved and quite prepared if left to herself to continue the pregnancy.

(e) *Reduction in essential earnings*. Especially in the case of older single women, the applicant's earnings may make a vital contribution to the family budget. A widowed mother or an invalid father with numerous younger siblings might have to be supported and a pregnancy could result in the loss of a valued job with little future prospect of a similar one.

(f) *Adverse living conditions*. Having to look after a young baby would make the present overcrowded accommodation intolerable for the applicant or her family. Alternatively, they might be forced out of their present lodgings into impossibly expensive or even more unsatisfactory housing as a result of the pregnancy.

(g) *Applicant is too young.* The pregnant girl and perhaps also the putative father may be considered as too young or economically dependent to marry and too emotionally immature to tolerate childbirth or rear a child. Pregnancies in school children and especially in girls under 16 years generally cause great concern in modern Western society. The number of such pregnancies increased in the early 1970s in the UK, possibly as a response to earlier puberty, greater social freedom and sexual permissiveness, but in recent years have declined. In fact, during the period 1970–80 there was a reduction of 8% in the conception rate for girls under 16 years of age. However, in the UK a high proportion of under 16s presenting for termination will be granted the operation. These abortions form some 2–3% of the total legal abortions and amount to some 5000 yearly, in England and Wales, out of a total of 8500 conceptions for the under 16s (Office of Population Census and Surveys, 1984).

Many such girls come from large families and broken homes with disturbed interpersonal relationships, lack of understanding and erratic discipline. Minimal knowledge of contraception, and sometimes of sexual matters in general, are frequent findings. They may feel starved of affection by their parents and develop a morbid craving for a loving relationship. The pregnancy may be preceded by disturbed rebellious behaviour and a deteriorating academic record. A minority continue to manifest disorganized antisocial behaviour and personality traits leading on to drug and alcohol abuse, further illegitimate pregnancies, abortions, increased infection and suicidal attempts.

It should be noted that considerable pressure may be applied by parents on young pregnant teenagers to have an abortion even when they are themselves prepared to continue with the pregnancy.

Young applicants, possibly due to unfamiliarity with the symptoms of pregnancy, a reluctance to approach parents or a general practitioner, and a tendency to denial ('it could never happen to me') are often referred at a comparatively late stage of pregnancy, possibly even too late for an abortion to be performed.

(2) THE EVER-MARRIED WOMAN WITH A LEGITIMATE PREGNANCY. This group, pregnant by their husbands, are often older multiparous mothers, with poor health or adverse social and financial circumstances, with contraceptive techniques that have failed and who are frequently requesting subsequent sterilization. The pattern of principal reasons for seeking termination differs from the unmarried group.

(a) *Marital problems.* Many applicants have a strained, unsatisfactory relationship with their husband, perhaps amounting to open hostility. He may be cruel, unfaithful, abuse alcohol, be economically and emotionally unsupportive or absent for long periods, possibly in prison. A pregnancy may be perceived as likely to precipitate a total breakdown of the marriage or, alternatively, to hinder an intended separation from the husband, and she may find the prospect of bearing his child totally repugnant.

(b) *Adverse socio-economic conditions.* Poverty and cramped inadequate accommodation may be associated with marital disharmony, but may also occur in united families beset by unemployment, low wages and ill health. An extra child to rear may be considered as a burden that would stretch the already extended family resources beyond the acceptable limit, and lead to serious deterioration in health and living conditions. The family may rely heavily on the pregnant woman's wage packet to survive economically.

(c) *Applicant too old.* Women in their late thirties, possibly in poor health, with teenage or older children and who themselves may be grandmothers, may become apprehensive at the prospect of going through the process of pregnancy and child-rearing all over again after a gap of so many years. Some confess to being ashamed at being pregnant at 'their advanced age', and have concealed the fact from their teenage children lest they be regarded by them as 'sex maniacs'!

(d) *Family complete.* Younger, comparatively fit women with several existing children and a settled planned way of life, perhaps involving extensive financial commitments requiring them to work, may consider, together with their husband, that they do not wish to increase the size of their family.

(e) *Health problems.* The applicant may have a previous history of serious obstetric complications or mental physical illness that can be aggravated by a further pregnancy. She may be currently suffering from a major illness, e.g. cardiac disease, rheumatoid arthritis, ulcerative colitis, manic depressive illness, or she may have been debilitated by a series of recently closely-spaced pregnancies. There could be a specific fear of further pregnancy and labour. Some women, despite their illness, dearly wish to continue with the pregnancy, although appreciating the potential danger to their health, but may be coerced by their relatives and medical advisers to have an abortion. Other family members may be so sick or dependent on the applicant that the family unit would break down if she had to cope with a further pregnancy.

(f) *Risk of serious fetal abnormality.* Frequently this involves women exposed to rubella in early pregnancy, but is also relevant to those with a family history of serious genetically-transmitted illness such as Huntington's chorea or a personal history of previous fetal abnormality such as Down's syndrome. Amniocentesis may help to clarify the actual risk.

In the ever-married group, clear medical indications for termination are generally more frequent than in the unmarried. The question of future sterilization has frequently to be considered in the ever-married group, but rarely in the unmarried, although on occasion it may be undertaken, for example in vulnerable unmarried mentally subnormal girls recurrently liable to sexual exploitation.

(3) EVER-MARRIED WOMEN WITH ILLEGITIMATE PREGNANCIES. In the Aberdeen series (Olley, 1973), 18% of the ever-married group admitted at referral to being pregnant by a man other than their husband. This situation was most frequent in the under 30 age group of applicants. Some of these women had marriages that they wished to preserve, but on impulse had had sexual intercourse with a casual acquaintance or sometimes a family friend at a party, during the husband's prolonged absence, for example at sea, or during a period of temporary estrangement from him. On occasion, the husband had been previously vasectomized.

The majority in this group were however separated, divorced or widowed. Most had become pregnant to a man they could not or would not wish to marry, while a few had a steady relationship with the putative father and were awaiting the outcome of divorce proceedings before marrying him. Widows in particular seemed to react with particularly intense guilt. Some of them had hoped for a second marriage, but had been let down by their sexual partners. Others had coped perfectly well with their sexuality in the context of marriage, but had become illegitimately pregnant on more than one occasion following their husband's death. A number of these ever-married women felt too embarrassed and ashamed to approach their general practitioner for contraception, although continuing to put themselves at risk of pregnancy. The group as a whole was characterized by frequent complete neglect of contraception, compared with the ever-married legitimate pregnancy group, and conformed much more closely to the pattern of the unmarried applicants, not only in this respect, but also in their youthfulness, parity and the presence of personality disorder.

(4) REPEAT ABORTERS. It was reported that 8.6% of women obtaining termination via the British Pregnancy Advisory Service in 1975 had previously had one or more legal abortions. Statistics from NHS hospitals are generally much lower, in the region of 3–5%. Despite these figures there is little evidence that abortion is used deliberately by many individuals in the UK as a form of birth control substituting for contraception, as has been the practice in Japan and Hungary.

Concern has been expressed that induced abortion might lead to obstetric complications in later pregnancies such as spontaneous abortion, low birth weight and prematurity and that these complications are likely to be even more prevalent in repeat aborters.

In the Aberdeen series of abortion applicants (Olley, 1973), 20% of the unmarried women were illegitimately pregnant for the second or further time and were, despite their previous experience, even more generally neglectful of contraception than those presenting with their first pregnancy.

Beard et al. (1974), however, reported in their follow-up study of outpatient abortion 81% of women some 1 or 2 years after termination using reliable contraceptive methods, compared with 41% of their cohort using any form of contraception immediately before conception. Schneider and Thompson (1976), however, considered that motivation for contraception waned steadily after an initial improvement following the first abortion.

About one-half of the second abortion pregnancies can be ascribed to contraceptive failure rather than neglect. There seem to be few definite distinguishing characteristics between those who have had one and those who have experienced two induced abortions. Brewer (1977a) studied a group who had had three abortions, in the hope of finding distinctive characteristics. He related their erratic use of contraception to previous unsettled relationships, poor education and a history of psychiatric illness. In the USA, patients on welfare have been reported as showing little improvement in their contraceptive regime following successive abortions (Shepard and Bracken, 1979).

These women clearly merit special attention if any reduction in the rate of repeat abortion is to be effected. The use of an IUD rather than oral contraceptives and continued counselling to maintain motivation for contraception might reduce the need for repeat abortions.

The chain of referral
Attaining a legal abortion can be viewed as an obstacle race, with a series of hurdles to be surmounted by the applicant before the goal is reached. Initially, she must convince herself that this is what is required, or at any rate feel that an interview with a doctor about the decision is indicated. In the process she may have to overcome attitudes implanted by her family and social background against such a course. She may not in fact consult significant others, such as husband, parents or putative father. Alternatively, they may be aware of her predicament, allow her to make her own decision or try to strongly influence her judgement for or against termination.

The process may stop at this point and the general practitioner be approached only for the purpose of arranging ante-natal care. However, the abortion application may progress via general practitioner, to the gynaecologist, with thereafter other professionals such as psychiatrist or social worker being implicated. It is now necessary to convince a series of professionals who themselves have to operate within the existing legal framework. Ingram (1971) comments on the various strategies that may be employed by both patients and doctors in his witty and penetrating article on 'Abortion games'.

Rejection of the application may occur at one of several points, or during the process the applicant may herself change or clarify her mind and decide to continue the pregnancy.

Those who change their minds

Aitken-Swann (1973), in a retrospective Aberdeen cohort of some 3000 applicants gathered over a nine-year period, showed that 5% had changed their minds and decided to continue with the pregnancy. Often this was before a clinical decision had been made, but occasionally it occurred after they had been accepted for termination. Change of mind might occur after interview with the general practitioner but before assessment by a gynaecologist, or after discussion with the latter, and occasionally even after admission to hospital for the abortion! Ever-married women and those in a more advanced stage of gestation were much more likely to reconsider their initial decision. On occasion, the application was proceeded with merely to placate husband or parents.

A husband may in fact play an important part in stiffening an ambivalent woman's resolve for abortion. If he falters, she may then take the opportunity to decline the operation. Sometimes after a full explanation of what is entailed in termination, a discussion of the various options and a chance to think over the general situation, many wavering applicants will opt for continuation of the pregnancy. Especially in the case of unmarried women the social situation may have changed in the interim, the putative father may have offered marriage or her family offered support, thus swaying the balance away from abortion.

Clearly, it is important to allow sufficient time for reflection and discussion before proceeding with an operation, although in some instances only minimal delay is possible before an abortion becomes impracticable.

THE HUSBAND OR THE PUTATIVE FATHER

The male sexual partner may or may not know of the pregnancy or the abortion application. If he is aware of the situation he is likely to have definite views and feelings about the pregnancy and its proposed termination. With unmarried applicants, consent from the putative father for abortion is not necessary. Generally, if the applicant is married and living with her husband he should be brought into a full discussion if time and circumstances permit, especially where the health of existing children is involved. Where a risk to the life or mental or physical health of the wife is concerned in the application it is not essential in the UK for consent of the husband to be obtained. Clearly, support from husband or putative father for the decision, whether this be continuation or termination of the pregnancy, is likely to improve the outcome as long as there is a consensus and it is not a case of coercion. Where feasible, it is important to involve him in the subsequent management. Research on the attitudes of the putative fathers of unmarried abortion applicants is sadly lacking and we know very little about their characteristics.

THE GENERAL PRACTITIONER

Inevitably, general practitioners develop attitudes about the desirability and availability of induced abortion in certain circumstances. They are an important link in the chain of referral and may block or facilitate referral to a specialist for the next stage of the process. Some may allow their own views of appropriate sexual behaviour or morality to unduly influence their abortion decision. Despite the law they may, for example, believe that abortion is only indicated in situations where the woman's life is at risk. General practitioners may filter out certain types of applicants, especially unmarried women from lower socio-economic groups. Certainly, the Aberdeen experience is that a much lower proportion of pregnant unmarried unskilled workers are referred to gynaecologists for termination than those from student or professional groups. The latter are likely to resemble more nearly their own daughters and the doctor can empathize more closely with their predicament. Furthermore, it is widely held (with little objective evidence to substantiate the view) that a lower social class family is less distressed by and more easily able to cope with an illegitimate birth. By contrast, referrals of married women for abortion show no clear social class bias.

General practitioners with a conscientious objection to abortion often refer the applicant to a colleague who is able to take a more objective attitude. However, it is also possible for the practitioner to refer patients selectively to 'conservative' gynaecologists who are unlikely to abort or to 'liberal' gynaecologists who almost certainly recommend termination, thereby effectively prejudging the issue. Clearly, the general practitioner can have a vital role in helping the applicant to clarify her own views, to initiate further referral and mobilize appropriate support. For some women suspecting themselves to be illegitimately pregnant, contact with their family practitioner, who may ordinarily have a close and trusting relationship and be 'a friend of the family', will be avoided. They will prefer to go to independent pregnancy testing and advisory services where they are relatively anonymous. Such patients may deter private clinics from contacting their general practitioner after an abortion, with obvious risks to efficient after-care.

THE GYNAECOLOGIST

No less than with general practitioners, attitudes towards abortion practice vary widely among gynaecologists. The great disparities between the availability of abortion in various parts of the UK and in the proportion of referrals that are terminated largely reflect these differences in attitude. The phenomenon of 'the Great White Chief' (Ingram, 1971), whereby a senior consultant or professor of obstetrics may influence junior staff towards his own bias about abortion (whether conservative or liberal) and engineer the appointment of like-minded colleagues in his area, can also account for some regional variations. However, even in Aberdeen, where a moderately liberal abortion policy had been carried out for more than 20 years, 'liberal' and 'conservative' operators were readily discernible among the senior gynaecologists. Variation in their abortion practice, however, mainly focused on unmarried women with prominent social reasons for seeking termination who were more frequently refused by the 'conservatives' (Horobin, 1973).

Unmarried girls from the upper socio-economic groups are still most likely to be accepted, possibly because they are able to elicit greater empathy from the specialist and have greater knowledge of the medical system, and present their case more skilfully.

Some gynaecologists are reluctant to abort a woman more than once, especially if she is unmarried, and feel that after one chance they are no longer 'deserving', particularly if they have neglected contraception. The gynaecologists under these circumstances tend to feel manipulated and exploited by their patients. However, the recurrent maladaptive behaviour displayed by some of these women is often indicative of serious underlying personality abnormalities and difficulties in interpersonal relationships that ill-equip her for responsible motherhood. The 'punishment' of having to continue the unwanted pregnancy is unlikely to teach her new, constructive ways of coping with life and, if anything, will compound her present instability.

THE PSYCHIATRIST

In comparison with the years prior to and immediately following the implementation of the Abortion Act, there are now very few referrals to psychiatrists for opinion about abortion. Gynaecologists seem to have learned in the interim to assess adequately, in consultation with the general practitioner, the psychological pros and cons and legal aspects of pregnancy termination in most applications.

Psychiatrist referral from gynaecologists is now generally confined to those abortion applicants where: (a) there has been a definite previous history of serious mental illness, especially in relation to pregnancy or childbirth; (b) the patient's present mental state is suggestive of a serious psychiatric illness and needs specialist assessment; (c) considerable uncertainty exists about the decision, for example where the applicant is threatening suicide if refused, and a second opinion is needed for protection of the medical practitioner.

Nowadays, psychiatric referral tends to focus mainly on help with management rather than aid in decision-making.

THE NURSES

Contact with the nursing profession occurs principally around the time of termination in the clinic or hospital. Their attitude to the woman undergoing abortion can have a supportive or a deleterious effect. Such might be their distaste of the whole process of induced abortion that they may behave punitively towards the applicant or at least transmit their hostility towards her, possibly indirectly in non-verbal ways, thereby intensifying her guilt feelings. It may be very difficult for some nurses working for most of the time in labour wards or gynaecological theatres, intent on preserving life, to assist in an operation which essentially is involved with the destruction of life. They may themselves dearly wish for a child of their own and resent another woman who has deliberately avoided continuing a precious pregnancy.

If necessary, nursing staff can invoke the conscience clause in the Abortion Act and opt out of assisting in termination operations. One of the arguments advanced in favour of units specializing in abortion has been the possibility of recruiting staff who will not be in serious psychological conflict about their work and can respond more therapeutically to their patients.

THE SOCIAL WORKER

The decision-making clinicians can be greatly assisted by an expert social worker's prior assessment of the applicant's social and family background, the circumstances leading up to the pregnancy and exploration of her feelings about termination. Social workers can appropriately carry out post-abortion counselling and, where the pregnancy is to be continued, can help in providing both social and psychological support measures, e.g. admission to a mother and baby home and, where necessary, initiate adoption procedures.

THE APPLICANT'S FAMILY

In many instances, the family is an important factor in the process of seeking abortion. It may have been because of illness or problems in the family, or because of its likely effect on existing children, that the pregnancy has been deemed 'unwanted'. Alternatively, and especially in the case of unmarried applicants, they may have pressured the applicant towards abortion as a solution. Where the pregnant woman is a young teenager, the parents tend to loom particularly large in the decision-making process. With under 16s it is important to consult the parents and if possible obtain written consent from them if abortion is proposed. If the parents refuse and the patient herself consents, a termination would be lawful if in the gynaecologist's opinion it is clinically necessary. If the girl herself was opposed to termination, then it should not be carried out even if the parents demanded it.

On the other hand, the pregnancy and the abortion application may have been concealed from the rest of the family, especially so in the case of unmarried women and their parents. The patient's wishes in the end must be respected, but wherever possible disclosure by the patient should be encouraged with a view to mobilizing support from the family and reducing emotional barriers stemming from guilty secrets. This may require a series of joint interviews delicately exploring and defusing some of the emotive issues involved. Not infrequently, the family may be a great source of support for the applicant and the crisis of the abortion application may result, once the situation is clarified, in a closer relationship with them.

The technique and setting of the abortion

If induced abortion is to take place, it is highly desirable that it be early rather than late. The type of technique that can be used is largely dictated by the stage of gestation, and those appropriate to the first trimester tend to be less traumatic both physically and psychologically than those procedures that must be applied in the second trimester. Late abortions entail a greater immediate risk to the woman's life and health and might be associated with obstetric complications in subsequent pregnancies such as spontaneous abortion, prematurity and low birth weight.

Several major medical procedures are currently widely used in abortions.

Instrumental evacuation via the vagina

MENSTRUAL REGULATION

Menstrual regulation (MR) involves aspiration of the uterine contents by a hand-held syringe within 6 weeks of the last menstrual period, using a flexible plastic Karman catheter. As a rule neither anaesthesia nor cervical dilatation is required. In effect, this procedure is undertaken before a definite diagnosis of pregnancy can be made. One drawback to this simple and convenient method is the risk of incomplete evacuation. Although not popular in the UK, where general practitioners are not allowed to use the technique, it is more widely used in the USA and in certain Third World countries.

VACUUM ASPIRATION

Vacuum aspiration (VA) can be employed up to 14 weeks, although with increasing danger. Cervical dilatation is required, a metal or a plastic cannula is introduced and the uterus evacuated by vacuum pump. Prior to 10 weeks, local analgesia via a paracervical block is sufficient for the operation. Compared to curettage, blood loss and operation time are reduced and this tends to be nowadays the procedure of choice in first trimester abortion.

DILATATION AND CURETTAGE

Under general anaesthesia the cervix is dilated with graduated metal dilators, sponge forceps introduced, the conceptus removed piecemeal and the uterus curetted to remove any remaining small pieces. An oxytocin preparation is vital to reduce haemorrhage. There is risk of uterine perforation and damage leading to cervical incompetence. Dilatation and curettage (D and C) is contra-indicated after the 12th week and is now being supplanted by VA.

DILATATION AND EVACUATION

Dilatation and evacuation (D and E) is a method increasingly applied to early second trimester abortions at 13–15 weeks' gestation. General anaesthesia is required and dilatation of the cervix is effected by the use of laminaria to reduce the risk of laceration. A small forceps is used to remove the fetus, and suction then applied followed by surgical curettage to ensure complete evacuation. The procedure requires a high degree of skill and is considered to be emotionally stressful by many staff. For the patients it has the advantage that they do not have to go into labour and has a much lower mortality rate than saline or prostaglandin abortion.

Stimulation of uterine contractions

In the following methods, essentially a premature labour is induced and the fetus and placenta expelled. They are thus understandably more frequently emotionally traumatic to the patient than the other procedures.

HYPERTONIC SALINE INSTILLATION

An intra-uterine injection into the amniotic fluid or between the amnion and the uterine wall will evacuate the uterus, usually within 36 h. This is effective from 16–20 weeks, but carries the appreciable risk of infection and blood-clotting problems and is much less frequently used nowadays. Oxytocin may have to be used to supplement its action.

PROSTAGLANDINS

Intra-amniotic injections or vaginal inserts can produce abortion more rapidly than saline and without significant disturbances in blood clotting, or the risk of hypernatraemia or myometrial necrosis. Major side effects are vomiting and diarrhoea. Repeat instillation may be necessary.

Major surgery

HYSTEROTOMY

Essentially, a caesarean section is carried out. The uterine scar may mean that any future pregnancy will have also to be born by this route. It may be performed at any stage of gestation and can be combined with sterilization. Sepsis and haemorrhage are usually minimal, although a comparatively long stay in hospital is required.

HYSTERECTOMY

Removal of the uterus is indicated where a need for termination of pregnancy and sterilization is coupled with a serious abnormality or disease of the cervix or uterus or a history of severe menstrual bleeding. Late abortions where fetal movements may have already been felt might be supposed to be more psychologically stressful.

Early abortions using MR or VA not only involve reduced risk to the woman's health, but also require less time and expense. They can frequently be performed on an outpatient basis, thereby reducing pressure on hospital beds (Lewis *et al.*, 1971).

Late applicants tend to be young, unmarried, childless or with one child, lower social class and an early school leaver, materially unsupported, totally neglecting contraception and estranged from the putative father (Johnstone and Vincent, 1973). They may not have recognized the early signs of pregnancy, or could not face up to their implication, had hesitated to approach parents or general practitioners and may have changed their mind after initially deciding to continue the pregnancy.

A late abortion refused by one clinician may lead to referral to a different gynaecologist, consuming more scarce time. Having been accepted, there may be significant delay in being admitted to hospital for the operation, possibly of 2 weeks or more (Chalmers and Anderson, 1972).

Clearly, some extra attention to administrative matters might significantly reduce the incidence of late aborters.

The reduction of the proportion of second trimester legal abortions for residents in England and Wales from 38% in 1968 to 17.9% in 1980 is an encouraging sign of progress.

Sequelae of abortion

Medical sequelae

Serious immediate complications within a few hours of abortion include instrumental perforation of the uterus or laceration of the cervix, major haemorrhage, hypernatraemia and severe blood coagulation disturbances from saline induction, water intoxication from the use of oxytocin, and adverse anaesthetic effects. They are rare in medical settings.

Delayed complications in the first month comprise infection, retention of placental fragments leading to post-abortal bleeding and venous thrombophlebitis which may result in pulmonary embolism. Endometriosis in hysterotomy scars and rhesus sensitization may also occur as late somatic sequelae. Complications tend to relate to specific methods of abortion. For instance, it has been suggested, although not yet definitely proved, that dilatation of the cervix and surgical curettage in late abortions can lead to obstetric complications in later pregnancies resulting from damage to the cervix and placental insufficiency from trauma to the basal endometrium. Sterility and ectopic pregnancy can be late sequelae of pelvic infection, especially from abortion by self-induction or unskilled operations.

Psychological sequelae

Earlier studies of the psychosocial aftermath of induced abortion frequently reported a high proportion of women with serious regrets, adverse sequelae and episodes of frank psychiatric illness. However, Simon and Senturia (1966), reviewing this type of research published in the years 1935–64, drew attention to several major methodological shortcomings in the research designs during this period. Small and unrepresentative cohorts of abortion applicants, retrospective rather than prospective studies, vague criteria for assessing outcome, absence of comparison groups of women continuing the pregnancy and relatively short periods of follow-up were cited as serious drawbacks. Many of the US studies, in particular, were heavily biased in terms of candidates with serious psychiatric disorder, reflecting the legal restrictions of that period.

The study by Ekblad (1955) of 479 Swedish women aborted on 'psychiatric grounds' broadly corresponding to those applied in the British Abortion Act 1967, was deemed the most satisfactory of the period and remains a classic in the field. Sixty-one per cent of his cohort were married women, and 58% were considered to have abnormal personalities, associated in the majority with chronic neurotic symptoms. At follow-up, between two and three and a half years after abortion, 64% had no reproach about the operation and 10% also felt no regrets but considered the abortion was unpleasant. Mild and serious regrets and guilt were reported, respectively, by 14% and 11% of the cohort, but in only 1% was there serious incapacity. All of these 5 cases had previously suffered from severe chronic neurosis.

In the past two decades, several prospective studies of the psychosocial sequelae of abortion have been carried out with sizeable cohorts of women, presenting with a wider range of indications – not only psychiatric, but also medical, eugenic and social (Illsley and Hall, 1976). The composition of the cohorts reflected the passing of more liberal abortion laws in several parts of the world. Methodology was more precise, with subjective reports of outcome often being supplemented by objective psychological tests, e.g. Pare and Raven (1970); Brody, Meikle and Gerritse (1971); Niswander, Singer and Singer (1972); McCance, Olley and Edward (1973); Greer et al. (1976); Ashton (1980); Greenglass (1981); Schmidt and Priest (1981).

Most studies encountered difficulties in tracing women a year or more after termination. The Aberdeen series, probably the most comprehensive of these studies (McCance, Olley and Edward, 1973), traced 72% of the cohort of 163 unmarried applicants and 90% of the 207 ever-married group some 18 months after the first interview. Cohorts comprised some 90% of the total NHS abortion referrals from an urban community during a 14-month period. Students were the group most difficult to locate for follow-up. Applicants who continued their pregnancy as well as those who aborted were included in the study.

Six per cent of both unmarried and ever-married aborted groups reported severe regrets at 18 months follow-up and a further 15% had mixed feelings or mild regrets. In many instances, guilt and regrets centred principally on the situation that led to the abortion rather than on the operation *per se*. Only 2% were found to be severely depressed at follow-up, although prior to the abortion psychological tests indicated 60% of the unmarried and 40% of the ever-married were in this category. Significant improvement in mental state had taken place in both groups, although the ever-married aborted women were rather more disturbed at follow-up than the unmarried, with 25% and 10% reporting minor depressive symptoms. It should be noted that frequently these were related to the continuing adverse environmental conditions and poor interpersonal relationships that necessitated the abortion in the first place. Both early and late abortions were included in the series.

Another detailed study of abortion sequelae, that of Greer *et al.* (1976) at King's College, London, consisted of 360 women with first trimester outpatient abortions carried out by vacuum aspiration, with brief counselling prior to termination. Significant improvement had occurred at 3 month and 18 month follow-up with respect to psychiatric symptoms, guilt feelings and interpersonal and sexual adjustment, although not in marital relationships. Ninety-six per cent were able to resume work or their normal activities satisfactorily after three months. After eighteen months, 4% of the 60% who could be contacted had severe guilt feelings and regretted the termination.

Thus, recent research has not confirmed the earlier fears of frequent serious mental illness following induced abortion. Brewer (1977b) reported an incidence of 0.3 per 1000 legal abortions for post-abortion psychosis, compared with 1.7 per 1000 deliveries for puerperal psychosis. Many patients, and particularly the unmarried, react quite quickly with a feeling of instant relief. Mild regrets and doubts prevalent in the first few months seem largely to remit by the 18 months stage.

Having a termination of pregnancy is psychologically doubly stressful; first the loss of a fetus and secondly the violation of the body's integrity by the operation. It is perhaps hardly surprising that a mild degree of emotional disturbance is not uncommon in the two or three months following abortion. In the main, this takes the form of a transient reactive depression with nervousness and sleep disturbance. Fears may be expressed about future sterility, giving birth to an abnormal child, becoming pregnant again or a worry that the fetus may not have been completely aborted.

A high proportion of the unmarried applicants later marry in the few years following the abortion, some to the putative father. An appreciable number of the married women with marital disharmony change their marital status following termination, frequently separating or being divorced from their spouse.

There seems to be no evidence that abortion predisposes to later frigidity; indeed if anything the subsequent sexual adjustment is often improved. Greer *et al.* (1976) reported satisfactory sexual adjustment rating increasing from 59% to 74% of their cohort at 3 months post-abortion. However, some unmarried girls are deterred by the unwanted pregnancy from further sexual encounters, and may be restricted socially by their families.

A minority become pregnant again shortly afterwards, although this time it may be in, as opposed to out of, wedlock. Some speculation has been made that there is an urgent need in some of these women to replace the lost fetus.

Although only a small minority experience serious mental sequelae, it is nevertheless important to predict and identify this group of women so that appropriate treatment can be administered at an early stage.

The outcome for women refused abortion

Abortion on request or 'demand' does not generally obtain in the UK under the present legal framework, especially in NHS hospitals, although considerable variation in abortion availability is found.

In the Aberdeen series (Olley, 1973), 37% and 30% of the unmarried and ever-married applicants, respectively, were refused an abortion by the gynaecologist and their pregnancies continued to term, 2% and 5% of these groups changed their minds and decided not to seek abortion, and 6% and 8%, respectively, reported a 'spontaneous abortion', although in at least one case it was probably self-induced. This particular study was exceptional in that only 1 of the 370 applicants obtained a legal abortion elsewhere after having been refused. It is doubtful whether nowadays, some 13 years later, with the subsequent national growth of the private sector, this virtual total acceptance of the initial decision would occur.

Beazley and Haeri (1971), who reported a series where 15% of 1034 applicants were initially refused abortion, found that some 40% of those refused subsequently obtained a termination elsewhere. In the study of Pare and Raven (1970), where 52% of 321 applicants were advised not to proceed to abortion, 37% of those refused were eventually terminated elsewhere. Inevitably, this process leads to the increased probability of second trimester abortions being performed, with increased risk of morbidity and mortality for the applicant. Maternal mortality from term childbirth is exceeded by that from termination only after the 16th week of gestation.

What then of the effect of continuing the pregnancy to term? McCance, Olley and Edward (1973) compared the outcome at follow-up some 18 months after application of aborted and non-aborted groups of unmarried and ever-married women. Severe regrets at the continuation of the pregnancy were found in 20% of the unmarried and 10% of the ever-married groups, and mixed feelings or mild regrets among 22% and 25%, respectively. About 2% of each group were found to be clinically severely depressed at follow-up. Thus, although the women who were eventually aborted demonstrated a much greater degree of depression prior to the abortion decision, there was no significant difference with the non-aborted groups at follow-up.

Profound dissatisfaction at having to continue to term was particularly evident among the unmarried women. At the same time it should be noted that around two-thirds of the women (58% and 65% of the unmarried and ever-married groups) were glad they had their baby. Höök (1963) reported that only 24% of 249 women who were refused an abortion were poorly adjusted several years later, although 13% had experienced periodic difficulty in working because of mental disturbance and 11% secured an illegal abortion. Adverse mental reactions in the mother are thus a recognized feature of a minority of women continuing unwanted pregnancies to term. Adoption or fostering seems to be an increasingly unpopular measure for women with an unwanted pregnancy. In the Aberdeen study, 16 of the unmarried women, 36% of those who continued the pregnancy to term, had their babies adopted.

Seven of these women had severe regrets and two mild regrets at having to bear the child. Proportionally fewer regrets at continuing the pregnancy were found among those who had kept their child, whether they had or had not remained unmarried. Of the 29 unmarried and 59 ever-married applicants who kept their baby, 2 (7%) and 5 (8%), respectively, felt they had not developed normal feelings towards it, and experienced hostility and rejection. There is a close association between the 'battered baby' syndrome, unwanted pregnancy and rejection of the baby after birth.

Forssman and Thuwe (1966), in a 21-year follow-up of 120 children born after an abortion application had been refused, found an increased incidence of delinquency and psychiatric disturbance compared with a matched control group. These children also tended to under-achieve, be generally insecure and were more often dependent on public assistance.

Decision-making and predicting the outcome

Predicting the outcome

Only a small minority of women experience serious adverse psychosocial sequelae following induced abortion, although a somewhat greater proportion do so after continuing an unwanted pregnancy to term. It is nevertheless important to predict who is likely to react in this way, so that the optimum decision can be taken and special arrangements made to support vulnerable women in the post-abortion or post-delivery phase.

Prediction is far from precise with termination of pregnancy. Only general guidelines can be stated and each case must be individually considered in detail.

PREVIOUS PSYCHOSOCIAL INSTABILITY

One important general principle is that a woman with a long history of mental instability prior to abortion is likely to continue in this way after the abortion. A general style of coping with crises is unlikely to be radically altered by the experience of termination or continuation of an unwanted pregnancy, although in younger women it is possible that some maturing of personality may occur. A chronically disturbed mental state is unlikely to be relieved by an abortion, although its intensification may be thereby prevented.

SEVERE AMBIVALENCE

Mixed feelings and uncertainty about proceeding with an abortion seem to be associated with later guilt, preoccupation with fantasies of the fetus, including its sex, awareness of the term delivery date and being upset at seeing other women with babies.

Conflict-free decisions about abortion are often correlated with general relief after the operation. Those who regard the fetus already as a baby may be more liable to post-abortion distress.

DECISION NOT HER OWN

Women who have been pressured into seeking abortion against their own better judgement and feelings, by spouse, putative father, parents or medical advisers, are vulnerable to later adverse reactions. Abortion is contra-indicated where the decision to apply is solely due to coercion.

MEDICAL INDICATIONS

A particularly high proportion of women who are aborted for medical or eugenic reasons experience unfavourable psychological sequelae. Despite serious risk to their health they may dearly wish to have a child. Ashton (1980), among several researchers, has reported that post-abortion guilt was common in women with physical grounds for abortion and those with a history of previous spontaneous abortion, stillbirth and post-partum depression.

POOR INTERPERSONAL RELATIONSHIPS

A history of tenuous family ties and relationships, few friends, poor work pattern, poor marital adjustment and support before abortion correlate with emotional disturbance after the operation (Belsey et al., 1977).

Making the decisions

In deciding whether or not induced abortion should be granted to the applicant, the clinician must assess the woman's present mental and physical state and circumstances and weigh up the likely risks of one or other of the courses of action that are legally permissible, often on the basis of limited information. Hard and fast rules cannot be laid down to deal precisely with every situation. Multiple factors operate in most cases and, although there are a few guidelines, the unique features of each woman's predicament must also be taken into account in arriving at a decision.

Essentially, the basic questions are:

1. What are the risks of physical and psychiatric morbidity of this woman after an abortion at this time?
2. What are the risks for her if the pregnancy is continued to term?
3. What is the risk to the child of being seriously handicapped?
4. What effect will continuing the pregnancy or an abortion have on the rest of the family?

Absolute medical indications are rare, although there are many conditions such as cardiac disease, ulcerative colitis and multiple sclerosis where it will be judged that in the circumstances pregnancy will promote deterioration. There are no absolute psychiatric indications, although severe reactive depression, especially where there is a risk of suicide, certain obsessional states, schizophrenia and mental subnormality were considered by the British Medical Association Committee on Therapeutic Abortion as possible indications.

Many patients with major mental illness such as schizophrenia or manic depressive psychosis can be treated and supported throughout pregnancy and the post-partum period and do not of necessity require termination.

For instance, women who have had a puerperal psychosis, have only a 20% likelihood of developing a similar condition in the next pregnancy. Usually, the prognosis for such an illness with appropriate treatment is quite good and disability is unlikely to last more than 2 or 3 months.

Schizophrenic women do not necessarily deteriorate mentally when pregnant. It is not so much the condition itself during pregnancy and the immediate post-partum period that usually gives concern in these patients, but the long-continued stress and problems associated with child-rearing, possibly in an adverse environment. The ability to respond to the newborn baby may be impaired and bonding interrupted. Possibility of breakdown of the family unit with the advent of an extra child has often to be considered, as has the genetic transmission of the patient's illness to her offspring.

Most patients with these 'medical psychiatric' indications for termination are mentally disturbed at the time of assessment and are likely to continue with their mental instability afterwards. Many of them will, nevertheless, have no regrets about termination and an operation may well have prevented serious decompensation.

The majority of patients with psychiatric difficulties come into the category of the so-called minor mental disorders, labelled as neuroses or personality disorders. These will often be women whose life adjustment is precariously balanced and who are possibly functioning to their limit in difficult socio-economic circumstances, with onerous responsibilities and poor marital or family support. Continuing a pregnancy may prove to be an unsupportable extra burden which will cause the onset of serious depression or anxiety and a breakdown in coping mechanisms.

Determination of the risk of suicide may be an important feature of the assessment. Not infrequently, the applicant may hint at, or overtly express, that she is contemplating suicide or illegal abortion if her request for legal abortion is refused. Although suicide during pregnancy is rare, it does occasionally happen, and with any such statement the possibility should be carefully evaluated and not dismissed out of hand. For women under 25 years, the suicide risk is in fact increased in pregnancy, and parasuicide is not uncommon.

Attention must also be given to the possibility of suicide or parasuicide following termination. Patients whose religious and cultural background places strong sanctions against abortion might be expected to be at greater risk. Some abortion applicants may deliberately exaggerate the mental distress that they are suffering in order to obtain termination, especially where social factors tend to be downgraded compared with psychiatric distress – 'the psychiatric case' of the 'Abortion games' of Ingram (1971).

The decision to abort or not may depend as much on the level of available support as the particular medical or psychiatric condition.

Principles of assessment for termination of pregnancy

Taking into account our present, rather limited knowledge and predictive principles, it is possible to lay down a pattern for the assessment process and management:

1. Early on, it should be confirmed that the patient is pregnant and what stage the pregnancy has reached.
2. It is important to ensure speedy referral and eliminate any unnecessary delay in assessment by specialists. Arrangements should be made so that, if at all possible, a first trimester abortion by vacuum aspiration is feasible. Strenuous

efforts to reduce the time between acceptance for termination and the operation should be made.

3. An understanding of the social background, the state of relationships with significant others, including spouse, parents or putative father, the circumstances leading up to the pregnancy and contraceptive practice is vital to the decision-making. It may be convenient for a social worker to assemble some of this information prior to an interview with the gynaecologist.

4. Previous menstrual and obstetric history with complications, previous unwanted pregnancies and abortions, together with past medical and psychiatric history, should be collected.

5. It is essential to convey a non-judgemental attitude to the applicant, to set her at ease wherever possible and to allow her to ventilate her worries and concerns about the pregnancy. Why is the pregnancy 'unwanted'? What does she think about abortion? Are there strong religious objections to abortion in her background? The opportunity should be provided to allow her to say if she really wants a termination or is undecided. Interview should take place alone, away from individuals who might be coercing the patient. The question 'Is it really her own decision?' must be decided by the clinician. The applicant must be allowed to put her case. It is usually desirable later to interview relations that accompany the applicant, but to respect her wishes if she does not wish them to know.

6. An appropriate explanation of what is entailed by termination and what the other options are, should always be given. If uncertainty about abortion is prominent, she should be given a chance to reconsider the situation and give a more definite opinion later, possibly after further counselling, for example by a social worker or psychiatrist.

7. An assessment of her current mental and physical state should be made and any treatment that she is currently receiving noted. Personality strengths and weaknesses and the degree of emotional support available in her environment require careful evaluation. Is she suicidal, is she likely to try self-induction, illegal abortion or harm a child?

8. What will she do if the abortion is refused? The applicant should be given the chance to discuss her feelings about this.

9. Wherever possible, and with the patient's permission, the spouse or putative father should be involved. Is there a consensus between them about the action to be taken?

10. Any further necessary referrals, e.g. to physician or psychiatrist, should be initiated rapidly.

11. Taking the above factors into account, the decision should be made and communicated to the applicant and if necessary her general practitioner as soon as possible. If pregnancy is to be continued, appropriate arrangements for ante-natal care and social support should be made. If there is to be an abortion, then this should be arranged as speedily as possible.

After the abortion

It is highly desirable that further unwanted pregnancies should not occur in the future. The opportunity should therefore be taken around the time of the abortion to give contraceptive advice and supplies. For the non-compliant, an IUD may be more suitable than oral contraception. Special counselling may be necessary to maintain motivation for contraception.

Wherever possible, a clinical follow-up should be arranged to determine any early physical or psychological complications of the abortion.

For many of the older married women, sterilization either of themselves or their spouse may be appropriate and this would now be generally carried out electively sometime after the termination, often by laparoscopy. In the Aberdeen series, the married group tolerated this procedure very well indeed and almost without exception were glad about it. Considerable improvement in sexual relationship with husband was reported following sterilization, whether or not they had been aborted. Post-abortion counselling for those women considered as vulnerable or relatively unsupported is to be encouraged and may be appropriately carried out by skilled social workers. This may reduce the incidence of long-term psychological reactions.

Apart from help with practical matters such as finance, housing or job, it may be important to allow such patients to express guilt feelings and work through any mourning process for the fetus. Opportunity may be given to discuss and modify the life-styles and motivations that resulted in the unwanted pregnancy and strengthen family and marital relationships, possibly through conjoint family or marital therapy and continued support for consistent contraception.

Induced abortion and the future

What of the future? Will abortion as we know it be a thing of the past? Better education in contraception, coupled with simpler, safer, more effective techniques, might considerably reduce the incidence of unplanned and unwanted pregnancies. A 'retrospective contraception pill' to be taken following intercourse would be a further significant advance, although not without potential problems. Despite these possible technological improvements, knowledge of human nature suggests that a number of individuals will still present with an 'unwanted' pregnancy and request abortion, having neglected to use the current technology. Possibly predictors of adverse effects might be refined and the techniques improved and made safer. But for the foreseeable future, induced abortion is likely to remain with us, although hopefully with a steadily decreasing incidence.

References

AITKEN-SWANN, J. (1973) Epidemiological background, in *Experience with Abortion* (Horobin, G., Ed.). London; Cambridge University Press

ASHTON, J. R. (1980) The psychosocial outcome of induced abortion. *British Journal of Obstetrics and Gynaecology,* **87,** 1115–1122

ASHTON, J. R., DENNIS, K. J., ROWE, R. G., WATERS, W. E. and WHEELER, M. (1980) The Wessex abortion studies: I. Interdistrict variation in provision of abortion services. *Lancet,* **1,** 82–85

ASHTON, J. R., MACHIN, D., OSMOND, C., BALJARAN, R., ADAM, S. A. and DONNAN, S. P. B. (1983) Trends in induced abortion in England and Wales. *Journal of Epidemiology and Community Health,* **37,** 105–110

BAIRD, D. (1967) Sterilisation and therapeutic abortion in Aberdeen. *British Journal of Psychiatry,* **113,** 701–709

BEARD, R. W., BELSEY, E. M., LAL, S., LEWIS, S. C. and GREER, H. S. (1974) King's Termination Study II: Contraception practice before and after out-patient termination of pregnancy. *British Medical Journal,* **1,** 418–421

BEAZLEY, J. M. and HAERI, A. D. (1971) Termination of pregnancy refused. *Lancet,* **1,** 1059–1061

BELSEY, E. M., GREER, H. S., LAL, S., LEWIS, S. C. and BEARD, R. W. (1977) King's Termination Study IV: Predictive factors in emotional response to abortion. *Social Science and Medicine,* **11,** 71–82

BONE, M. (1973) *Family Planning Services in England and Wales.* London; HMSO

BREWER, C. (1977a) Third time unlucky: a study of women who have three or more legal abortions. *Journal of Biosocial Science,* **9,** 99–105

BREWER, C. (1977b) Incidence of post-abortion psychosis: a prospective study. *British Medical Journal,* **1,** 476–477

BRODY, H., MEIKLE, S. and GERRITSE, R. (1971) Therapeutic abortion: a prospective study, 1. *American Journal of Obstetrics and Gynecology,* **109,** 347–353

CARTWRIGHT, A. (1976) *How Many Children?* London; Routledge and Kegan Paul

CHALMERS, I. and ANDERSON, A. (1972) Factors affecting gestational age at therapeutic abortion. *Lancet,* **1,** 1324–1326

CHERTOK, L., MONDZAIN, M. L. and BONNAUD, M. (1963) Vomiting and the wish to have a child. *Psychosomatic Medicine,* **25,** 13–18

DIGGORY, P. and SIMM, M. (1970) Two years after the Abortion Act. *New Scientist,* No. 48, 261–263

EKBLAD, M. (1955) Induced abortion on psychiatric grounds. A follow-up of 479 women. *Acta Psychiatrica Scandinavica,* Suppl. 99, 1–238

FORSSMAN, H. and THUWE, I. (1966) One hundred and twenty children born after application for therapeutic abortion refused. Their mental health, social adjustment and eucational level up to the age of 21. *Acta Psychiatrica Scandinavica,* **42,** 71–88

GREENGLASS, E. (1981) A Canadian study of psychological adjustment after abortion. In *Abortion. Readings and Research* (Sachdev, P., Ed.). Toronto; Butterworths

GREER, H. S., LAL, S., LEWIS, S. C., BELSEY, E. M. and BEARD, R. W. (1976) King's Termination Study III: Psychosocial consequences of therapeutic abortion. *British Journal of Psychiatry,* **128,** 74–79

HÖÖK, K. (1963) Refused abortion. A follow-up study of 249 women whose applications were refused by the National Board of Health of Sweden. *Acta Psychiatrica Scandinavica,* **39,** Suppl. 168

HOROBIN, G., Ed. (1973) *Experience with Abortion.* London; Cambridge University Press

ILLSLEY, R. and HALL, M. H. (1976) Psychosocial aspects of abortion. A review of issues and needed research. *Bulletin of the World Health Organization,* **53,** 83–106

INGRAM, I. M. (1971) Abortion games: an inquiry into the working of the Act. *Lancet,* **ii,** 969–970

JOHNSTONE, F. D. and VINCENT, L. (1973) Factors affecting gestational age at termination of pregnancy. *Lancet,* **ii,** 717–719

LEWIS, S. C., LAL, S., BRANCH, B. and BEARD, R. W. (1971) Out-patient termination of pregnancy. *British Medical Journal,* **4,** 606–610

McCANCE, C., OLLEY, P. C. and EDWARD, V. (1973) Long-term psychiatric follow-up. In *Experience with Abortion* (Horobin, G., Ed.). London; Cambridge University Press

NISWANDER, K. R., SINGER, J. and SINGER, M. (1972) Psychological reaction to therapeutic abortion. II. Objective response. *American Journal of Obstetrics and Gynecology,* **114,** 29–33

OFFICE OF POPULATION CENSUS AND SURVEYS (1984) Conceptions inside and outside marriage, 1969 to 1981. *OPCS Monitor,* FMI 84/6. London; HMSO

OLLEY, P. C. (1973) Social and psychological characteristics at referral. In *Experience with Abortion* (Horobin, G., Ed.). London; Cambridge University Press

PARE, C. M. B. and RAVEN, H. (1970) Follow up of patients referred for termination of pregnancy. *Lancet,* **1,** 635–638

PRIEST, R. G. (1972) New trends in therapeutic abortion. *Lancet,* **2,** 1085

REPORT OF THE LANE COMMITTEE ON THE WORKING OF THE ABORTION ACT (1974). London; HMSO

RESNICK, R. J. (1970) Murder of the newborn: a psychiatric review of neonaticide. *American Journal of Psychiatry,* **126,** 1414

SANDBERG, E. C. and JACOBS, R. I. (1971) Psychology of the misuse and rejection of contraception. *American Journal of Obstetrics and Gynecology,* **110,** 227–242

SCHMIDT, R. and PRIEST, R. G. (1981) The effects of termination of pregnancy: a follow-up study of psychiatric referrals. *British Journal of Medical Psychology,* **54,** 267–276

SCHNEIDER, S. M. and THOMPSON, B. S. (1976) Repeat aborters. *American Journal of Obstetrics and Gynecology,* **26,** 316–320

SHEPARD, M. J. and BRACKEN, M. B. (1979) Contraceptive practice and repeat induced abortion: an epidemiological investigation. *Journal of Biosocial Science,* **11,** 289–302

SIMON, N. M. and SENTURIA, A. G. (1966) Psychiatric sequelae of abortion: review of the literature 1935–1964. *Archives of General Psychiatry,* **15,** 378–389

THOMPSON, B. (1977) Problems of abortion in Britain – Aberdeen, a case study. *Population Studies,* **31,** 143–154

TIETZE, C. (1983) *Induced Abortion: A World Review,* 5th edn. New York; The Population Council

WOODSIDE, M. (1963) Attitudes of women abortionists. *Howard Journal,* **2,** 93

Chapter 8

The menopause and the climacteric

C. Barbara Ballinger

Introduction

The menopause is identified as the time of the last menstrual period and is therefore a point in time that can be specified only in retrospect. The term climacteric or climacterium is derived from the Greek word for the rung of a ladder and is defined in *Chambers's Twentieth Century Dictionary* (Macdonald, 1972) as 'a critical period in human life in which some critical body change takes place'. This very adequately describes the immediately pre- and post-menopausal years, but unfortunately in both the medical and lay literature the word climacteric is now rarely used; instead the term menopause is used in a less precise fashion for the year or two before and after cessation of menstrual periods. As this now seems to be the generally accepted use of the term menopause it will be so used in this chapter, although it is regrettable that the term climacteric has not been retained.

In the gynaecological literature concerning the menopause there has been much emphasis on the occurrence of emotional or psychological disturbance at this time. Kroger and Freed (1951), in a textbook concerned with psychosomatic disorders, noted that of all gynaecological conditions the menopausal syndrome was the one most clearly associated with psychological factors. Psychological symptoms have become so closely associated with the menopause that they are included in the definition of climacteric as 'the syndrome of endocrine, somatic and psychic changes occurring at the termination of the reproductive period in the female' in *Dorland's Illustrated Medical Dictionary* (Daly, 1974).

The view that the time of the menopause is associated with emotional disturbance was proposed at an early date by Tilt (1857). He stated that many women became 'thoroughly unhinged' at this time, and in a series of 500 women 'at the change' 459 were said to be suffering from nervous irritability.

The association of psychological symptoms with the clinical features of the menopause has persisted in standard gynaecological textbooks. Klopper (1969) stated that the psychological changes of the menopause may be tempestuous and even the most stable of women could show outbursts of irritability, depression or hysteria. In a later edition of the same book, Macnaughton (1976) included psychological symptoms in his account of the clinical features of the menopause and ascribed them to fears of loss of femininity and reproductive potential.

Peel and Brudenell (1969), in a textbook for medical students, included

204

emotional problems such as depression and hysterical outbursts in a description of the clinical manifestations of the menopause and they emphasized the contribution of a constitutional predisposition to nervous irritability in the aetiology of these symptoms. Parsons and Sommers (1962), in their textbook of gynaecology, stated that the instability experienced by women at the time of the menopause was well documented and they attributed this emotional instability to the threat to personal security implied in this undeniable reminder of the aging process.

As for textbooks of gynaecology for postgraduate students, McClure Browne (1973) included irritability, palpitations, insomnia, depression, fatigue, emotional instability and a tendency to self-deprecation in a description of the clinical features of the menopause. Gold and Josimovich (1980) stated that irritability, emotional instability, depression and negativism are common manifestations of the menopause, but the relationship of these symptoms to hormonal changes is uncertain.

Llewelyn-Jones (1978) listed the symptoms presented by 500 patients attending a gynaecology clinic at the time of the menopause and included depression, insomnia and fatigue. However, he pointed out that these were the symptoms in women seeking medical aid at the time of the menopause and that they made up only 25% of the female population. He suggested that the psychological symptoms were related more to the individual's reaction to the realization of reaching the menopause rather than any direct effect of ovarian failure.

Jeffcoate (1975) presented a different view of the symptoms associated with the menopause. He maintained that psychological changes were few or insignificant in well-adjusted and well-informed women and suggested that symptoms arising from family problems and other issues were often wrongly attributed to the menopause, giving it an undeservedly bad reputation. Novak, Jones and Jones (1975) expressed a similar view that psychological symptoms occurring at this time of life were erroneously attributed to the menopause by many women, and their physicians acquiesced in this belief. Davey (1976) also advised caution in deciding what were the true clinical features of the menopause and stated that physicians should resist the temptation to attribute any symptoms occurring in women over the age of 40 to the menopause.

From this review of a sample of standard textbooks of gynaecology it would appear that the majority still express the opinion that a variety of psychological symptoms are associated with the menopause. It is therefore surprising that standard psychiatric textbooks make very little mention of the menopause and there is no evidence of a sudden increase in the rate of psychiatric referral around the age of 50 in women. The menopause is not mentioned in the works of Forrest, Affleck and Zealley (1978) or Hill, Murray and Thorley (1979) and receives but brief comment by Slater and Roth (1969), Kolb (1977) and Gelder, Gath and Mayou (1983). The one issue which has been debated at length in the psychiatric literature in relation to the menopause is the possible existence of a psychotic illness, involutional melancholia, which is characteristic of this time of life and distinct from depressive illness occurring at other times. This is a very different matter from the symptoms frequently mentioned in the gynaecology textbooks in relation to the menopause.

It would appear that views of the psychological impact of the menopause differ in gynaecological and psychiatric practice and this difference is reflected in the literature. Over the past decade the results of several epidemiological studies of symptoms reported by women at the time of the menopause, including cross-cultural studies, have been made available and give a clearer indication of what symptoms are directly related to the menopause. There have also been several studies of what factors other than menopausal status influence psychological symptoms in women at this time and the effects of various therapeutic agents on these symptoms.

Clinical features of the menopause

Clinical studies

There has been considerable debate in the literature about what symptoms are specific to the menopause and what conditions are specific to the physiological changes of the post-menopausal years. Prior to the results of the general population surveys becoming available, symptoms listed in the climacteric or menopausal syndrome were based on those symptoms presented by women attending gynaecology or menopause clinics. Kupperman, Wetchler and Blatt (1959) based their 'menopausal index' on the symptoms elicited from women attending a gynaecology clinic and they derived 11 factors for the calculation of this index. These 11 factors were vasomotor symptoms, paraesthesiae, insomnia, nervousness, melancholia, vertigo, weakness, arthralgia and myalgia, headache, palpitations and formication. This is an impressive list and it would now seem that very few of these symptoms are directly related to the physiological changes of the menopause. The menopausal syndrome remains a popular concept and the inclusion of such a large variety of symptoms, some with very dubious connection with the physiological changes of the menopause and post-menopausal years, has led to confusion in both clinical management and research.

The symptoms most consistently reported in studies of the menopause are the vasomotor symptoms such as hot flushes and episodic excessive sweating. Donovan (1951) questioned whether the association of even these symptoms with the menopause was an artefact, claiming that many women experienced episodic sensations of abnormal heat or cold throughout their life span, but these were only called hot flushes when the women were around the age of the menopause.

However, there is now good physiological evidence for the existence of the hot flush in menopausal women and the associated physiological changes were described in detail by Sturdee et al. (1978). It was found that the hot flush in menopausal women was associated with an acute rise in skin temperature, peripheral vasodilatation, transient increase in heart rate, fluctuations in the electrocardiographic base line and a marked decrease in the skin's electrical resistance. In contrast, artificial warming of pre-menopausal women produced a greater increase in skin temperature with peripheral vasodilatation, but a smaller decrease in the skin's electrical resistance and no change in the electrocardiographic base line or heart rate.

The aetiology of the vascular phenomena associated with the menopause is still uncertain. A study of 3 men who developed hot flushes following acute testicular insufficiency with high circulating levels of gonadotrophins suggested that FSH or LH may be involved in the genesis of hot flushes (Feldman, Postlethwaite and Glen, 1976). Tataryn et al. (1979) found a correlation between the pulsatile release of LH and hot flushes and suggested that hot flushes may be initiated by LH pulses or the mechanism triggering the pulsatile release of LH. Further studies (Caspar and Yen, 1981; De Fazio et al., 1983) showed that flushes still occur when the pulsatile release of LH is abolished, indicating that LH pulses do not directly trigger the flushes but the hypothalamic mechanism controlling the pulsatile release of LH may be involved.

The inclusion of various psychological symptoms in the menopausal index as described by Kupperman, Wetchler and Blatt (1959) implies that these are in some way related to the menopause and this view has been expressed by several authors. Wilson and Wilson (1963) strongly supported the concept of psychological disturbance directly related to the hormonal changes of the menopause. Malleson (1953) stated that long-term changes in mood with exaggeration of neurotic traits was directly related to the hormonal changes of the menopause and went on to describe menopausal depression, menopausal exhaustion, menopausal irritability and menopausal masochism. This view was questioned by Donovan (1951) and Jeffcoate (1960) and both authors suggested that the association of psychological symptoms with the menopause was an artefact.

Utian (1972a) endeavoured to define the true clinical features of the menopause in a group of women with a surgically induced menopause. He concluded that hot flushes and atrophic vaginitis were the only conditions directly resulting from the menopause and symptoms such as depression, irritability, insomnia and palpitations were probably independent and psychological in origin.

Some studies of menopausal symptoms appear to be based on the premise that all symptoms reported by women attending menopause clinics are related to the menopause and oestrogen deficiency. Jones, Marshall and Nordin (1977) devised a checklist of 'menopausal' symptoms by comparing a group of women over the age of 50 attending a menopause clinic with a group of normal women under the age of 40, and the assumption was made that the differences in psychological symptoms between these two groups were related to menopausal status. In the paper presented there was no evidence that any allowance was made for the age difference between the two groups or the fact that one group had been referred to a menopause clinic by themselves or by their general practitioners. Studd (1979) also stressed the presence of psychological symptoms in women attending menopause clinics and again seemed to accept that because women attending the clinics had a high level of psychological symptoms these were related to the menopause and oestrogen deficiency.

A working group at a conference concerned with the menopause attempted to bring order out of the confusion surrounding the term menopausal syndrome (Utian and Serr, 1976). It was decided that those symptoms which were almost certainly a result of oestrogen deficiency should be divided into two groups: an early group including hot flushes, sweats and atrophic vaginitis and a late group of conditions related to the long-term metabolic effects of oestrogen deficiency including such conditions as osteoporosis. It was then suggested that the symptoms commonly included in the climacteric or menopausal syndrome should be considered in three groups according to their *aetiology*. The first group would be those symptoms related to reduced oestrogen production, including vasomotor symptoms and atrophic vaginitis. The second group would be symptoms related to sociocultural factors and the third group those related to psychological factors dependent on the women's personality.

A similar view was expressed in a report by the World Health Organization (1981), in which it was concluded that vasomotor symptoms and vaginal dryness were the only conditions convincingly related to hormonal changes in the peri-menopause. It was also stated that no convincing relationship had been established between peri-menopausal hormonal changes and psychological symptoms or change in sexual interest.

General population studies

Most of the confusion concerning the true symptoms of the menopause has arisen because the majority of early studies were carried out on clinic populations and these are not representative of the normal population, particularly in relation to psychological symptoms. A much more accurate picture of the clinical features of the menopause has been obtained from symptom surveys of general population samples.

One of the first attempts to survey symptoms in women outside a clinic setting was reported by Neugarten and Kraines (1965). They studied a group of 460 women between the ages of 13 and 65 years using a symptom checklist of 28 items. The symptoms were considered in three groups – somatic, psychosomatic and psychological – and two symptom peaks were identified, one at puberty and one at the menopause. Although the majority of symptoms reported at puberty were in the psychological group, at the menopause the majority of symptoms were in the somatic group. This increase in reports of *somatic* symptoms in women at the time of the menopause was also reported by Priest and Crisp (1972).

Jaszmann, Van Lith and Zaat (1969), in a survey involving over 3000 women between 40 and 60 years of age, investigated a variety of symptoms in relation to 'biological age' as defined by menstrual pattern. They found that reports of hot flushes increased sharply from 17% of women who were still menstruating regularly to 65% of women whose last menstrual period was 1–2 years previously. In contrast, complaints of fatigue, headache, irritability, depression and mental imbalance were more common in women who were still menstruating than in women who were menopausal or post-menopausal. These symptoms reached a peak, although not a very dramatic peak, in those women who reported irregular menstruation and *could be considered to be immediately pre-menopausal*.

Thompson, Hart and Durno (1973), in a postal survey of 269 women between the ages of 40 and 60 years registered in one general practice in Scotland, also grouped their subjects according to menstrual pattern. They found that hot flushes were reported most frequently by women whose periods had stopped less than 2 years previously and least frequently by subjects who were still menstruating regularly. Reports of other symptoms including insomnia, fatigue and depression showed no such variation with menopausal status.

McKinlay and Jefferys (1974) reported a study of 638 women between the ages of 45 and 54 drawn from a group of 8 general practice units. A postal questionnaire including a checklist of symptoms such as hot flushes, headaches, dizzy spells, palpitations, sleeplessness, depression and night sweats was used and the subjects were grouped according to menstrual pattern. This study again showed that increased complaints of hot flushes and night sweats were clearly associated with the time of the natural menopause, but reports of other symptoms did not show any significant variation with menopausal status.

Some indirect evidence concerning the prevalence of psychological symptoms at the time of the menopause comes from a study of drug use by Dunnell and Cartwright (1972). It was found that while complaints of sleeplessness and aches and pains tended to increase with age, being most frequent in women aged 55 and over, reports of 'nerves', depression, irritability and headache were more common in women under 45 years of age. The findings reported in this study did not support the view that the menopause is a time of psychological crisis associated with an exacerbation of psychological symptoms.

More direct evidence concerning variation in reports of psychological symptoms with age was presented by Wood (1979). He reported a survey of 948 women from the general population between the ages of 20 and 65 years, including an assessment of what symptoms the women associated with the menopause. Symptoms were assessed using structured interviews carried out by medical students and the findings studied in 5-year age groups. It was found that symptoms of sleeplessness, joint pains, numbness, palpitations, dizziness and weakness tended to increase with age, while headaches, skin problems and irritability decreased with age. Symptoms of tiredness, fainting, loss of appetite, nervousness, backache, urinary frequency, depression, restlessness, tension and weight gain showed no significant trend with age and there was no evidence of any exacerbation of symptoms around the age of the natural menopause. When post-menopausal women were asked directly about problems they had experienced at the time of the menopause, the only consistently reported symptom was the hot flush, and 64% of the subjects reported that they were symptom free at the time of the menopause. This study again stressed the lack of any clear evidence to support the hypothesis that the menopause is a time of psychological crisis and that psychological symptoms elicited from women attending menopause clinics should be interpreted with caution.

Bungay, Vessey and McPherson (1980) carried out a survey of 1120 women and 510 men between the ages of 30 and 64 years using postal questionnaires. The symptom checklists included the symptoms listed in the menopausal index (Kupperman, Wetchler and Blatt, 1959). The prevalence of flushes and sweats in women showed a peak associated with the mean age of the menopause, while 'minor mental symptoms' showed a less impressive peak at an age just preceding the mean age of the menopause. Prevalence of other symptoms (including loss of appetite, crawling or tingling sensations under the skin, headaches, difficulty with intercourse, difficulty sleeping, loss of interest in sexual relations and urinary problems) showed no fluctuation related to the menopause.

Most of the studies mentioned so far used symptom checklists based on the views of menopausal symptomatology derived from clinic populations and not developed specifically for the detection of psychiatric morbidity. Hallström (1973) used detailed psychiatric interviews in the screening of a random sample of 800 women in four age strata: 38, 46, 50 and 54 years. He found no significant variation in the prevalence of mental illness with menopausal status, but women with irregular periods who were defined as peri-menopausal had a higher frequency of mental deterioration than the rest. This suggestion of an excess of psychiatric morbidity in women *just prior to the menopause* is also found in the surveys of Jaszmann, Van Lith and Zaat (1969) and Bungay, Vessey and McPherson (1980).

An increase in psychiatric morbidity in women just prior to the cessation of menstrual periods was also reported by Ballinger (1975). In this study, 539 women from the general population between the ages of 40 and 55 years were screened for psychiatric morbidity using the General Health Questionnaire. This questionnaire was developed by Goldberg (1972) to be used in community surveys for the detection of current emotional disturbance. The women were considered in three groups, 40–44, 45–49 and 50–54 years, and it was found that the group aged 45–49 years inclusive contained the highest proportion of women with evidence of emotional disturbance. When the women were subdivided according to both menopausal status and chronological age it was the pre-menopausal women in the 45–49 year age group, or those women who were still menstruating but very near to the menopause, who showed most evidence of emotional disturbance. The post-menopausal women over the age of 50 years showed least evidence of emotional disturbance.

Krüskemper (1975) also commented that once the menopause was past, the crisis seemed to be resolved. He based this opinion on the results of psychological testing using a personality inventory in a group of 59 women between 40 and 50 years of age. The 25 pre-menopausal women in this group had a greater tendency to report minor symptoms and higher scores for social introversion compared with the women whose menstrual periods had ceased.

These studies refute the view that the post-menopausal years, when oestrogen levels are lowest and reports of hot flushes most frequent, are a time of increased risk of psychological disturbance. Many of the studies would indeed suggest that there is a lower level of emotional disturbance in the post-menopausal years.

Insomnia

One symptom which may be related to the menopause and which is often included with the psychological symptoms is that of insomnia. McGhie and Russell (1962), in a study of a general population sample, found that reported sleep disturbance increased with increasing age but the pattern of change was different in the two sexes. In women, the increase commenced in 'middle age' but, in men, there was no significant change until after the age of 65 years. Jaszmann, Van Lith and Zaat (1969) found that complaints of insomnia increased from 20% in pre-menopausal women to 40% in women whose last menstrual period was between 2 and 5 years previously. Ballinger (1976a) found that difficulty getting off to sleep and difficulty staying asleep for the duration of the night were reported more frequently by post-menopausal women than pre-menopausal women, but reports of early morning wakening did not vary significantly with menopausal status.

This change in reported sleep disturbance with the menopause was not merely a reflection of change in psychiatric morbidity which is also known to be a factor in sleep disturbance (Orme, 1972). It was not possible in Ballinger's study (Ballinger, 1976a) to examine the effects of increasing age and menopausal status separately as the subgroups were too small, and since sleep disturbance is known to increase with age it was difficult to assess the effect of menopausal status alone. However, studies of the effect of oestrogen on sleep pattern (Thomson and Oswald, 1977a, 1977b) have further emphasized the possibility of a link between the endocrine changes of the menopause and sleep disturbance.

Sexual behaviour

Another issue which is frequently mentioned in relation to the menopause is that of a change in sexual responsiveness. Sexual problems presenting at the time of the menopause can be considered in two main groups, those relating to dyspareunia resulting from vaginal atrophy and vaginitis and the much larger and less specific group of problems relating to reduction in sexual responsiveness with no local symptoms.

Studies of vaginal cytology in the post-menopausal years have confirmed the changes produced by diminished oestrogen production. Utian (1978) stated that vaginal smears can be used to assess response to oestrogen therapy, as oestrogen has such a specific effect on the parabasal cell count. In a study of a group of women after oophorectomy, those women who had both hot flushes and symptoms of vaginal atrophy had significantly lower circulating oestradiol levels than the rest (Hutton *et al.*, 1978). Where the sexual difficulties are related to vaginal atrophy the problem is therefore very likely one of oestrogen deficiency.

Complaints of general loss of interest in sexual activity without any local symptoms are much more frequent than dyspareunia. Of 300 women presenting at a menopause clinic, only 19 complained of dyspareunia alone compared with 59 complaining of loss of libido without dyspareunia and 58 complaining of both (Studd *et al.*, 1977). In a study of a general population sample of 800 women, Hallström (1977) found that a large number of women complained of general reduction in sexual responsiveness, but relatively few suffered from dyspareunia.

Complaints of loss of libido in relation to the menopause need to be considered against a background of change in sexual responsiveness with age, as the majority of post-menopausal women are older than pre-menopausal women. Priest and Crisp (1972), in a general population survey, found that positive responses to the question 'has your sexual interest altered?' increased from around 25% in the early 40s to over 75% in the early 60s. This tendency to decreasing sexual interest with age was shown by both sexes, but was most marked in women.

Pfeiffer, Verwoerdt and Davis (1972) reported a similar finding from America, in that 7% of a sample of women aged 46–50 years reported no sexual interest, compared with 51% in the age range 61–65 years. In contrast to this finding in women, no men reported absent sexual interest in the 46–50 year age group and only 11% of men in the 61–65 year age group reported no sexual interest. There would appear to be a very definite decline in sexual interest with age in women and there is no objective evidence to support the view based on anecdotal material and discussed by Masters and Johnson (1966) that many women experience an increase in sexual drive at the time of menopause.

Hallström (1977) reported the findings in relation to sexual interest in 800 women in a general population sample in four age strata: 38, 46, 50 and 54 years of age. Sexual interest, capacity for orgasm and coital frequency declined markedly between the ages of 38 and 54 years, and when the findings were studied in relation to menopausal status it was found that the post-menopausal years were associated with a decline in sexual interest independent of the effect of increasing age. It was also found that decreasing sexual interest and activity were associated with an increased prevalence of mental illness, particularly depression, and problems in marital relationships such as insufficient support from husband. Hallström commented that the change in sexual behaviour with menopausal status may not necessarily be due to biological factors, because women may 'use' the menopause as an acceptable reason for opting out of sexual relations, without having to look at the problems in the marital relationship which may be more closely related to the wish to avoid sexual contact.

These studies indicate that the general level of sexual interest and activity is affected by many psychosocial factors and shows a decline with age in both sexes. In women, diminution in libido without pelvic symptoms is a much more complex issue than that of dyspareunia and there is no evidence of any direct relationship between declining sexual interest and circulating hormone levels, as has been demonstrated with dyspareunia. There is, however, evidence of decline in sexual interest in the post-menopausal years independent of aging, but this may be to some extent an artefact. None of the studies reviewed here supports the view that there is an increase in sexual interest at the time of the menopause.

Treatment

The most striking hormonal change of the menopausal and post-menopausal years is the fall in level of circulating oestrogen of ovarian origin and the raised levels of circulating gonadotrophic hormones (Jones, 1979). There has been great emphasis on the use of oestrogen therapy in the prevention and treatment of those conditions which have been attributed to oestrogen deficiency, in particular osteoporosis (Cooke, 1983). The most extreme view of the importance of oestrogen therapy for psychological symptoms in the post-menopausal age group was expounded by Wilson and Wilson (1963) who discussed at length the emotional symptoms which they considered specific to the post-menopausal oestrogen deficiency state. Malleson (1953, 1956) and Greenblatt (1965) expressed similar views that oestrogen replacement therapy was the only sound basis of treatment for emotional symptoms occurring at the time of the menopause, as these symptoms were directly attributable to the oestrogen deficiency. This opinion was challenged by Jeffcoate (1960) who considered that there was as little argument for giving hormones at the menopause as there was for the emotional problems of puberty.

Although many symptoms have been attributed to an oestrogen deficiency state in the post-menopausal years, this cannot be compared directly with conditions such as hypothyroidism where a definite diagnosis can be made by estimation of circulating hormone levels. As yet a definite relationship between circulating oestrogen levels and symptoms has been established only for those symptoms related to vaginal atrophy (Hutton et al., 1978). It is not surprising therefore that it is this group of symptoms which is consistently relieved by oestrogen therapy, local or systemic. There have been few studies of hormone metabolism in relation to psychiatric symptoms, but one study reported by Nikula-Baumann (1971) of levels of urinary excretion of various hormones in relation to psychiatric illness was essentially negative.

Almost 50 years ago, Pratt and Thomas (1937) stated that although a variety of symptoms were attributed to the menopause, a causal relationship to the physiological changes of the menopause had rarely been established. They reported a study of the effect of several parenteral and oral preparations on symptoms attributed to the menopause with high rates of improvement on all preparations, including lactose and plain oil injections. Hemphill and Reiss (1940) stated that follicular hormones produced improvement in a group of women admitted to mental hospital with a diagnosis of involutional depression, but no control group was included in this study. In another study without controls, reported by Palmer, Hastings and Sherman (1941), no improvement was detected in 11 patients with a diagnosis of involutional melancholia treated with an oestrogen preparation for 3 months. Ripley, Shorr and Papanicolaou (1940) reported an investigation of the effect of oestrogen on depressive symptoms in 20 women between the ages of 39 and 58 years presenting at a psychiatric outpatient clinic. They found that the benefit of oestrogen was confined to the relief of vasomotor symptoms and there was no evidence that depressive illness as such was influenced specifically by oestrogen or the course of the illness shortened.

Initially encouraging results about the effect of oestrogen on emotional symptoms came from studies carried out on women presenting at gynaecology clinics at the time of the menopause. However, no attempt was made to include control or placebo groups in these studies and some included subjects who were still menstruating regularly. Tramont (1966) reported a study of 305 women between the ages of 31 and 70 years, 51 of whom were still menstruating regularly and 176 of whom had irregular menstruation. He stated that oestrogen therapy produced marked relief of all psychiatric symptoms, but did not quote any results to support this statement. There was no control group in this study and the relationship of the psychiatric symptoms to the menopause in some of these patients is obviously questionable, as many were still menstruating regularly. Kaufman (1967) reported a study of 200 private patients and commented that it was difficult to decide which symptoms were related to the hormonal changes of the menopause and which were due to the problems of 'middle age'. He found that whereas hot flushes, sweats and symptoms related to vaginal atrophy were relieved in more than 90% of patients by oestrogen therapy, depression was relieved in only 49%, insomnia in 48%, fatigue in 40% and headaches in 52%. Again no controls were included in this study, so there was no additional indication of the level of placebo response.

Further studies of the efficacy of oestrogen therapy have shown an impressive placebo response. Coope, Thomson and Poller (1975), in a study of the effect of oestrogen on blood clotting and hot flushes, commented that the marked effect of the placebo on all symptoms made it difficult to assess the value of treatment. Mulley and Mitchell (1976) questioned the evidence for the efficacy of oestrogen in relation to hot flushes, one of the few symptoms now considered to be clearly related to the hormonal changes of the menopause (Utian, 1976), and the evidence for any effect on psychiatric symptoms is very much weaker. As the placebo response is so marked it is obviously essential that well-controlled double-blind studies are used to assess the efficacy of oestrogen in the treatment of emotional symptoms.

Another difficulty encountered in assessing the effect of different types of treatment on symptoms in women at the time of the menopause is the tendency to group symptoms together under the term 'menopausal syndrome' and judge the effect of treatment on change in overall scores. The use of this type of index means that the response of those items which may be oestrogen dependent will be diluted by those items which are not directly influenced by oestrogen. It also means that individual items which have not changed significantly with treatment may be reported as having improved because of the change in overall score. Despite this major deficiency, this type of index continues to be used (Jones, Marshall and Nordin, 1977), although the results of such studies are at best of limited value and at worst positively misleading.

The differential effect of various forms of treatment on separate symptoms included in the menopausal index was demonstrated in a study reported by Sheffery, Wilson and Walsh (1969). It was found that chlordiazepoxide was superior to an oestrogen preparation in the relief of anxiety and vertigo, but oestrogen was superior to chlordiazepoxide in the relief of vasomotor symptoms. There have now been several well-conducted studies of the effects of oestrogen on anxiety and depression in women presenting with symptoms at the time of the menopause (George, Utian and Beumont, 1973; Campbell, 1976; Thomson and Oswald, 1977b; Strickler et al., 1977) and none of these studies confirms any direct effect of oestrogen on either anxiety or depression. These symptoms are not directly oestrogen dependent, but may well show some improvement if other symptoms such as hot flushes are relieved. This probably accounts for the 'mental tonic' effect of oestrogen as described by Utian (1972b) and the 'domino effect' as described by Campbell (1976).

There are two psychological symptoms which may respond to treatment with oestrogen. Sheffery, Wilson and Walsh (1969) reported that subjective complaints of insomnia responded significantly better to a combination of oestrogen and chlordiazepoxide than either oestrogen or chlordiazepoxide alone. Campbell (1976) reported that subjective complaints of insomnia were significantly improved by oestrogen compared with placebo on a 6-month cross-over study. In the 2-month cross-over study reported in the same paper the improvement in complaints of insomnia appeared to be linked to the change in frequency of hot flushes. Although vasomotor symptoms were less severe in patients on the 6-month cross-over study, the effect on insomnia was maintained suggesting a direct effect of oestrogen on insomnia. Thomson and Oswald (1977a, 1977b) investigated 34 subjects using the facilities of a sleep laboratory to obtain an objective measure of changes in sleep pattern. They found that, compared with placebo, an oestrogen preparation significantly reduced the number of episodes of wakefulness. Considering the grave problems which may arise from prescribing anxiolytic drugs as hypnotics, the further investigation of the use of oestrogen as a hypnotic in women who first complain of insomnia at the time of the menopause is obviously of importance.

Another psychological function which has appeared to respond to oestrogen in some studies is that of memory. Subjective complaints of memory loss are difficult to evaluate as they may be related more to a concentration defect secondary to other symptoms than to impaired retention or recall of information. Campbell (1976) reported that, in his study, subjective assessment of memory improved significantly on oestrogen compared with placebo, but as this was not accompanied by any objective assessment of memory function the clinical significance of this finding is difficult to evaluate.

Kantor, Michael and Shore (1973) studied a group of older women between the ages of 60 and 91 years. They found that over a 3-year period scores for formal memory testing fell in both an oestrogen-treated and placebo group, but the rate of fall was slower in the oestrogen group. Rauramo et al. (1975) investigated the effects of hysterectomy and bilateral oophorectomy on several psychological functions and found no change in attention, memory or cognitive functions on formal psychological testing after operation. They also found no significant difference in these tests between the group treated with oestrogen replacement after operation and the untreated group. An interesting reversal of the findings of Campbell (1976) and Rauramo et al. (1975) was reported by Hackman and Galbraith (1977). In a 6-month pilot study including only 18 patients, the 9 patients on oestrogen therapy showed a significant improvement in test scores for memory over the 6 months and there was no such improvement in the placebo group. Despite this improvement in the test results there was no significant difference between the placebo and treatment groups in their subjective assessment of memory function.

The findings so far in relation to memory function and oestrogen therapy are contradictory, but in view of the considerable difficulties in relation to failing memory function with age, this is an important area for further investigation.

There have now been several studies of the effects of psychotropic drugs on symptoms reported by women at the time of the menopause. Kerr (1970) reported a placebo-controlled study of the effect of amitriptyline on emotional symptoms in 50 women who presented for treatment at the time of the menopause. All 50 patients received oestrogen therapy titrated on the basis of their hot flush counts and 25 of the patients also received amitriptyline and the other 25 received placebo tablets. Amitriptyline was significantly more effective than placebo in relieving the symptoms of anxiety and depression and also produced more improvement than placebo in the symptoms of insomnia, headache, apathy and palpitations.

Wheatley (1972) reported a study from general practice comparing the effect of an antidepressant with stilboestrol on menopausal symptoms. When all the symptoms were considered together there was no significant difference in the effect of these two drugs on symptom relief. When individual symptoms were studied separately it was found that the antidepressant was significantly better than stilboestrol in the relief of fatigue, depression and vertigo, while stilboestrol was superior in the relief of insomnia and joint and muscle pains. Foldes (1972) reported a placebo-controlled study of the use of an antidepressant in the treatment of menopausal symptoms and found it superior to placebo in overall symptom relief. When individual symptoms were studied it was found that the antidepressant was most effective in the relief of insomnia, headache, irritability and depression, but the hot flushes were very resistant to treatment.

These studies would suggest that some of the women attending menopause clinics are indeed depressed and some require antidepressant medication. The studies again emphasize that symptoms must be studied separately and considered separately in the clinical setting. Hot flushes and dyspareunia or discharge due to vaginal atrophy will respond to oestrogen, while symptoms of depression and anxiety may respond adequately to the psychotherapeutic effect of attending the clinic (Strickler et al., 1977), but some women may require psychotropic medication. There is certainly no evidence to suggest that oestrogen is an effective treatment for anxiety or depression, but there may be a place for oestrogen preparations in the treatment of insomnia in the post-menopausal years.

With so much information available emphasizing the differential response of various so-called 'menopausal' symptoms to oestrogen therapy, it is difficult to understand why the use of the menopausal index should be perpetuated. Craig (1983) suggests that suitability for hormone replacement therapy be assessed using a checklist of 18 items based on the menopausal index, only two of which (vasomotor symptoms and difficulty with intercourse) have been shown to respond better to oestrogen than to placebo.

Psychosocial and cultural factors

Although psychological symptoms were frequently described in women attending menopause clinics, many authors expressed Utian's opinion (Utian, 1976) that vasomotor symptoms and atrophic vaginitis were the only conditions directly related to changes in the level of circulating oestrogen and various views were expressed about the aetiology of emotional symptoms displayed at this time of life.

English (1954) suggested that the multitude of vague psychological symptoms seen in these women could be attributed to the sociological problems of adjustment at this time of life. He emphasized that this was a time of change in family structure with children reaching independence, the woman's social aspirations may not have been achieved and her husband may have failed to give her prestige. The woman may not have returned to a career of her own and her reproductive career is at an end. English suggested that improved education and changes in attitude in wider social terms were necessary to make any impact on these problems at the time of the menopause. Rogers (1956) commented on the unfortunate practice of attributing any symptoms in middle-aged women to the menopause and he again emphasized the influence of changing family structure resulting in women feeling that they were no longer needed at the same time as they lost their reproductive potential.

The loss of reproductive potential and its significance has been highlighted by psychoanalytic writers as an important factor in the aetiology of psychological symptoms at this time of life. Deutsch (1945) presented a very bleak picture of the menopause, claiming that almost every woman at this time goes through a period of depression related to the loss of all that was received during puberty in terms of femininity and reproductive potential. She felt that psychotherapy had little to offer and resignation without compensation was the only solution.

This very pessimistic view of mental health of women at the time of the menopause is given no support in the results of the general health population surveys, but in certain individuals the fear of loss of femininity and sexual attraction with increasing age may be significant issues. Fessler (1950) also presented a very negative view of the menopause, stating that the conduct of the majority of women during the climacteric was not normal and disappointment was at the core of menopausal depression. He considered that the deprivation of potential for child bearing at the time of the menopause resulted psychodynamically in a resurgence of 'penis envy' which had been compensated for by reproductive potential in the pre-menopausal years.

Of all the psychoanalysts, Benedek (1950) took the most optimistic view of the menopause. She described it as a time of intrapersonal reorganization with desexualization of emotional needs resulting in release of psychic energy for integration of the personality and planning of an active life with much ego gratification.

Prados (1967) was also optimistic about the post-menopausal years, saying that this could be a time of serenity, but he also stated that women showed behaviour change preceding, accompanying and following the critical age period of the menopause. He considered that the biological events of the menopause were a precipitating factor rather than the underlying cause of whatever emotional disturbance appeared.

Achte (1970) stressed the role of *fear* in relation to emotional disturbance at the time of the menopause: fear of aging, of which the menopause is a very clear reminder, fears of loss of youth and beauty and possibly of sexual partner. He also emphasized the loss of self-esteem associated with loss of reproductive potential and femininity which was previously reinforced by regular menstrual flow. He stressed the importance of a woman's personality in coping with the menopausal crisis which he described as a crisis of human existence.

Benedek (1950) suggested that culturally determined attitudes may influence how a woman approached the menopause and what symptoms she developed. Mannes (1968) discussed the difficulties of coping with this reminder of aging in a society where youth was 'worshipped' and old age was not something to look forward to. Flint (1975, 1979) presented some fascinating information on the effect of culturally determined attitudes on the number and nature of symptoms reported by women at the time of the menopause. She found that in a society where a woman's standing and self-esteem improved after the menopause, the only symptoms associated with the menopause were menstrual cycle changes. These women anticipated the menopause with enthusiasm and the menopause was seen as a reward, whereas in modern Western culture the menopause is anticipated with apprehension and seen more as a punishment.

A study reported by Neugarten *et al.* (1968) supported the view that in Western culture the menopause was worse in anticipation than in reality. Several groups of women in different age groups were asked to indicate what they expected would happen at the time of the menopause or, if they were post-menopausal, what changes they attributed to the menopause. A wide range of views was expressed, but when the group was considered as a whole about 50% of the women stated that the menopause was disagreeable, troublesome and unpleasant. However, there were marked differences between the age groups in their attitudes to the post-menopausal years. Women over 45 years of age expressed very much more positive views than the younger women and post-menopausal women tended to the view that the menopause created no major discontinuity in their lives, whereas the younger women were clearly expecting the worst.

Maoz *et al.* (1970) carried out a cross-cultural study in Israel where different ethnic groups lived in the same geographical area. They studied 11 independent sociocultural factors in relation to attitudes to the menopause and found that only one factor was associated with a positive response to the menopause and that was lack of desire for additional children in women of the Oriental Arab group. A variety of other factors were associated with negative attitudes to the menopause in the European group, including dissatisfaction with sexual relationships and being emotionally disturbed. This finding may to some extent account for the apparent excess of the emotionally disturbed women with sexual problems attending the menopause clinics, as those with negative expectations of the menopause are presumably more likely to present themselves at a clinic for treatment.

As well as cultural differences in attitudes to the menopause, English (1954) and Rogers (1956) stressed the influence of changes in family structure and social factors on the way in which a woman adapted at this time. The family change which has been mentioned most frequently is that of children growing up and leaving home and the effect this has on a woman's self-esteem as she becomes partially or wholly redundant in the role of mother. The emotive term 'empty nest' was introduced to describe this phenomenon in middle-aged women with psychiatric symptoms (Deykin *et al.*, 1966).

Ballinger (1975) presented some evidence from a general population survey to support the view that changes in family structure are a relevant issue at this time. Women between 40 and 55 years of age who reported that a child had married or left home within the year prior to taking part in the survey were significantly more likely than the rest to show evidence of emotional disturbance, as detected by the General Health Questionnaire. The personal impact of these events and the individual problems of readjustment are described in detail in a study involving lengthy interviews with 160 married women between 34 and 54 years of age (Rubin, 1979).

Other sociological issues which have been studied in relation to symptoms in women at the time of the menopause are marital status, social class and working outside the home. Jaszmann, Van Lith and Zaat (1969) found that married women reported symptoms at the time of the menopause significantly more frequently than single women. He also found that women from higher income groups and those who had had higher education reported fewer complaints than women from the low income groups and those who had only a primary education. This is contrary to the frequently quoted view that middle class women have more menopausal complaints because they have nothing else to worry about.

Severne (1979) described a complex interaction between the factors of social class and outside work in relation to menopausal symptoms. In a sample of 922 married Belgian women between the ages of 46 and 55 years, it was found that peri-menopausal women showed the highest level of symptoms with considerable improvement in the post-menopausal group. This recovery effect was least prominent in housewives who were generally at a disadvantage throughout. However, the difference between housewives and women working outside the home was most apparent in the upper socio-economic groups and least apparent in the lower socio-economic groups. It was suggested that in the latter group work outside the home was unlikely to be of a particularly satisfying nature and indeed may have been yet another stress for the woman rather than any positive contribution to self-esteem.

Severne (1979) concluded that the physical effects of the menopause appeared to be of little importance in the opinion of her subjects and problems at the time of the menopause were more likely to be due to difficulties in adaptation to new roles at this time of life rather than to the physical changes of the menopause. This opinion was supported by a study of symptoms in relation to stressful life-events in a sample of 131 women between the ages of 25 and 64 years drawn from the general population and reported by Greene and Cooke (1980). It was found that life stresses had a significantly more powerful influence on the elevation of symptom counts than did the menopause.

From the cross-cultural and sociological studies it is apparent that a multiplicity of factors influence how a woman anticipates and adapts to the changes both in family structure and physiology that occur at this time. These studies also demonstrate again the problems of using a measure such as the menopausal index which groups together symptoms such as hot flushes, which will almost certainly be influenced by the hormonal changes of the menopause, with emotional symptoms which are more likely to be related to the family and social issues.

Having discussed some of the physiological, sociological and cultural factors which influence how a woman copes at this time, the other most significant issue is that of personality. Achte (1970) discussed the importance of personality in relation to how a woman copes with the stresses related to the menopause. A crude indication of how a woman coped with stress in the past may be obtained from her previous medical history. Ballinger (1976b) found that women who showed evidence of emotional disturbance between the ages of 40 and 55 years had attended their general practitioners more frequently with 'nerves', had been prescribed more psychotropic drugs in the past and a higher proportion of these women had a past history of admission to psychiatric hospital when compared with controls who were not emotionally disturbed. Women displaying emotional disturbance at the time of the natural menopause would appear to be an emotionally vulnerable population who have previously developed symptoms in relation to various stresses.

These studies suggest that many factors, including culturally and socially determined attitudes to the menopause, changes in family structure, social class, marital status, satisfying work outside the home and pattern of reaction to stress in the past all influence the likelihood of developing emotional symptoms around the time of the menopause. The physiological changes of the menopause are probably of little significance in the aetiology of psychological symptoms at this time, but the menopause remains a convenient scapegoat for the symptoms and the menopause clinic an acceptable route for obtaining support and treatment.

Comparison of clinical and general population studies

The studies carried out in gynaecology or menopause clinics (Kupperman, Wetchler and Blatt, 1959; Jones, Marshall and Nordin, 1977) suggest that the time of the menopause is associated with a particularly high rate of psychological disturbance, to such an extent that psychological symptoms are included in some definitions of the menopausal syndrome (Utian and Serr, 1976). However, this view is not supported by information from the general population surveys (Neugarten and Kraines, 1965; Jaszmann, Van Lith and Zaat, 1969; Hallström, 1973; Thompson, Hart and Durno, 1973; McKinlay and Jefferys, 1974; Ballinger, 1975; Wood, 1979). One possible explanation for this discrepancy is that the clinics attract a selected group of women, not representative of the general population in terms of psychiatric morbidity. The high level of psychiatric symptoms reported in the clinic setting could therefore be a spurious finding related more to the selective use of clinic facilities than to the menopause.

There are several studies suggesting that women with psychiatric problems, particularly those diagnosed as having neurotic disorders, have an increased likelihood of contact with gynaecological services, including outpatient clinics. Gregory (1957), in a survey of menstrual disturbance in psychiatric inpatients, found that 48% of 52 patients with a diagnosis of neurotic illness had had a previous gynaecological procedure compared with 4% in 46 psychotic patients. Coppen (1965) reported a similar finding that 20.4% of female inpatients with a diagnosis of neurotic illness had had a previous dilatation and curettage compared with 14.6% of inpatients with a diagnosis of affective disorder and 6.5% of those diagnosed as having schizophrenia.

Further evidence of this association comes from several studies of subjects attending outpatient clinics. Sainsbury (1960), in a study of psychosomatic and neurotic disorders in outpatients attending a general hospital, found that of 79 women attending the gynaecology outpatient clinic 47% scored above the median value on the neuroticism scale of the Maudsley Personality Inventory (Eysenck, 1959) compared with 23% of the total sample attending all clinics. The diagnostic categories related to high neuroticism scores in the gynaecology clinics were dysmenorrhoea, leucorrhoea, menorrhagia and sterility. Sainsbury commented on this association and on the need for further investigation of the relationship between abnormality of personality and common menstrual disorders.

Munro (1969), in a study of 164 first attenders at a gynaecology outpatient clinic, found that 10% of these women were 'psychiatrically unwell' as defined by the Foulds Personal Illness Inventory (Foulds, 1962). In the psychiatrically unwell group, 25% of the subjects had demonstrable physical illness compared with 50% of the psychiatrically well subjects. He also commented that excessive menstrual bleeding was a particularly common complaint in the psychiatrically unwell group and 50% of this group were in the menopausal age range.

Worsley, Walters and Wood (1977), using the General Health Questionnaire (GHQ) as described by Goldberg (1972) as a screening instrument, reported that 48% of 97 women attending a gynaecology outpatient clinic obtained high scores on the GHQ, indicating the presence of significant emotional disturbance. The high scorers had an increased prevalence of complaints of menstrual dysfunction, a relatively low prevalence of organic diagnoses and were less likely than low scorers to be subjected to orthodox gynaecological procedures. The subjects in this study also completed a checklist relating to problems in social roles such as those of wife, mother, daughter or worker. From this information it was found that most problems were family centred and were mainly in relation to husband and children.

In a recent study, Byrne (1984) screened 211 women between 18 and 65 years of age attending a gynaecology outpatient clinic and found high rates of psychiatric disturbance compared with general population studies. Psychiatric disorder was more common in women who were divorced or separated and in married women who reported marital difficulties. The gynaecological symptoms most commonly associated with psychiatric disorder were disturbance of menstruation and complaints of pelvic pain.

An association between high scores on the GHQ and attendance at the gynaecological outpatient clinic has been found for women around the age of the menopause (Ballinger, 1977). Of 217 first attenders at the gynaecology outpatient clinic between the ages of 40 and 55 years, 53% obtained high scores on the GHQ. This was significantly higher than the 29% of high scorers in a general population survey drawn from the same area (Ballinger, 1975). Also, in comparison with the general population sample the clinic subjects were more likely to be separated or divorced, less likely to be single and more likely either to have had previous or to have subsequent contact with the local psychiatric services.

This apparent excess of women with emotional disturbance in the population attending outpatient clinics and in particular gynaecology clinics may, in part, be due to the stress of the physical condition for which they have been referred. This explanation seems unlikely in view of Sainsbury's finding (Sainsbury, 1960) that those subjects who were attending outpatient clinics with clearly diagnosed chronic debilitating illness showed no excess of psychological disturbance.

Another possible explanation for the excess of women with neurotic disorders in the clinic populations is that subjects with these disorders are more aware of any change in body function and perhaps less tolerant of that change. In support of this view, Tyrer, Lee and Alexander (1980) found that anxious, phobic and hypochondriacal subjects were more aware of body function in terms of pulse rate than were controls. However, there have been no studies of this issue in relation to gynaecological complaints.

Another factor influencing the character of the population attending the outpatient clinic is the selective use of medical services. Mechanic (1966) suggested that clinic populations would be biased in relation to the general population of individuals with the same symptoms because of the difference in attitudes to the use of medical facilities. He stated that this effect would be most marked in relation to conditions of high prevalence, which are easily recognized and have a benign course. This description would apply very well to menopausal symptoms. Mechanic also pointed out that the more subjective were the symptoms the greater would be the selection bias, and most of the symptoms attributed to the menopause are subjective in nature.

Life-events quite unrelated to the physical illness may influence the use of clinical services. Mechanic and Volkart (1960) reported a study of the use of college medical services by students and the findings supported the view that some students used attendance at the clinic as a way of coping with stressful events. Mechanic commented that complaints of trivial illness may be one way of seeking reassurance and support in a socially acceptable manner when it would be difficult for the individual to present the underlying problem directly. This view is certainly supported by the findings in a gynaecology clinic population (Worsley, Walters and Wood, 1977).

These studies of subjects attending various hospital outpatient clinics suggest that the finding of multiple psychological symptoms in women attending menopause clinics could be accounted for by the selected nature of the population attending the clinic rather than any deleterious effects of the menopause on mental health. There are several possible reasons for this selection process such as variation in the use of medical services and perhaps a variation in awareness of changes in body function and tolerance of these changes.

The pre-menopausal years

Several of the general population surveys already described have indicated that, although reports of vasomotor symptoms increase sharply at the time of the natural menopause, reports of psychological symptoms or the onset of psychiatric disorder are more frequent in the immediately pre-menopausal years (Jaszmann, Van Lith and Zaat, 1969; Hallstrom, 1973; Ballinger, 1975; Krüskemper, 1975; Bungay, Vessey and McPherson, 1980). It may be that this tendency to an increase in psychological symptoms is related to the hormonal changes that precede the menopause or even to the anxiety about what will happen at the menopause, since this time of life has had such negative publicity.

Although the hormonal changes found in the post-menopausal years and after oophorectomy have been described in some detail (Chakravarti *et al.*, 1977), the change in the pattern of reproductive hormones during the transition from regular menstrual cycles to the cessation of menstruation has received less attention. Sherman, West and Korenman (1976) studied 10 women between the ages of 46 and 56 years who were still menstruating. They concluded that the endocrinological findings could be interpreted in the context of depletion in numbers of ovarian follicles with diminished potential for hormone secretion by the residual follicles. Pre-menopausal women who were still menstruating regularly showed cyclical hormonal changes similar to those of younger women, except that they had lower levels of oestradiol, higher levels of FSH and a shorter interval from the onset of menstruation to the mid-cycle gonadotrophin peak.

Another feature which was specific to women in the immediate pre-menopausal years was the dissociation of changes in circulating FSH and LH. Although LH was in the normal range for each stage of the menstrual cycle, FSH levels were consistently elevated and it was suggested that these elevated FSH levels could be responsible for the initiation of follicular maturation at more frequent intervals, resulting in the general reduction in menstrual cycle length in older women. Sherman, West and Korenman (1976) stated that this difference in change in FSH and LH levels in pre-menopausal women emphasized the complexity of the systems involved in the control of circulating levels of reproductive hormones.

There have been two studies of symptoms in pre-menopausal women which have included hormone estimations. Abe *et al.* (1977) investigated serum levels of oestradiol, progesterone, FSH and LH in relation to a group of symptoms based on the menopausal index described by Kupperman, Wetchler and Blatt (1959). In a sub-group of women aged 35–39 years, elevated symptom counts as measured on this index correlated with low oestradiol levels and elevated LH levels. As all the symptoms were grouped together it is not possible to comment on the psychological symptoms separately from items such as vasomotor symptoms which may well be expected to vary in relation to hormonal levels.

Chakravarti *et al.* (1979) reported a study of 82 pre-menopausal women who presented at a menopause clinic. There was a wide age range in this sample, with 16 of the patients less than 40 years old and 18 over 50 years old, and reported symptoms were studied in relation to circulating levels of FSH and LH, oestradiol and testosterone. It was found that an elevated hot flush count was associated with low levels of circulating oestradiol, but psychological symptoms were not related to any particular pattern of circulating hormone levels.

The most obvious clinical manifestation of the transitional phase prior to the menopause is the change in menstrual cycle pattern. Treloar *et al.* (1967) described how the menstrual cycle became shorter with increasing age, and variability in cycle length was marked just before the menopause, with long intervals alternating with unusually short cycles. It has also been shown that menstrual blood loss tends to increase with age, and complaints of irregular or excessive menstruation are common in the immediately pre-menopausal years (Hallberg *et al.*, 1966). Ballinger (1977) found that the presenting complaint in 39% of 76 pre-menopausal women aged 40 and 44 years at a gynaecology clinic was excessive menstrual blood loss, increasing to 62% of 48 women aged 45–49 years.

In the gynaecological literature, menorrhagia in the absence of obvious pathology, or dysfunctional uterine bleeding, is often ascribed to anovulatory cycles in the years just prior to the menopause (Davey, 1976). In a study of endometrial biopsies from women presenting with dysfunctional uterine bleeding, Gambrell (1974) found that 23% were in the secretory phase, consistent with ovulatory cycles. However, in a total of 667 biopsies the ratio of proliferative to secretory phase endometrial tissue rose from approximately 1 to 1 in women in their 30s to 3 to 1 in the late 40s, indicating that anovulatory cycles are a more frequent cause of dysfunctional uterine bleeding in women just prior to the menopause.

Any association of psychological disturbance with complaints of menorrhagia in the pre-menopausal years is rarely mentioned in the gynaecological literature, in sharp contrast with the impressive list of psychological symptoms said to be associated with the menopause. In a general population study of women between 40 and 55 years of age (Ballinger, 1975), it was found that a significantly higher proportion of women with evidence of emotional disturbance complained of heavier than usual menstrual periods compared with women without evidence of emotional disturbance. In several clinic studies (Sainsbury, 1960; Munro, 1969; Worsley, Walters and Wood, 1977) it was found that vague complaints of menstrual dysfunction or menorrhagia were frequently presented by emotionally disturbed women.

Subjective assessment of menstrual blood loss is notoriously inaccurate and this was demonstrated by Hallberg *et al.* (1966) by comparing subjective assessment with measured blood loss. Menorrhagia is the sort of vague subjective complaint which Mechanic (1966) discussed in relation to a form of illness behaviour where a relatively trivial physical complaint may be used as a way of obtaining reassurance and sympathy in a socially acceptable way. This would seem to apply to some of the women described by Worsley, Walters and Wood (1977) and Byrne (1984), who had evidence of emotional disturbance in relation to problems with their husbands and families and presented at the gynaecology outpatient clinic with complaints such as menorrhagia in the absence of pathological findings.

Although the association of emotional disturbance with complaints of menorrhagia is not emphasized in current gynaecology textbooks, it was discussed at some length in an earlier textbook of psychosomatic gynaecology (Kroger and Freed, 1951). Various hypotheses were discussed relating to the effects of the emotions on the hypothalamus producing changes in secretion of gonadotrophic hormones, resulting in menorrhagia, or even a direct effect of the emotions on the vascular system of the uterus.

Other authors have suggested that emotional problems could induce menorrhagia. Hamilton (1955) stated that excessive menstruation could be produced by emotional disturbance. Blaikley (1949) considered emotional problems to be a common cause of menorrhagia, but presented only 8 cases by way of evidence, and O'Neill (1952) described only 12 cases where complaints of menorrhagia appeared to be precipitated by emotional crises. Levy (1967) stated that autonomic dysfunction in relation to depression of mood was often localized in the pelvis in women, resulting in menstrual irregularities, but he presented no factual evidence for this statement.

One type of psychiatric disorder which commonly presents with physical symptoms is that of depression. The general problem of depressive illness presenting with physical symptoms was discussed by Stoeckle and Davidson (1962) in relation to a medical clinic. They described several cases where individuals presenting with bodily symptoms for which no organic cause could be detected were suffering from depressive reactions following life-events characterized by loss.

In a gynaecology clinic survey (Ballinger, 1977), it was found that not only was there a higher proportion of women with emotional disturbance in the clinic attenders compared with the general population sample, but the emotional disturbance was more severe and more depressive in nature. Greenberg (1983) reported that 31 out of 50 women presenting in a gynaecology clinic with a complaint of menorrhagia showed evidence of depression and he suggested that the complaint menorrhagia may be a manifestation of psychological disturbance.

Dowling and Knox (1964) concentrated on the dilemma for the general practitioner of patients with depressive illness presenting with physical symptoms and the choice of direction of hospital referral. They noticed that a history of unrelated physical illness in the past 5 years increased the likelihood of a referral to a 'physical' clinic. A similar finding was reported in relation to gynaecology outpatients (Ballinger, 1977), in that patients who were referred back to the gynaecology clinic after having a hysterectomy had the highest incidence of psychiatric disorder and also the most severe psychiatric disorder. The direction of referral was clearly influenced by the previous gynaecological surgery.

Another aspect of the association between psychiatric and gynaecological symptoms has been investigated in studies of the prevalence of psychiatric disorder following hysterectomy. Melody (1962) found that 4% of 267 women developed depression in the 3 months following hysterectomy and the best predictive factor of depression after operation was a history of an episode of depression some time prior to hysterectomy.

Barker (1968) compared 729 women who had had a hysterectomy with 280 women who had had a cholecystectomy. The average age of the first group was 44 years and of the second 55 years. There was a significantly higher level of psychiatric referral following surgery in the hysterectomy group, reaching a peak two years after the operation. Women were more likely to be referred to the psychiatric services following hysterectomy if they had a history of psychiatric referral prior to operation, if they had a presenting symptom of menorrhagia with no significant uterine pathology or anaemia and if they had a history of divorce or marital disruption prior to hysterectomy.

The findings in both these studies of an excess of psychiatric morbidity in those women who had had psychiatric illness prior to hysterectomy suggests that some women may be developing psychiatric illness just prior to surgery when they present with the symptoms that lead to hysterectomy.

More direct evidence of an excess of psychiatric morbidity in patients prior to hysterectomy comes from recent studies. Ballinger (1977), in the study of peri-menopausal women presenting at a gynaecological outpatient clinic, found that of the 29 women who went on to have a hysterectomy 19 (65%) obtained high scores on the GHQ prior to surgery compared with 29% of the subjects in the same age range in the local population. Twenty of these 29 patients responded to follow-up one year after surgery and only 6 (30%) obtained high scores on the GHQ at that time.

A similar finding of high levels of psychiatric symptoms prior to hysterectomy was reported by Martin et al. (1977). They screened 49 patients for psychiatric symptoms prior to hysterectomy and 28 (57%) of these women were diagnosed as psychiatrically ill. It was noted that women under 40 years of age had a high risk of psychiatric symptoms prior to surgery and it was felt that, in this group particularly, women were being considered for hysterectomy for psychiatric rather than gynaecological illness. It was also noted in this study that some of the symptoms seen in the women prior to surgery were very similar to those labelled as 'post hysterectomy syndrome' by Richards (1974).

Gath, Cooper and Day (1982) investigated 156 women with menorrhagia of benign origin who underwent hysterectomy. Psychiatric morbidity in this group of women was significantly higher before hysterectomy than after, but the level of psychiatric morbidity was higher than that found in women from the general population both before and after hysterectomy. It is clear that hysterectomy does not precipitate psychiatric morbidity as previously suggested (Richards, 1974), but rather that there is a high level of psychiatric disturbance in women presenting with menorrhagia and being considered for hysterectomy.

Gynaecologists' views on the indications for hysterectomy show considerable variation. Gusberg (1969), in a discussion of the indications for hysterectomy, commented that the uterus was the focus for many psycho-emotional ills and surgery should be avoided where there was no clear pathological lesion requiring surgery. In contrast, Davey (1976), in a discussion of dysfunctional uterine bleeding, suggested that for women over 40 hysterectomy is the treatment of choice in all cases where bleeding is persistent or severe and he commented that in this age group the uterus is less important psychologically. This second approach could well lead to a considerable number of emotionally disturbed women being subjected to hysterectomy in the immediately pre-menopausal years in view of the findings of high levels of emotional disturbance in women presenting at gynaecology clinics with complaints of menorrhagia in the absence of obvious pathology on examination.

In conclusion, the years immediately prior to the menopause are characterized by changes in menstrual cycle and possibly associated with an increased level of emotional disturbance. Both general population surveys and gynaecology clinic studies have indicated an association between complaints of menorrhagia and evidence of emotional disturbance, particularly depression. It is possible that the hormonal changes of this time produce both these changes or that the emotional disturbance has a direct effect on menstrual bleeding pattern. There is, as yet, no evidence to support either of these hypotheses. The limited evidence at present available supports the sociological view that women presenting with vague menstrual complaints are often suffering from emotional disturbance in relation to situational stress, and presenting gynaecological symptoms is a particularly acceptable and effective way of obtaining sympathy and support at this time of life. The association of emotional disturbance and complaints of menorrhagia may well account for the reported excess of psychiatric morbidity following hysterectomy.

Involutional melancholia

Rosenthal (1968) reviewed in detail the extensive psychiatric literature concerning the possible existence of a type of depressive illness, termed involutional melancholia, which occurred for the first time in the involutional years and was clinically distinct from depressive illness commencing at other times of life. Involutional melancholia was said to be characterized by hypochondriasis and pessimism accompanied by severe agitation and restlessness, but in a review of the clinical features of depressive illness Lewis (1936) considered that there was no clinical reason for classifying involutional melancholia separately from psychotic depressive illness.

Several clinical studies of depressive illness have now been reported and none of these indicates any clinical grounds for making a diagnosis of involutional melancholia separate from psychotic depression (Stenstedt, 1959; Stenback, 1963). Kendell (1968), in a systematic study of patients admitted to hospital with psychiatric illness, reported that those patients with a diagnosis of involutional melancholia were identical with patients with a diagnosis of psychotic depression on the variables of symptoms, treatment and outcome.

When ovarian extracts were first introduced, the concept of involutional melancholia as a separate entity, related to the involutional changes of later life, was still popular and attempts were made to use these new substances in the treatment of this condition. Enthusiastic claims were made for the use of ovarian extracts in the treatment of involutional melancholia and it was even suggested by Werner *et al.* (1934) that this condition was merely an extreme manifestation of the symptomatology of the menopause caused by ovarian failure. Further studies of oestrogen therapy in involutional melancholia did not confirm Werner's work (Hemphill and Reiss, 1940; Palmer, Hastings and Sherman, 1941).

If the hormonal changes of the menopause do, indeed, have any significance in the aetiology of mental illness, particularly depression, there should be an increase in mental illness and perhaps admission to mental hospital around the time of the menopause. Several studies have been reported in which this issue has been investigated in different ways.

Tait, Harper and McClatchey (1957) carried out a prospective study of women patients first admitted to mental hospital between the ages of 40 and 55 years. They found no evidence of the traditional clinical picture of involutional melancholia and the most common diagnoses were psychotic depression, neurotic illness and late onset schizophrenia. They also investigated the timing of onset of the illness in relation to the time of the natural menopause and found no evidence to suggest an increased risk of any of these disorders in relation to the time of cessation of menstrual periods.

Smith (1971) reported a study in which several life-events, including developmental events such as the menopause, menarche and pregnancy, were investigated in relation to admission to mental hospital. The occurrence of these events in the year prior to admission to hospital was noted and the same information was obtained from a general population sample. It was found that whereas events such as divorce and problems with the police were more common in that year in the group admitted to mental hospital than in the general population sample, the reverse was true for reaching the natural menopause. This finding was quite contrary to the view that the hormonal change of the menopause would put a woman at increased risk of mental illness.

Another study, restricted to an assessment of the risk of onset of depressive illness, was reported by Winokur (1973). He calculated the risk for suffering an attack of depressive illness requiring admission to hospital for a group of 71 women admitted to hospital with a depressive illness between the ages of 20 and 80 years. He then calculated the risk for 28 post-menopausal women in the sample who were within 3 years of the natural menopause. There was no significant difference in risk between the whole group, age range 20–80 years, and the women in the 3 years after the cessation of menstrual periods.

In conclusion, there is no evidence from this limited number of studies to suggest that the menopause is associated with an increased risk of serious mental illness requiring admission to mental hospital. There is now very little support for the concept of a specific type of involutional psychotic illness, previously termed involutional melancholia, which can be distinguished from depressive illness occurring at other times of life on clinical features.

Conclusions

Early studies of the clinical features of the menopause were based on symptoms elicited from clinic attenders and suggested that a variety of emotional symptoms were associated with the menopause as well as vasomotor symptoms and symptoms of vaginal atrophy. Further studies, carried out on samples of women drawn from the general population, confirmed the association of vasomotor symptoms and symptoms of vaginal atrophy with the menopause, but provided no evidence of a significant increase in emotional symptoms at the time of cessation of menstrual periods. These studies did, however, indicate that insomnia and reduced sexual interest were more frequent in the post-menopausal years.

The discrepancy between the clinic findings and the general population studies in relation to emotional symptoms is probably related to selective use of clinic facilities by women with evidence of emotional disturbance. This finding emphasizes that information from the clinic populations should be applied to the general population only with caution.

Several of the general population studies indicate that although there is no increase in emotional disturbance in the post-menopausal years there may be some increased risk of emotional disturbance in the years just prior to the menopause. This is the time of transition from regular menstrual cycles to the cessation of menstrual periods, and the changes in reproductive hormones at this time have only recently been investigated in any detail. Complaints of excessive menstrual blood loss are frequent at this time and appear to be more common in women with evidence of emotional disturbance. Emotionally disturbed women may therefore be more at risk for having a hysterectomy at this time, which could account to some extent for the excess of psychiatric morbidity following this operation.

With the introduction of several potent oestrogen preparations there has been considerable interest in the possibility of using these preparations in the treatment of emotional disturbance at the time of the menopause. There is no evidence from extensive clinical studies that oestrogen preparations have any place in the treatment of anxiety or depression. Oestrogen may have a place in the treatment of insomnia in menopausal and post-menopausal women and the effect of oestrogen on memory function is still being investigated, although the results so far are conflicting.

In recent studies of psychological disturbance at the time of the menopause, there has been more emphasis on the influence of psychosocial and cultural factors. Wide cultural variation in attitudes to the menopause have been shown and the influence of these attitudes on the number and nature of symptoms reported by women at the time of the menopause investigated. From studies of social factors and life stresses, particularly in relation to family changes, it seems that these issues have significantly more effect on a woman's mental health at this time than do the physiological changes of the menopause.

As for the more severe types of mental illness requiring admission to hospital, there is no evidence of any increased risk of developing these disorders at the time of the menopause. The concept of a distinct type of psychotic illness, involutional melancholia, specific to the involutional years, has not been upheld in studies of clinical features, treatment or outcome.

Despite all these essentially negative findings concerning the influence of the menopause on mental health, the menopause remains a popular explanation for many emotional problems with both lay and medical opinion. In this way the women, their doctors and their families avoid the need to examine in more detail the issues which give rise to the emotional disturbance. The menopause is thus a convenient, and sometimes comforting, scapegoat.

References

ABE, T., FURUHASHI, N., YAMAYA, Y., WADA, Y., HOSHIAI, A. and SUZUKI, M. (1977) Correlation between climacteric symptoms and serum levels of oestradiol, progesterone, follicle-stimulating hormone and luteinizing hormone. *American Journal of Obstetrics and Gynecology*, **129**, 65–67

ACHTE, K. (1970) Menopause from the psychiatrist's point of view. *Acta Obstetrica et Gynaecologica Scandinavica*, **49**, Suppl. 1, 7–17

BALLINGER, C. B. (1975) Psychiatric morbidity and the menopause: screening of general population sample. *British Medical Journal*, **3**, 344–346

BALLINGER, C. B. (1976a) Subjective sleep disturbance at the menopause. *Journal of Psychosomatic Research*, **20**, 509–513

BALLINGER, C. B. (1976b) Psychiatric morbidity and the menopause: clinical features. *British Medical Journal*, **1**, 1183–1185

BALLINGER, C. B. (1977) Psychiatric morbidity and the menopause: survey of gynaecological out-patient clinic. *British Journal of Psychiatry*, **131**, 83–89

BARKER, M. (1968) Psychiatric illness after hysterectomy. *British Medical Journal*, **2**, 91–95

BENEDEK, T. (1950). Climacterium: a developmental phase. *Psychoanalytic Quarterly*, **19**, 1–27

BLAIKLEY, J. B. (1949) Menorrhagia of emotional origin. *Lancet*, **2**, 691–694

BUNGAY, G. T., VESSEY, M. P. and McPHERSON, C. K. (1980) Study of symptoms in middle life with special reference to the menopause. *British Medical Journal*, **2**, 181–183

BYRNE, P. (1984) Psychiatric morbidity in a gynaecology clinic: an epidemiological survey. *British Journal of Psychiatry*, **144**, 28–34

CAMPBELL, S. (1976) Double blind psychometric studies on the effects of natural oestrogens on post-menopausal women. In *The Management of the Menopause and Post-Menopausal Years* (Campbell, S., Ed.), pp. 149–158. Lancaster, UK; MTP Press

CASPAR, R. F. and YEN, S. S. C. (1981) Menopausal flushes: effect of pituitary gonadotrophin desensitization by a potent luteinizing hormone-releasing factor agonist. *Journal of Clinical Endocrinology and Metabolism*, **53**, 1056–1058

CHAKRAVARTI, S., COLLINS, W. P., FORECAST, J. D., NEWTON, J. R., ORAM, D. H. and STUDD, J. W. W. (1976) Hormonal profiles after the menopause. *British Medical Journal*, **2**, 784–787

CHAKRAVARTI, S., COLLINS, W. P., NEWTON, J. R., ORAM, D. H. and STUDD, J. W. W. (1977) Endocrine changes and symptomatology after oophorectomy in premenopausal women. *British Journal of Obstetrics and Gynaecology*, **8**, 769–775

CHAKRAVARTI, S., COLLINS, W. P., THOM, M. H. and STUDD, J. W. W. (1979) Relation between plasma hormone profiles, symptoms, and response to oestrogen treatment in women approaching the menopause. *British Medical Journal*, **1**, 983–985

COOKE, I. D. (1983) Treating the menopause. *British Medical Journal*, **1**, 2001–2002

COOPE, J., THOMSON, J. M. and POLLER, L. (1975) Effects of 'natural oestrogen' replacement therapy on menopausal symptoms and blood clotting. *British Medical Journal*, **4**, 139–143

COPPEN, A. (1965) The prevalence of menstrual disorders in psychiatric patients. *British Journal of Psychiatry*, **111**, 155–167

CRAIG, G. M. (1983) Guidelines for community menopausal clinics. *British Medical Journal*, **1**, 2033–2036

DALY, L. W., Ed. (1974) *Dorland's Illustrated Medical Dictionary*, 25th edn. Philadelphia and London; W. B. Saunders

DAVEY, D. A. (1976) Dysfunctional uterine bleeding. In *Integrated Obstetrics and Gynaecology for Postgraduates* (Dewhurst, C. J., Ed.), 2nd edn, pp. 606–634. Oxford; Blackwell Scientific Publications

DE FAZIO, J., MELDRUM, D. R., LAUFER, L., VALE, W., RIVIER, J., LU, J. K. H. and JUDD, H. L. (1983) Induction of hot flashes in premenopausal women treated with a long-acting GnRH agonist. *Journal of Clinical Endocrinology and Metabolism*, **56**, 445–448

DEUTSCH, H. (1945) Epilogue. The climacterium. In *The Psychology of Women*, Vol. 2, pp. 456–487. New York; Grune and Stratton

DEYKIN, E. Y., JACOBSON, S., KLERMAN, G. and SOLOMON, M. (1966) The empty nest: psychosocial aspects of conflict between depressed women and their grown children. *American Journal of Psychiatry*, **122**, 1422–1426

DONOVAN, J. C. (1951) The menopausal syndrome: a study of case histories. *American Journal of Obstetrics and Gynecology*, **62**, 1281–1291

DOWLING, R. H. and KNOX, S. J. (1964) Somatic symptoms in depressive illness: a problem of referral for general practitioners. *British Journal of Psychiatry*, **110**, 720–722

DUNNELL, K. and CARTWRIGHT, A. (1972) *Medicine Takers, Prescribers and Hoarders*. London and Boston; Routledge and Kegan Paul

ENGLISH, O. S. (1954) Climacteric neuroses and their management. *Geriatrics*, **9**, 139–145

EYSENCK, H. J. (1959) *The Manual of the Maudsley Personality Inventory*. London; University of London Press

FELDMAN, J. M., POSTLETHWAITE, R. W. and GLEN, J. F. (1976) Hot flashes and sweats in men with testicular insufficiency. *Archives of Internal Medicine*, **136**, 606–608

FESSLER, L. (1950) The psychopathology of climacteric depression. *Psychoanalytic Quarterly*, **19**, 28–42

FLINT, M. P. (1975) The menopause: reward or punishment. *Psychosomatics*, **16**, 161–163

FLINT, M. P. (1979) Transcultural influences in peri-menopause. In *Psychosomatics in Peri-Menopause* (Haspels, A. A. and Musaph, H., Eds), pp. 41–56. Lancaster, UK; MTP Press Ltd

FOLDES, J. J. (1972) Psychosomatic approach to the menopausal syndrome. Treatment with Opipramol. In *Psychosomatic Medicine in Obstetrics and Gynaecology* (Morris, N., Ed.), pp. 617–621. Basel; Karger

FORREST, A. D., AFFLECK, J. W. and ZEALLEY, A. K. (1978) *Companion to Psychiatric Studies*, 2nd edn. Edinburgh; Churchill Livingstone

FOULDS, G. A. (1962) A quantification of diagnostic differentiae. *Journal of Mental Science*, **108**, 389–405

GAMBRELL, R. D. (1974) Perimenopausal and postmenopausal bleeding: mechanism, pathology, management with progestational agents. In *The Menopausal Syndrome* (Greenblatt, R. B., Mahesh, V. B. and McDonough, P.G., Eds.). New York; Medicom Press

GATH, D., COOPER, P. and DAY, A. (1982) Hysterectomy and psychiatric disorder: I. Levels of morbidity before and after hysterectomy. *British Journal of Psychiatry,* **140,** 335–350

GELDER, M., GATH, D. and MAYOU, R. (1983) *Oxford Textbook of Psychiatry,* pp. 393–394. London; Oxford University Press

GEORGE, G. C. W., UTIAN, W. H. and BEUMONT, P. J. V. (1973) Effect of exogenous oestrogens on minor psychiatric symptoms in postmenopausal women. *South African Medical Journal,* **47,** 2387–2388

GOLD, J. J. and JOSIMOVICH, J. B. (1980) *Gynecologic Endocrinology,* 3rd edn. Hagerstown; Harper Row

GOLDBERG, D. P. (1972) *The Detection of Psychiatric Illness by Questionnaire.* Oxford; Oxford University Press

GREENBERG, M. (1983) The meaning of menorrhagia: an investigation into the association between the complaint of menorrhagia and depression. *Journal of Psychosomatic Research,* **27,** 209–214

GREENBLATT, R. B. (1965) Estrogen therapy for postmenopausal females. *New England Journal of Medicine,* **272,** 305–308

GREENE, J. G. and COOKE, D. J. (1980) Life stress and symptoms at the climacterium. *British Journal of Psychiatry,* **136,** 486–491

GREGORY, B. A. J. C. (1957) The menstrual cycle and its disturbance in psychiatric patients – II. *Journal of Psychosomatic Research,* **2,** 199–224

GUSBERG, S. B. (1969) Indications for hysterectomy. In *Controversy in Obstetrics and Gynecology* (Reid, D. E. and Barton, T. C., Eds.), pp. 315–319. Philadelphia and London; W. B. Saunders and Company

HACKMAN, B. W. and GALBRAITH, D. (1977) Six month pilot study of oestrogen replacement therapy with piperazine oestrone sulphate and its effect on memory. *Current Medical Research and Opinion,* **4,** Suppl. 3, 21–27

HALLBERG, L., HOGDAHL, A. M., NILSSON, L. and RYBO, G. (1966) Menstrual blood loss – a population study. *Acta Obstetrica et Gynaecologica Scandinavica,* **45,** 320–351

HALLSTRÖM, T. (1973) *Mental Disorder and Sexuality in the Climacteric.* Gothenburg; Scandinavian University Books

HALLSTRÖM, T. (1977) Sexuality in the climacteric. *Clinical Obstetrics and Gynecology,* **4,** 227–239

HAMILTON, M. (1955) *Psychosomatics.* London; Chapman and Hall

HEMPHILL, R. E. and REISS, J. (1940) Investigations into the significance of endocrines in involutional melancholia. *Journal of Mental Science,* **86,** 1065–1077

HILL, P., MURRAY, R. and THORLEY, A. (1979) *Essentials of Postgraduate Psychiatry.* London; Academic Press

HUTTON, J. D., JACOBS, H. S., JAMES, V. H. T. and MURRAY, M. A. F. (1978) Relation between plasma oestrone and oestradiol and climacteric symptoms. *Lancet,* **1,** 678–681

JASZMANN, L., VAN LITH, N. D. and ZAAT, J. C. A. (1969) The perimenopausal symptoms: the statistical analysis of a survey. *Medical Gynecology and Sociology,* **4,** 268–277

JEFFCOATE, T. N. A. (1960) Drugs for menopausal symptoms. *British Medical Journal,* **1,** 340–342

JEFFCOATE, T. N. A. (1975) *Principles of Gynaecology,* 4th edn, p. 90. London; Butterworths

JONES, E. C. (1979) The post-fertile life of non-human primates and other mammals. In *Psychosomatics in Peri-Menopause* (Haspels, A. A. and Musaph, H., Eds.), pp. 13–19. Lancaster, UK; MTP Press

JONES, M. J., MARSHALL, D. H. and NORDIN, B. E. C. (1977) Quantitation of menopausal symptomatology and its response to ethinyl oestradiol and piperazine oestrone sulphate. *Current Medical Research and Opinion,* **4,** Suppl. 3, 12–20

KANTOR, H. I., MICHAEL, C. M. and SHORE, H. (1973) Estrogen for older women. A three year study. *American Journal of Obstetrics and Gynecology,* **116,** 115–118

KAUFMAN, S. A. (1967) Limited relationship of maturation index to estrogen therapy for menopausal symptoms. *Obstetrics and Gynecology,* **30,** 399–407

KENDELL, R. E. (1968) *The Classification of Depressive Illness,* Maudsley Monograph 18. London; Oxford University Press

KERR, M. (1970) Amitriptyline in emotional states at the menopause. *New Zealand Medical Journal,* **72,** 243–245

KLOPPER, A. (1969) Physiology of the reproductive system, in *Combined Textbook of Obstetrics and Gynaecology* (Baird, Sir Dugald, Ed.), 8th edn, pp. 41–81. Edinburgh; Livingstone

KOLB, L. L. (1977) *Modern Clinical Psychiatry,* 9th edn. Philadelphia and London; W. B. Saunders

KROGER, W. S. and FREED, S. C. (1951) *Psychosomatic Gynecology.* Philadelphia and London; W. B. Saunders

KRÜSKEMPER, G. (1975) Results of psychological testing (MMPI) in climacteric women. In *Estrogens in the Post-Menopause: Frontiers in Hormone Research* (Van Keep, P. and Lauritzen, C., Eds.), pp. 105–111. Basel; Karger

KUPPERMAN, H. S., WETCHLER, B. B. and BLATT, M. H. G. (1959) Contemporary therapy of the menopausal syndrome. *Journal of the American Medical Association,* **171,** 1627–1637

LEVY, S. (1967) Depressive reaction. Its diagnosis and treatment with special reference to the 'Somatic Mask' and the newer psychopharmacologic agents. In *Psychosomatic Medicine* (Dunlop, E. and Weisman, M. N., Eds.), pp. 33–41. Amsterdam; Excerpta Medica Foundation

LEWIS, A. (1936) Melancholia: prognostic study and case material. *Journal of Mental Science,* **82,** 488–558

LLEWELLYN-JONES, D. (1978) *Fundamentals of Obstetrics and Gynaecology,* Vol. II, *Gynaecology,* 2nd edn. London and Boston; Faber and Faber

McCLURE BROWNE, J. C. (1973) *Postgraduate Obstetrics and Gynaecology,* 4th edn. London; Butterworths

MACDONALD, A. M., Ed. (1972). *Chambers's Twentieth Century Dictionary.* Edinburgh; W. & R. Chambers

McGHIE, A. and RUSSELL, S. M. (1962) The subjective assessment of normal sleep patterns. *Journal of Mental Science,* **108,** 642–654

McKINLAY, S. M. and JEFFERYS, M. (1974) The menopausal syndrome. *British Journal of Preventative and Social Medicine,* **28,** 108–115

MACNAUGHTON, M. C. (1976) The menopause and post-menopause. In *Combined Textbook of Obstetrics and Gynaecology* (Walker, J., MacGillivray, I. and Macnaughton, M. C., Eds.), 9th edn, pp. 671–676. Edinburgh; Churchill Livingstone

MALLESON, J. (1953) An endocrine factor in certain affective disorders. *Lancet,* **2,** 158–164

MALLESON, J. (1956) Climacteric stress: its empirical management. *British Medical Journal,* **2,** 1422–1425

MANNES, M. (1968) Of time and the woman. *Psychosomatics,* **9,** Suppl., 8–11

MAOZ, B., DOWTY, N., ANTONOVSKY, A. and WIJSENBEEK, H. (1970) Female attitudes to menopause. *Social Psychiatry,* **5,** 35–40

MARTIN, R. L., ROBERTS, W. V., CLAYTON, P. J. and WETZEL, R. (1977) Psychiatric illness and non-cancer hysterectomy. *Diseases of the Nervous System,* **38,** 974–980

MASTERS, V. H. and JOHNSON, V. E. (1966) *Human Sexual Response.* Boston; Little, Brown

MECHANIC, D. (1966) Response factors in illness: the study of illness behaviour. *Social Psychiatry,* **1,** 11–20

MECHANIC, D. and VOLKART, E. H. (1960) Illness behaviour and medical diagnoses. *Journal of Health and Human Behaviour,* **1,** 86–94

MELODY, G. F. (1962) Depressive reactions following hysterectomy. *American Journal of Obstetrics and Gynecology,* **83,** 410–413

MULLEY, G. and MITCHELL, J. R. A. (1976) Menopausal flushing: does oestrogen therapy make sense? *Lancet,* **1,** 1397–1399

MUNRO, A. (1969) Psychiatric illness in gynaecological outpatients: a preliminary study. *British Journal of Psychiatry,* **115,** 807–809

NEUGARTEN, B. L. and KRAINES, R. J. (1965) 'Menopausal symptoms' in women of various ages. *Psychosomatic Medicine,* **27,** 266–273

NEUGARTEN, B. L., WOOD, V., KRAINES, R. J. and LOOMIS, B. (1968) Women's attitudes towards the menopause. In *Middle Age and Ageing* (Neugarten, B. L., Ed.), pp. 195–200. Chicago and London; University of Chicago Press

NIKULA-BAUMANN, L. (1971) Endocrinological studies on subjects with involutional melancholia. *Acta Psychiatrica Scandinavica,* Suppl. 226

NOVAK, E. R., JONES, G. S. and JONES, H. W. (1975) *Novak's Textbook of Gynecology,* 9th edn. Baltimore; Williams and Wilkins

O'NEILL, D. (1952) Uterine bleeding in tension states. *Journal of Obstetrics and Gynaecology of the British Empire,* **59,** 234–239

ORME, J. E. (1972) Duration of sleep and its relationship to age, personality and psychiatric illness. *British Journal of Social and Clinical Psychology,* **11,** 70–72

PALMER, H. D., HASTINGS, D. W. and SHERMAN, S. H. (1941) Therapy in involutional melancholia. *American Journal of Psychiatry,* **97,** 1086–1115

PARSONS, L. and SOMMERS, S. C. (1962) *Gynaecology.* Philadelphia and London; W. B. Saunders

PEEL, J. and BRUDENELL, J. M. (1969) *Textbook of Gynaecology,* 6th edn. London; Heinemann

PFEIFFER, E., VERWOERDT, A. and DAVIS, G. C. (1972) Sexual behaviour in middle life. *American Journal of Psychiatry,* **128,** 1262–1267

PRADOS, M. (1967) Emotional factors in the climacterium of women. *Psychotherapy and Psychosomatics,* **15,** 231–244

PRATT, J. P. and THOMAS, W. L. (1937) The endocrine treatment of menopausal phenomena. *Journal of the American Medical Association,* **109,** 1875–1877

PRIEST, R. G. and CRISP, A. H. (1972) The menopause and its relationship with reported somatic experiences. In *Psychosomatic Medicine in Obstetrics and Gynaecology* (Morris, N., Ed.), pp. 605–607. Basel; Karger

RAURAMO, L., LAGERSPETZ, K., ENGBLOM, P. and PUNNONEN, R. (1975) The effect of castration and peroral estrogen therapy on some psychological factors. In *Estrogens in the Post-Menopause: Frontiers of Hormone Research* (Van Keep, P. A. and Lauritzen, C., Eds.), Vol. 3, pp. 94–104. Basel; Karger

RICHARDS, D. H. (1974) A post-hysterectomy syndrome. *Lancet*, **2**, 983–985

RIPLEY, H. S., SHORR, E. and PAPANICOLAOU, G. N. (1940) The effect of treatment of depression in the menopause with estrogenic hormone. *American Journal of Psychiatry*, **96**, 905–911

ROGERS, J. (1956) The menopause. *New England Journal of Medicine*, **254**, 697–703, 750–756

ROSENTHAL, S. H. (1968) The involutional depressive syndrome. *American Journal of Psychiatry*, **124**, Suppl., 21–35

RUBIN, L. B. (1979) *Women of a Certain Age. The Midlife Search for Self.* New York; Harper, Colophon Books/Harper and Row

SAINSBURY, P. (1960) Psychosomatic disorders and neurosis in outpatients attending a general hospital. *Journal of Psychosomatic Research*, **4**, 261–273

SEVERNE, L. (1979) Psychosocial aspects of the menopause. In *Psychosomatics in Peri-Menopause* (Haspels, A. A. and Musaph, H., Eds.), pp. 101–120. Lancaster, UK; MTP Press

SHEFFERY, J. B., WILSON, T. A. and WALSH, J. C. (1969) Double-blind cross-over study comparing chlordiazepoxide, conjugated estrogens, combined chlordiazepoxide and conjugated estrogens, and placebo in treatment of the menopause. *Medical Annals of the District of Columbia*, **38**, 433–436

SHERMAN, B. M., WEST, J. H. and KORENMAN, S. G. (1976) The menopausal transition: analysis of LH, FSH, estradiol and progesterone concentrations during menstrual cycles of older women. *Journal of Clinical Endocrinology and Metabolism*, **42**, 629–636

SLATER, E. and ROTH, M. (1969) *Clinical Psychiatry.* London; Baillière, Tindall and Cassell

SMITH, W. G. (1971) Critical life-events and prevention strategies in mental health. *Archives of General Psychiatry*, **25**, 103–109

STENBACK, A. (1963) On involutional and middle age depressions. *Acta Psychiatrica Scandinavica*, **39**, Suppl. 169, 14–32

STENSTEDT, A. (1959) Involutional melancholia. *Acta Psychiatrica et Neurologica Scandinavica*, **34**, Suppl. 127

STOECKLE, J. D. and DAVIDSON, G. E. (1962) Bodily complaints and other symptoms of depressive reaction. *Journal of the American Medical Association*, **180**, 134–139

STRICKLER, R. C., BORTH, R., CECUTTI, A., COOKSON, B. A., HARPER, J. A., POTVIN, R., RIFFEL, P., SORBARA, V. J. and WOOLEVER, C. A. (1977) The role of oestrogen replacement in the climacteric syndrome. *Psychological Medicine*, **7**, 631–639

STUDD, J. W. W. (1979) The climacteric syndrome. In *Female and Male Climacteric* (Van Keep, P. A., Serr, D. M. and Greenblatt, R. B., Eds.), pp. 23–33. Lancaster, UK; MTP Press

STUDD, J. W. W., COLLINS, W. P., CHAKRAVARTI, S., NEWTON, J. R., ORAM, D. H. and PARSONS, A. (1977) Oestradiol and testosterone implants in the treatment of psychosexual problems in the postmenopausal woman. *British Journal of Obstetrics and Gynaecology*, **84**, 314–315

STURDEE, D. W., WILSON, K. A., PIPILI, E. and CROCKER, A. D. (1978) Physiological aspects of menopausal hot flush. *British Medical Journal*, **2**, 79–80

TAIT, A. C., HARPER, J. and McCLATCHEY, W. T. (1957) Initial psychiatric illness in involutional women. 1. Clinic aspects. *Journal of Mental Science*, **103**, 132–145

TATARYN, I. V., MELDRUM, D. R., LU, K. H., FRUMAR, A. M. and JUDD, H. L. (1979) LH, FSH and skin temperature during the menopausal hot flush. *Journal of Clinical Endocrinology and Metabolism*, **49**, 152–154

THOMPSON, B., HART, S. A. and DURNO, D. (1973) Menopausal age and symptomatology in a general practice. *Journal of Biosocial Science*, **5**, 71–82

THOMSON, J. and OSWALD, I. (1977a) Hormones and sleep. *Current Medical Research and Opinion*, **4**, Suppl. 3, 67–72

THOMSON, J. and OSWALD, I. (1977b) Effect of oestrogen on the sleep, mood and anxiety of menopausal women. *British Medical Journal*, **2**, 1317–1319

TILT, E. J. (1857) *The Change of Life in Health and Disease*, 2nd edn. London; Churchill

TRAMONT, C. B. (1966) Cyclic hormone therapy: a report on 305 cases. *Geriatrics*, **21**, 212–215

TRELOAR, A. E., BOYNTON, R. E., BENN, B. G. and BROWN, B. W. (1967) Variation of the human menstrual cycle through reproductive life. *International Journal of Fertility*, **12**, 77–126

TYRER, P., LEE, I. and ALEXANDER, J. (1980) Awareness of cardiac function in anxious, phobic and hypochondriacal patients. *Psychological Medicine*, **10**, 171–174

UTIAN, W. H. (1972a) The true clinical features of postmenopause and oophorectomy and their response to oestrogen therapy. *South African Medical Journal,* **46,** 732–737

UTIAN, W. H. (1972b) The mental tonic effect of oestrogens administered to oophorectomized females. *South African Medical Journal,* **46,** 1079–1082

UTIAN, W. H. (1976) Scientific basis for post-menopausal oestrogen therapy: the management of specific symptoms and rationale for long-term replacement. In *The Menopause. A Guide to Current Research and Practice* (Beard, R. J., Ed.), pp. 175–201. Lancaster, UK; MTP Press

UTIAN, W. H. (1978) Plasma-oestrogens and climacteric symptoms. *Lancet,* **1,** 1099–1100

UTIAN, W. H. and SERR, D. (1976) The climacteric syndrome. In *Consensus on Menopause Research* (Van Keep, P. A., Greenblatt, R. B. and Albeaux-Fernet, M., Eds.), pp. 1–4. Lancaster, UK; MTP Press

WERNER, A. A., JOHNS, G. A., HOCTOR, E. F., AULT, C. C., KOHLER, L. H. and WEIS, M. W. (1934) Involutional melancholia. Probable etiology and treatment. *Journal of the American Medical Association,* **103,** 13–16

WHEATLEY, D. (1972) The use of psychotropic drugs in the female climacteric. In *Psychosomatic Medicine in Obstetrics and Gynaecology* (Morris, N., Ed.), pp. 612–616. Basel; Karger

WILSON, R. A. and WILSON, T. A. (1963) The fate of the nontreated postmenopausal woman: a plea for the maintenance of adequate estrogen from puberty to the grave. *Journal of the American Geriatrics Society,* **11,** 347–362

WINOKUR, G. (1973) Depression in the menopause. *American Journal of Psychiatry,* **130,** 92–93

WOOD, C. (1979) Menopausal myths. *Medical Journal of Australia,* **1,** 496–499

WORLD HEALTH ORGANIZATION (1981) *Research on the Menopause.* Report of a WHO Scientific Group. Technical Report Series 670. Geneva; WHO

WORSLEY, A., WALTERS, W. A. W. and WOOD, E. C. (1977) Screening for psychological disturbance amongst gynaecology patients. *Australia and New Zealand Journal of Obstetrics and Gynaecology,* **17,** 214–219

Index